Engineering a Learning Healthcare System

A Look at the Future

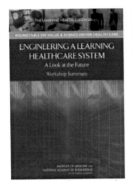

Lessons from engineering have the potential to drive positive change in both the efficiency and quality of healthcare delivery. Working cooperatively with the National Academy of Engineering (NAE), the Institute of Medicine (IOM) hosted a workshop on applying knowledge from systems and operations engineering to improve the organization, delivery, and process of health care.

This report, *Engineering a Learning Healthcare System: A Look at the Future*, summarizes participants views on the promise of, and strategies necessary to implement, engineering approaches to continuous improvement in quality, safety, knowledge, and value in health care. Highlighted below are key discussion elements, with the full version available at www.iom.edu/vsrt.

Learning from Practice
Engineering Continuous Improvement into Care

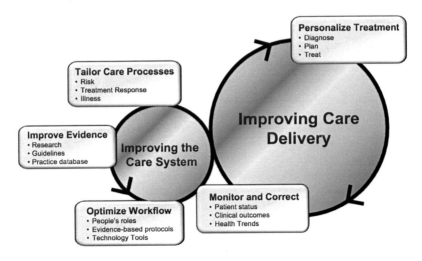

Engineering a Learning Healthcare System
Workshop Common Themes

Center the system's processes on the right target—the patient. Throughout several sessions, workshop participants emphasized the need to ensure that processes support patients—and patients are not forced into processes. Patient needs and perspectives must be at the center of all process design, technology application, and clinician engagement.

System excellence is created by the reliable delivery of established best practice. Participants often cited the need to better integrate the development and dissemination of best practices, in addition to using data systems to improve patient care and clinical outcomes.

Expect errors in the performance of individuals, perfection in the performance of systems. Human error is inevitable in any system and should be assumed. On the other hand, safeguards and designed redundancies can deliver perfection in system performance. Mapping processes, embedding prompts, cross-checks, and information loops can assure best outcomes, and allow human capacity to focus on what can not be programmed—compassion and individual patient needs.

Learning is a non-linear process. The focus on an established hierarchy of scientific evidence as a basis for evaluation and decision making cannot accommodate the fact that much of the sound learning in complex systems occurs in local and individual settings. Participants cited the need to bridge the gap between dependence on formal trials and the experience of local improvement, in order to speed learning and avoid impractical costs.

Align rewards on the key elements of continuous improvement. Incentives, standards, and measurement requirements can serve as powerful change agents. Participants noted that it is vital that incentives be carefully considered and directed to the targets most important to improving the efficiency, effectiveness and safety of the system (patient outcomes), as well as taking into consideration the patient and provider experiences.

Development of education and research to facilitate understanding and partnerships between engineering and the health professions. The relevance of systems engineering principles to health care and the impressive transformation brought to other industries speaks to the merits of developing common vocabularies, concepts, and ongoing joint education and research activities.

Teamwork and cross-checks trump command and control. Especially in systems designed to guarantee safety, system performance that is effective and efficient requires careful coordination and teamwork, as well as a culture that encourages parity among all with established responsibilities.

Bringing Engineering to Health Care
Example Applications of Engineering Principles

Strategy	Examples
• Evidence-based protocols	• Data mining and analysis of past treatments can point to effective protocols, including minimization of false positives linking diseases and DNA genes
• Adaptive clinical trials	• Design/success criteria adjusted as results are obtained
• E-care	• Biomarkers/diagnostic tools allow for predictive care
• Personalized care	• Genomics-based adaptive, customized care
• Reducing errors	• Dash board displays to ensure that steps are taken to reduce ventilator-associate pneumonia and central line infections

---

Foster a leadership culture, language, and style that reinforce teamwork and results. Positive leadership cultures foster and celebrate consensus goals, teamwork, multidisciplinary efforts, transparency, and continuous monitoring and improvement. In citing examples of successful learning systems, participants highlighted the need for a supportive and integrated leadership.

Emphasize interdependence and tend to the process interfaces. A system is most vulnerable at links between critical processes. In health care, attention to the nature of relationships and hand-offs between elements of the patient care and administrative processes is therefore vital, and a crucial component of focusing the process on patient satisfaction and improved outcomes.

Performance, transparency, and feedback serve as the engine for improvement. Continuous learning and improvement in patient care requires transparency in processes and outcomes, as well as capacity to capture feedback and make adjustments.

Complexity compels reasoned allowance for tailored adjustments. Mass customization and other engineering practices can help accelerate the recognition of the need for tailoring and delivering the most appropriate care, with the best prospects for improved outcomes, for the patient.

Clarify terms. The ability of healthcare professionals to draw upon relevant and helpful engineering principles for system improvement could be facilitated by a better mutual understanding of the terminology.

Identify best practices. Three areas of systems orientation are particularly important to improving the efficiency and effectiveness of health care: 1) focusing the system elements more directly on patient experience; 2) ensuring transparency in the performance of the system; and 3) establishing a culture that emphasizes teamwork, consistency, and excellence. Progress could be accelerated by identifying and disseminating examples of best practices from health care and from engineering on each of these dimensions.

Explore health professions education change. In the face of a rapidly changing environment in health care, changes to the education of health professionals can advance caregiver skills in knowledge navigation, teamwork, patient/provider partnership, and process awareness.

Advance the science of payment for value. Progress on increasing value could be achieved with a stronger focus on understanding, measuring, and providing incentives for value in health care.

Explore fostering the development of a science of waste assessment and engagement. Similarly, an exploration of the elements of inefficiency in health care, how to define and measure waste, and how to mobilize responses to eliminating waste could contribute to increasing value within healthcare systems.

Support the development of a robust health information technology system. Much work remains in order to achieve a health information technology system that allows for continuous learning, permits data sharing, employs consistent standards, and addresses privacy and security concerns.

STAFF CONTACT: Robert Saunders, Ph.D, Program Officer
202-334-2747 / rsaunders@nas.edu

ENGINEERING A LEARNING HEALTHCARE SYSTEM

A Look at the Future

Workshop Summary

Claudia Grossmann, W. Alexander Goolsby, LeighAnne Olsen,
and J. Michael McGinnis

INSTITUTE OF MEDICINE *AND*
NATIONAL ACADEMY OF ENGINEERING
OF THE NATIONAL ACADEMIES

THE NATIONAL ACADEMIES PRESS
Washington, D.C.
www.nap.edu

THE NATIONAL ACADEMIES PRESS   500 Fifth Street, N.W.   Washington, DC 20001

NOTICE: The project that is the subject of this report was approved by the Governing Board of the National Research Council, whose members are drawn from the councils of the National Academy of Sciences, the National Academy of Engineering, and the Institute of Medicine.

This project was supported by the Agency for Healthcare Research and Quality, America's Health Insurance Plans, AstraZeneca, Blue Shield of California Foundation, Burroughs Wellcome Fund, California Health Care Foundation, Centers for Medicare & Medicaid Services, Charina Endowment Fund, Department of Veterans Affairs, Food and Drug Administration, Johnson & Johnson, Gordon and Betty Moore Foundation, National Institutes of Health, the Peter G. Peterson Foundation, sanofi-aventis, and Stryker. Any opinions, findings, conclusions, or recommendations expressed in this publication are those of the author(s) and do not necessarily reflect the view of the organizations or agencies that provided support for this project.

International Standard Book Number-13:   0-978-0-309-12064-7
International Standard Book Number-10:   0-309-12064-0

Additional copies of this report are available from The National Academies Press, 500 Fifth Street, N.W., Lockbox 285, Washington, DC 20055; (800) 624-6242 or (202) 334-3313 (in the Washington metropolitan area); Internet, http://www.nap.edu.

For more information about the Institute of Medicine, visit the IOM home page at: **www.iom.edu.**

Copyright 2011 by the National Academy of Sciences. All rights reserved.

Printed in the United States of America

The serpent has been a symbol of long life, healing, and knowledge among almost all cultures and religions since the beginning of recorded history. The serpent adopted as a logotype by the Institute of Medicine is a relief carving from ancient Greece, now held by the Staatliche Museen in Berlin.

Suggested citation: IOM (Institute of Medicine). 2011. *Engineering a learning healthcare system: A look at the future: Workshop summary.* Washington, DC: The National Academies Press.

THE NATIONAL ACADEMIES
Advisers to the Nation on Science, Engineering, and Medicine

The **National Academy of Sciences** is a private, nonprofit, self-perpetuating society of distinguished scholars engaged in scientific and engineering research, dedicated to the furtherance of science and technology and to their use for the general welfare. Upon the authority of the charter granted to it by the Congress in 1863, the Academy has a mandate that requires it to advise the federal government on scientific and technical matters. Dr. Ralph J. Cicerone is president of the National Academy of Sciences.

The **National Academy of Engineering** was established in 1964, under the charter of the National Academy of Sciences, as a parallel organization of outstanding engineers. It is autonomous in its administration and in the selection of its members, sharing with the National Academy of Sciences the responsibility for advising the federal government. The National Academy of Engineering also sponsors engineering programs aimed at meeting national needs, encourages education and research, and recognizes the superior achievements of engineers. Dr. Charles M. Vest is president of the National Academy of Engineering.

The **Institute of Medicine** was established in 1970 by the National Academy of Sciences to secure the services of eminent members of appropriate professions in the examination of policy matters pertaining to the health of the public. The Institute acts under the responsibility given to the National Academy of Sciences by its congressional charter to be an adviser to the federal government and, upon its own initiative, to identify issues of medical care, research, and education. Dr. Harvey V. Fineberg is president of the Institute of Medicine.

The **National Research Council** was organized by the National Academy of Sciences in 1916 to associate the broad community of science and technology with the Academy's purposes of furthering knowledge and advising the federal government. Functioning in accordance with general policies determined by the Academy, the Council has become the principal operating agency of both the National Academy of Sciences and the National Academy of Engineering in providing services to the government, the public, and the scientific and engineering communities. The Council is administered jointly by both Academies and the Institute of Medicine. Dr. Ralph J. Cicerone and Dr. Charles M. Vest are chair and vice chair, respectively, of the National Research Council.

www.national-academies.org

This workshop summary is dedicated to Jerome H. Grossman, M.D., a long-time member, friend, and leader in the work of the National Academies. Bridging by nature and by profession, Jerry Grossman served as the liaison between the Institute of Medicine and the National Academy of Engineering and was a key motivator and intellectual compass for this workshop and its focus on bringing the insights of engineering principles to the benefit of the complex and vital activities of health care. He passed away suddenly on April 1, 2008.

ROUNDTABLE ON VALUE & SCIENCE-DRIVEN HEALTH CARE*

Denis A. Cortese (*Chair*), Emeritus President and Chief Executive Officer, Mayo Clinic; Foundation Professor, ASU

Donald Berwick, Administrator, Centers for Medicare & Medicaid Services (*ex officio*)

David Blumenthal, National Coordinator, Office of the National Coordinator for Health IT (*ex officio*)

Bruce G. Bodaken, Chairman, President, and Chief Executive Officer, Blue Shield of California

David R. Brennan, Chief Executive Officer, AstraZeneca PLC

Paul Chew, Chief Science Officer and CMO, sanofi-aventis U.S., Inc.

Carolyn M. Clancy, Director, Agency for Healthcare Research and Quality (*ex officio*)

Michael J. Critelli, Former Executive Chairman, Pitney Bowes, Inc.

Helen Darling, President, National Business Group on Health

Thomas R. Frieden, Director, Centers for Disease Control and Prevention (*designee*: **Chesley Richards**) (*ex officio*)

Gary L. Gottlieb, President and CEO, Partners HealthCare System

James A. Guest, President, Consumers Union

George C. Halvorson, Chairman and Chief Executive Officer, Kaiser Permanente

Margaret A. Hamburg, Commissioner, Food and Drug Administration (*ex officio*)

Carmen Hooker Odom, President, Milbank Memorial Fund Board

Ardis Hoven, Board Chair, American Medical Association

Brent James, Chief Quality Officer and Executive Director, Institute for Health Care Delivery Research, Intermountain Healthcare

Michael M. E. Johns, Chancellor, Emory University

Craig Jones, Director, Vermont Blueprint for Health

Cato T. Laurencin, Vice President for Health Affairs, Dean of the School of Medicine, University of Connecticut

Stephen P. MacMillan, President and Chief Executive Officer, Stryker

Mark B. McClellan, Director, Engelberg Center for Healthcare Reform, The Brookings Institution

Sheri S. McCoy, Worldwide Chairman, Johnson & Johnson Pharmaceuticals Group

Elizabeth G. Nabel, President, Brigham and Women's Hospital

---

*Formerly the Roundtable on Evidence-Based Medicine, Institute of Medicine forums and roundtables do not issue, review, or approve individual documents. The responsibility for the published workshop summary rests with the workshop rapporteurs and the institution.

Mary D. Naylor, Professor and Director of Center for Transitions in Health, University of Pennsylvania

Peter Neupert, Corporate Vice President, Health Solutions Group, Microsoft Corporation

William D. Novelli, Former CEO, AARP; Professor, Georgetown University

Jonathan B. Perlin, Chief Medical Officer and President, Clinical Services, HCA, Inc.

Robert A. Petzel, Under Secretary, Veterans Health Administration (*ex officio*)

Richard Platt, Professor and Chair, Harvard Medical School and Harvard Pilgrim Health Care

John C. Rother, Group Executive Officer, AARP

John W. Rowe, Professor, Mailman School of Public Health, Columbia University

Susan Shurin, Acting Director, National Heart, Lung, and Blood Institute (*ex officio*)

Mark D. Smith, President and CEO, California HealthCare Foundation

George P. Taylor, Assistant Secretary for Health Affairs (Acting), Department of Defense (*designee*: Michael Dinneen) (*ex officio*)

Reed D. Tuckson, Executive VP and Chief of Medical Affairs, UnitedHealth Group

Frances M. Visco, President, National Breast Cancer Coalition

Workshop Planning Committee

William B. Rouse (*Chair*), Georgia Institute of Technology
Jerome H. Grossman, Harvard University
Brent C. James, Intermountain Healthcare, Inc.
Helen S. Kim, Gordon and Betty Moore Foundation
Cato T. Laurencin, University of Virginia
The Honorable Paul H. O'Neill, Value Capture, LLC

Roundtable and National Academy of Engineering Staff

Christie Bell, Financial Associate
Katharine Bothner, Senior Program Assistant (through July 2008)
Patrick Burke, Financial Associate (through December 2009)
Andrea Cohen, Financial Associate (through December 2008)
W. Alexander Goolsby, Program Officer (through September 2008)
Claudia Grossmann, Program Officer
Kiran Gupta, Mirzayan Fellow (through May 2009)
J. Michael McGinnis, Senior Scholar and Executive Director

LeighAnne Olsen, Program Officer (through July 2010)
Daniel O'Neill, Research Associate (through January 2009)
Stephen Pelletier, Consultant
Laura Penny, Consultant
Brian Powers, Senior Program Assistant
Proctor Reid, Director, National Academy of Engineering Program Office
Valerie Rohrbach, Program Assistant
Julia Sanders, Program Assistant
Robert Saunders, Program Officer
Ruth Strommen, Intern (through August 2009)
Leigh Stuckhardt, Program Associate
Kate Vasconi, Senior Program Assistant (through January 2011)
Pierre L. Young, Program Officer (through May 2010)
Catherine Zweig, Senior Program Assistant (through June 2010)

Reviewers

This report has been reviewed in draft form by individuals chosen for their diverse perspectives and technical expertise, in accordance with procedures approved by the National Research Council's Report Review Committee. The purpose of this independent review is to provide candid and critical comments that will assist the institution in making its published report as sound as possible and to ensure that the report meets institutional standards for objectivity, evidence, and responsiveness to the study charge. The review comments and draft manuscript remain confidential to protect the integrity of the deliberative process. We wish to thank the following individuals for their review of this report:

Arthur Garson, University of Virginia
C. David Naylor, University of Toronto
David Pryor, Ascension Health
Ronald Rardin, University of Arkansas
Harold W. Sorenson, University of California, San Diego

Although the reviewers listed above have provided many constructive comments and suggestions, they were not asked to endorse the final draft of the report before its release. The review of this report was overseen by **Patricia F. Brennan,** University of Wisconsin, Madison. Appointed by the Institute of Medicine, she was responsible for making certain that an independent examination of this report was carried out in accordance with institutional procedures and that all review comments were carefully considered. Responsibility for the final content of this report rests entirely with the authoring committee and the institution.

Institute of Medicine
Roundtable on Value & Science-Driven Health Care
Charter and Vision Statement

The Institute of Medicine's Roundtable on Value & Science-Driven Health Care has been convened to help transform the way evidence on clinical effectiveness is generated and used to improve health and health care. Participants have set a goal that, by the year 2020, 90 percent of clinical decisions will be supported by accurate, timely, and up-to-date clinical information, and will reflect the best available evidence. Roundtable members will work with their colleagues to identify the issues not being adequately addressed, the nature of the barriers and possible solutions, and the priorities for action, and will marshal the resources of the sectors represented on the Roundtable to work for sustained public–private cooperation for change.

٭ ٭

The Institute of Medicine's Roundtable on Value & Science-Driven Health Care has been convened to help transform the way evidence on clinical effectiveness is generated and used to improve health and health care. We seek the development of a **learning health system** that is designed to generate and apply the best evidence for the collaborative healthcare choices of each patient and provider; to drive the process of discovery as a natural outgrowth of patient care; and to ensure innovation, quality, safety, and value in health care.

Vision: Our vision is for a healthcare system that draws on the best evidence to provide the care most appropriate to each patient, emphasizes prevention and health promotion, delivers the most value, adds to learning throughout the delivery of care, and leads to improvements in the nation's health.

Goal: By the year 2020, 90 percent of clinical decisions will be supported by accurate, timely, and up-to-date clinical information, and will reflect the best available evidence. We feel that this presents a tangible focus for progress toward our vision, that Americans ought to expect at least this level of performance, that it should be feasible with existing resources and emerging tools, and that measures can be developed to track and stimulate progress.

Context: As unprecedented developments in the diagnosis, treatment, and long-term management of disease bring Americans closer than ever to the promise of personalized health care, we are faced with similarly unprecedented challenges to identify and deliver the care most appropriate for individual needs and conditions. Care that is important is often not delivered. Care that is delivered is often not important. In part, this is due to our failure to apply the evidence we have about the medical care that is most effective—a failure related to shortfalls in provider knowledge and accountability, inadequate care coordination and support, lack of insurance, poorly aligned payment incentives, and misplaced patient expectations. Increasingly, it is also a result of our limited capacity for timely generation of evidence on the relative effectiveness, efficiency, and safety of available and emerging interventions. Improving the value of the return on our healthcare investment is a vital imperative that will require much greater capacity to evaluate high-priority clinical interventions, stronger links between clinical research and practice, and reorientation of the incentives to apply new insights. We must quicken our efforts to position evidence development and application as natural outgrowths of clinical care—to foster health care that learns.

Approach: The IOM Roundtable on Value & Science-Driven Health Care serves as a forum to facilitate the collaborative assessment and action around issues central to achieving the vision and goal stated. The challenges are myriad and include issues that must be addressed to improve evidence development, evidence application, and the capacity to advance progress on both dimensions. To address these challenges, as leaders in their fields, Roundtable members will work with their colleagues to identify the issues not being adequately addressed, the nature of the barriers and possible solutions, and the priorities for action, and will marshal the resources of the sectors represented on the Roundtable to work for sustained public–private cooperation for change.

Activities include collaborative exploration of new and expedited approaches to assessing the effectiveness of diagnostic and treatment interventions, better use of the patient care experience to generate evidence on effectiveness, identification of assessment priorities, and communication strategies to enhance provider and patient understanding and support for interventions proven to work best and deliver value in health care.

Core concepts and principles: For the purpose of the Roundtable activities, we define evidence-based medicine broadly to mean that, *to the greatest extent possible, the decisions that shape the health and health care of Americans—by patients, providers, payers, and policy makers alike—will be grounded on a reliable evidence base, will account appropriately for individual variation in patient needs, and will support the generation of new insights on clinical effectiveness.* Evidence is generally considered to be information from clinical experience that has met some established test of validity, and the appropriate standard is determined according to the requirements of the intervention and clinical circumstance. Processes that involve the development and use of evidence should be accessible and transparent to all stakeholders.

A common commitment to certain principles and priorities guides the activities of the Roundtable and its members, including the commitment to the right health care for each person; putting the best evidence into practice; establishing the effectiveness, efficiency, and safety of medical care delivered; building constant measurement into our healthcare investments; the establishment of healthcare data as a public good; shared responsibility distributed equitably across stakeholders, both public and private; collaborative stakeholder involvement in priority setting; transparency in the execution of activities and reporting of results; and subjugation of individual political or stakeholder perspectives in favor of the common good.

Foreword

The nation turns to the National Academies for sound advice on issues related to science, technology, and health. Accordingly, the Institute of Medicine (IOM), as the healthcare arm of the National Academies, is the advisor to the nation on matters of health and medicine. Similarly, the National Academy of Engineering (NAE) serves as the nation's preeminent advisor on matters of engineering and technology. Improving our nation's healthcare system is a challenge which, because of its scale and complexity, requires a creative approach and input from many different fields of expertise.

This publication summarizes presentations and discussions at Engineering a Learning Healthcare System: A Look at the Future, a meeting sponsored by the IOM's Roundtable on Value & Science-Driven Health Care (formerly the Roundtable on Evidence-Based Medicine) in cooperation with the NAE. The IOM Roundtable provides a neutral forum for engaging in key health issues through collaborative discussion, with a focus on improving evidence generation and its application in health care. The Roundtable membership has developed the concept of *a learning health system* with the stated goal that, by the year 2020, 90 percent of clinical decisions will be supported by accurate, timely, and up-to-date clinical information and will reflect the best available evidence.

Building on previous work done by the IOM and NAE in this area, including production of the report *Building a Better Delivery System: A New Engineering/Health Care Partnership*, the workshop convened leading engineering practitioners, health professionals, and scholars to explore how the field might learn from and apply systems engineering principles in the design of a learning healthcare system, one that embeds real-time learning for continuous improvement in the quality, safety, and efficiency of care, while generating new knowledge and evidence about what works best.

The following pages summarize the workshop discussions during which participants explored barriers to care delivery, lessons in transformation from other organizations, and harnessing the technical talent of the engineering field to inform the development of necessary decision support, feedback mechanisms, and infrastructure. Throughout the workshop, participants emphasized that health care is substantially underperforming on many dimensions and that significant opportunity remains for the system to learn and to develop into one that yields the best results and the highest value. Among the most important of these opportunities are the realignment of incentives to compel continuous improvement, fostering a leadership culture that reinforces teamwork, enhancing opportunities for sustained learning and research from different perspectives, accounting for human error but requiring perfection in system performance, and, most importantly, centering the system's processes on the major consideration—the patient experience. The engagement of diverse perspectives, including those of engineering and healthcare professionals, will be essential to designing such a system.

We would like to offer our thanks to the Roundtable members for the leadership that they bring to these important issues; to the members of the workshop planning committee, especially its chair, NAE member William B. Rouse, for the invaluable insight and guidance provided; to the Roundtable and NAE staff for their skill and dedication in coordinating and facilitating the activities; and, importantly, to the sponsors who make this work possible: Agency for Healthcare Research and Quality, America's Health Insurance Plans, AstraZeneca, Blue Shield of California Foundation, Burroughs Wellcome Fund, California Health Care Foundation, Centers for Medicare & Medicaid Services, Charina Endowment Fund, Department of Veterans Affairs, Food and Drug Administration, Johnson & Johnson, Gordon and Betty Moore Foundation, National Institutes of Health, the Peter G. Peterson Foundation, sanofi-aventis, and Stryker.

Harvey V. Fineberg, M.D., Ph.D.
President, Institute of Medicine

Charles M. Vest, Ph.D.
President, National Academy of Engineering

Preface

Engineering a Learning Healthcare System: A Look at the Future focuses on current major healthcare system challenges and what the field of engineering has to offer in the redesign of the system toward one of continuous improvement—a learning healthcare system. The Institute of Medicine's (IOM's) Roundtable on Value & Science-Driven Health Care (formerly the Roundtable on Evidence-Based Medicine) envisions that such a system will be the product of collaboration across major healthcare stakeholders and could draw significant benefits from insights from the field of engineering. Thus this workshop is a product of a collaboration between the IOM and the National Academy of Engineering (NAE) and investigates the interfaces and synergies between the engineering and medical sciences. The workshop convened experts to identify and discuss issues related to healthcare system improvement and how lessons learned from engineering might inform current thinking about the different components of healthcare delivery, from research and knowledge generation to clinical care at the bedside.

The Roundtable has outlined important crosscutting issues in healthcare system transformation through the *Learning Health System* set of workshops. These provide a framework for working toward the Roundtable's goal that by the year 2020, 90 percent of clinical decisions will reflect and be supported by accurate, timely, and up-to-date evidence. A reworking of the current healthcare delivery system to one that ensures that the right patient receives the right care at the right time is essential to this transformation, and insights from the systems engineering field, such as those discussed during these 2 days, will be crucial in making progress toward that goal.

Workshop presentations and discussions surveyed the potential for greater interaction between the disciplines of medicine and engineering. Presentations covered various opportunities for learning on the part of health care as well as teaching opportunities for engineering fields. Participants heard accounts of how engineering engages complex systems, such as health care; case studies of how systems engineering has transformed other industries and sectors; and ways in which the application of engineering principles can foster changes toward continuous learning in health care. Presentations and discussions also identified current healthcare system complexities, impediments, and failures; identified opportunities for capturing more value in health care; and considered ideas about how to initiate the necessary systems changes and align policies and leadership opportunities with them.

Numerous themes emerged over the course of the 2-day workshop, and they centered on the issue of how to transform the current healthcare system into one that learns throughout the continuum of care. These themes included the need to center the system's processes on the right target—the patient experience, the notion that system excellence is created by the reliable delivery of established best practices, the idea that complexity compels reasoned allowance for tailored adjustments, the need to emphasize interdependence of different components and to address the interfaces of the different components, the importance of communication through teamwork, the need for cross-checking, transparency and feedback as engines for system improvement, the acknowledgment and management of human error, the alignment of rewards to foster continuous improvement, the enhancement of opportunities for sustained learning and research from different perspectives, and the need to foster a leadership culture that reinforces teamwork and results.

In addition to these themes, a number of cross-sector follow-up actions were identified that may be pursued by the Roundtable. These actions may include further collaboration between the IOM Roundtable and the NAE to clarify terminology in order to prompt healthcare professionals to draw more naturally upon relevant and helpful engineering principles for system improvement. Actions may also include greater focus on identifying and disseminating best practices in order to improve patient outcomes; exploring the possibility of changing the education of health professionals to advance skills in knowledge navigation, teamwork, patient–provider partnerships, and process awareness; advancing the notion of paying for value; and exploring the elements of inefficiency in health care and developing a science of waste assessment and how to mobilize resources to eliminate it.

We would like to acknowledge those individuals and organizations that donated their valuable time toward the development of this workshop summary. In particular, we acknowledge the contributors to this volume for their presence at the workshop and their efforts to further develop their presentations into the manuscripts contained in this publication. We would also like to acknowledge those who provided counsel by serving on the planning committee for this workshop, including William B. Rouse (*Chair*) (Georgia Institute of Technology), the late Jerome H. Grossman (Harvard University), Brent C. James (Intermountain Health Care, Inc.), Helen S. Kim (Gordon and Betty Moore Foundation), Cato T. Laurencin (University of Virginia), and the Honorable Paul H. O'Neill (Value Capture, LLC).[*] Although not a formal member of the planning committee, Proctor Reid of the NAE contributed to the planning and execution of the workshop. Roundtable staff, including Katharine Bothner, Kiran Gupta, W. Alexander Goolsby, LeighAnne Olsen, Daniel O'Neill, Ruth Strommen, and Catherine Zweig, helped to translate the workshop proceedings and discussion into this workshop summary. Stephen Pelletier also contributed substantially to publication development. We would also like to thank Lara Andersen, Greta Gorman, Jackie Turner, Michele de la Menardiere, Vilija Teel, and Bronwyn Schrecker for helping to coordinate the various aspects of review, production, and publication. This book is dedicated to the memory of Jerry Grossman, who was a stellar planning committee member, with lifelong dedication to and leadership in the bridging of medicine and engineering.

Engineering a Learning Healthcare System: A Look at the Future offers important insights to the field of medicine from the field of engineering concerning the development of a learning healthcare system. It also provides an example of how collaboration across diverse disciplines can lead to vast improvements in healthcare delivery. The hope is that, by making major stakeholders more aware of the importance of the delivery system, it will prompt the development of strategies for applying the insights from this workshop to health system improvements and that these strategies will ultimately transform the current healthcare system into one that smoothly operates to both generate and apply evidence to improve the health of Americans.

Denis A. Cortese
Chair, Roundtable on Value & Science-Driven Health Care

J. Michael McGinnis
Executive Director, Roundtable on Value & Science-Driven Health Care

---

[*] Institute of Medicine planning committees are solely responsible for organizing the workshop, identifying topics, and choosing speakers. The responsibility for the published workshop summary rests with the workshop rapporteurs and the institution.

Contents

Summary

The fundamental notion of the learning healthcare system—continuous improvement in effectiveness, efficiency, safety, and quality—is rooted in principles that medicine shares with engineering. In particular, the fields of systems engineering, industrial engineering, and operations research have long experience in the systematic design, analysis, and improvement of complex systems, notably in such large sectors as the airline and automobile industries. Working cooperatively with the National Academy of Engineering (NAE), the Institute of Medicine (IOM) organized Engineering a Learning Healthcare System: A Look at the Future to bring together leaders from the fields of health care and engineering to identify particularly promising areas for application of engineering principles to the design of more effective and efficient health care—a learning healthcare system. This report presents the summary of the meeting's discussions.

Currently, the organization, management, and delivery of health care in the United States falls short of delivering quality health care reliably, consistently, and affordably. As health care continues to increase in scope and complexity, so will the challenges to efficiency. In part, the capacity to address these challenges will depend on the ability to develop information about the relative effectiveness of interventions in a fashion that is more timely and practical than is typically the case for individually designed prospective studies, such as randomized clinical trials. It will also depend on the ability to design delivery systems in which the dynamics at the component interfaces are much more efficient. In both cases, the adaptation of engineering principles to facilitate continuous learning will be key.

The goal of a learning healthcare system is to deliver the best care every time, and to learn and improve with each care experience. This goal is attainable only through system-wide changes of the sort that have been successfully undertaken in certain activities of the manufacturing sectors. In these cases significant benefits have been realized through organization-wide transformations guided by principles of systems and process engineering and the practices of structured data feedback for process improvement. Data collection and monitoring are increasingly important components of health care, but much remains to be done in their application for continuous improvement. Engineering sciences associated with system design could contribute to a learning healthcare system that applies the best-known evidence, encourages continuous learning, and allows for knowledge generation as a natural by-product of patient care delivery. A fully functional system of this sort would advance quality; improve patient and provider safety, in turn delivering increasing value to consumers; and ensure that the care that is delivered is centered on the best outcome for each patient.

With these issues in focus, Engineering a Learning Healthcare System: A Look at the Future was organized by the National Academies to take stock of lessons from engineering that might be applicable to health, to investigate examples of efforts completed or under way in that respect, and to examine prospects for increasing the level of interdisciplinary, cooperative activity. The workshop was one of a series of workshops sponsored by the IOM Roundtable on Value & Science-Driven Health Care (then, the Roundtable on Evidence-Based Medicine) and focused on the development of a learning healthcare system. Because the workshop aimed to identify learning opportunities from health care, and teaching opportunities from engineering, it was structured both to review already well-established examples of activities in which engineering principles—in particular, systems engineering—have been adapted for use in healthcare settings, as well as to encourage discussion of additional opportunities and approaches to fostering ongoing progress in communication between the two fields.

An overview of the premises of the workshop identified by the workshop planning committee is found in Box S-1. Throughout the meeting's discussions, frequent mention was made of the cross-relevance of the concepts, and participants observed that even some of the terminology and reference points were similar—e.g., the discussions of Harold W. Sorenson and William W. Stead who addressed, respectively, how to engage health as a complex system, and approaches to adjusting to a more complex clinical decision environment. Case studies illustrated achievements in health care that have drawn upon systems engineering, and breakout sessions challenged workshop participants to identify opportunities and actions for generating additional value in health care through application of engineering concepts. Neither the case studies nor the breakout sessions yielded

> **BOX S-1**
> **Workshop Premises**
>
> - Health care is substantially underperforming on most dimensions: effectiveness, appropriateness, safety, cost, efficiency, and value.
> - Increasing complexity in health care is likely to accentuate current problems unless reform efforts go beyond financing to foster significant changes in the culture, practice, and delivery of health care.
> - Extensive administrative and clinical data collected in healthcare settings are largely unused for new insights on the effectiveness of healthcare interventions and systems of care.
> - If the effectiveness of health care is to keep pace with the opportunity of diagnostic and treatment innovation, system design and information technology must be structured to ensure application of the best evidence, continuous learning, and research insights generated as a natural by-product of the care process.
> - Engineering principles are at the core of a learning healthcare system—one structured to keep the patient constantly in focus, while continuously improving quality, safety, knowledge, and value in health care.
> - Impressive transformations have occurred through systems and process engineering in service and manufacturing sectors—e.g., banking, airline safety, automobile manufacturing.
> - Despite the obvious differences that exist in the dynamics of mechanical vs. biological and social systems, the current challenges in health care necessitate an entirely fresh view of the organization, structure, and function of the delivery and monitoring processes in health care.
> - Taking on the challenges in health care offers the engineering sciences an opportunity to test, learn, and refine approaches to understanding and improving innovation in complex adaptive systems.

breakthrough insights, but that fact itself is testament to the need for more systematic engagement of terms, education, and opportunities for jointly targeted projects.

THE ROUNDTABLE AND THE LEARNING HEALTHCARE SYSTEM

Convened in 2006 under the auspices of the IOM, the Roundtable on Value & Science-Driven Health Care provides a trusted setting for healthcare stakeholders—patients, employers, manufacturers, payers, policy makers, providers, and researchers—to discuss strategies to improve the effectiveness and efficiency of the nation's healthcare system. The Roundtable is therefore aimed at exploring ways in which health care may be improved through the systematic and routine capture and analysis of clinical data for point-of-care learning, the seamless application of insights to improve the effectiveness and efficiency of care processes, and the outcomes and value optimized for each patient and the system as a whole. It has devoted substantial attention to prospects and strategies for substantially expanded use of clinical data, with careful attention to security and privacy protection, as a basic resource for the generation of new knowledge.

Roundtable participants established a goal that, *by the year 2020, 90 percent of clinical decisions will be supported by accurate, timely, and up-to-date clinical information, and will reflect the best available evidence* (IOM Roundtable on Evidence-Based Medicine, 2005). Members are committed to identifying, prioritizing, and addressing opportunities through ongoing public–private initiatives, including convening the Learning Health System series of workshops and resulting publications. To date, the workshop series has included

- The Learning Healthcare System (July 2006)
- Judging the Evidence: Standards for Determining Clinical Effectiveness (February 2007)
- Leadership Commitments to Improve Value in Healthcare: Finding Common Ground (July 2007)
- Redesigning the Clinical Effectiveness Research Paradigm: Innovation and Practice-Based Approaches (December 2007)
- Clinical Data as the Basic Staple of Health Learning: Creating and Protecting a Public Good (February 2008)
- Engineering a Learning Healthcare System: A Look at the Future (April 2008)
- Learning What Works: Infrastructure Required for Comparative Effectiveness Research (July 2008)
- Value in Health Care: Accounting for Cost, Quality, Safety, Outcomes, and Innovation (November 2008)
- The Healthcare Imperative: Lowering Costs and Improving Outcomes (May, July, September, and December 2009)
- Patients Charting the Course: Citizen Engagement and the Learning Health System (April 2010)
- Digital Infrastructure for the Learning Health System: The Foundation for Continuous Improvement in Health and Health Care (July, September, and October 2010)

Engineering a Learning Healthcare System: A Look at the Future was the sixth workshop in the Learning Health System series, and this chapter briefly summarizes the presentations, discussions, and recurring themes. The first day of the workshop provided insights into potential synergies between engineering disciplines and healthcare challenges (Chapter 1) and guided the audience through some of the processes by which engineering deals with systems complexity (Chapter 2). The afternoon sessions on the first day lent insight into the complexities of health care (Chapter 3) and the mechanisms through which other industries have addressed complexity (Chapter 4). The second day's presentations identified opportunities for systems improvement followed by a breakout session, and it concluded with observations on systems change (Chapter 5 and Berwick, Chapter 1, p. 53) and a discussion on opportunities to align policies with leadership opportunities. Chapter 6 explores the next steps for aligning policies with leadership opportunities and summarizes the common themes and issues for the Roundtable's attention. The workshop agenda, biographical sketches of participants, and a list of attendees can be found in the appendixes.

COMMON THEMES

The presentations and discussions within the workshop highlighted multiple opportunities for applying engineering principles in the establishment of a learning healthcare system. The presentations and discussions also provided insight into engineering approaches to systems complexity and identified critical areas that need attention in health care. Throughout the 2 days of the workshop, a set of common themes emerged as recurring elements of the discussion (Box S-2).

- *The system's processes must be centered on the right target—the patient.* Patient-centered care was defined in the 2001 IOM report *Crossing the Quality Chasm* as providing care that is respectful of and responsive to individual patient preferences, needs, and values and ensuring that patient values guide all clinical decisions (IOM, 2001). However, health care is by nature highly complex, involving multiple participants and parallel activities that sometimes take on a character of their own, independent of patient needs or desires. Throughout several sessions, workshop participants emphasized the need to ensure that processes support patients—and that patients are not forced into processes. Patient needs and perspectives must be at the center of all process design, technology application, and clinician engagement.
- *System excellence is created by the reliable delivery of established best practice.* Identifying and embedding practices that work best, and developing the system processes to ensure their delivery every time, help to define excellence in system performance and to focus the system on delivering the best possible care for patients. In health care, establishing practices from the best available evidence

and building them as routines into practice patterns, as well as developing systems to document results and update best practices as the evidence evolves, will integrate some of the best elements from the engineering disciplines into healthcare issues. Participants often cited the need for better integration of development and communication of best practices in healthcare systems, as well as the need for process systems to track healthcare details and outcomes, with feedback for practice refinement and better patient outcomes.

- *Complexity compels reasoned allowance for tailored adjustments.* Established routines may need circumstance-specific adjustments related to differences in the appropriateness of established healthcare regimens for various individuals, variations in caregiver skill, and the evolving nature of the science base—or all three. Mass customization and other engineering practices can help assure a consistency that can accelerate the recognition of the need for tailoring and delivering the most appropriate care—with the best prospects for improved outcomes—for the patient. Participants pointed to the need for the development of a system of care flexible enough to incorporate these considerations and to leverage the lessons learned from their employment in a process of continuous learning.

BOX S-2
Workshop Common Themes

- The system's processes must be centered on the right target—the patient.
- System excellence is created by the reliable delivery of established best practice.
- Complexity compels reasoned allowance for tailored adjustments.
- Learning is a non-linear process.
- Emphasize interdependence and tend to the process interfaces.
- Teamwork and cross-checks trump command and control.
- Performance, transparency, and feedback serve as the engine for improvement.
- Expect errors in the performance of individuals but perfection in the performance of systems.
- Align rewards on key elements of continuous improvement.
- Education and research can facilitate understanding and partnerships between engineering and the health professions.
- Foster a leadership culture, language, and style that reinforce teamwork and results.

- *Learning is a non-linear process.* The focus on an established hierarchy of scientific evidence as a basis for evaluation and decision making cannot fully accommodate the fact that much of the sound learning in complex systems occurs in local and individual settings. Participants cited the need to bridge the gap between dependence on formal trials, such as randomized clinical trials, and the experience of local improvement in order to speed learning and avoid impractical costs.
- *Emphasize interdependence and tend to the process interfaces.* A system is most vulnerable at links between critical processes. In health care, attention to the nature of relationships and hand-offs between elements of the patient care and administrative processes is therefore vital and a crucial component of focusing the process on the patient experience and improving outcomes.
- *Teamwork and cross-checks trump command and control.* Especially in systems designed to guarantee safety, system performance that is effective and efficient requires careful coordination and teamwork as well as a culture that encourages parity among all those with established responsibilities. During the workshop, several examples were cited of other industries that have used systems design and social engineering to better integrate and strengthen their systems processes with great improvements in efficiency and safety.
- *Performance, transparency, and feedback serve as the engine for improvement.* Continuous learning and improvement in patient care requires transparency in processes and outcomes as well as the ability to capture feedback and make adjustments.
- *Expect errors in the performance of individuals, but perfection in the performance of systems.* Human error is inevitable in any system and should be assumed. On the other hand, safeguards and designed redundancies can deliver perfection in system performance. Mapping processes and embedding prompts, cross-checks, and information loops can assure best outcomes and allow human capacity to focus on what can not be programmed—compassion and individual patient needs. Several workshop presentations shared success stories and lessons learned from other industries, such as the automotive and airline industries, that have effectively incorporated this strategy.
- *Align rewards on the key elements of continuous improvement.* Incentives, standards, and measurement requirements can serve as powerful change agents. Therefore, it is vital that they be carefully considered and directed to the targets most important to improving the patient and provider experiences. Participants noted that it

is vital that incentives be carefully considered and directed to the targets most important to improving the efficiency, effectiveness, and safety of the system—and ultimately patient outcomes—as well as taking into consideration the patient and provider experiences.

- *Education and research can facilitate understanding and partnerships between engineering and the health professions.* The relevance of systems engineering principles to health care and the impressive transformation brought to other industries speaks to the merits of developing common vocabularies, concepts, and ongoing joint education and research activities that help generate stronger questions and solutions. Workshop participants pointed to the dearth of training opportunities bridging these two professions and spoke of the need to encourage greater collaborative work between them.

- *Foster a leadership culture, language, and style that reinforce teamwork and results.* Positive leadership cultures foster and celebrate consensus goals, teamwork, multidisciplinary efforts, transparency, and continuous monitoring and improvement. In citing examples of successful learning systems, participants highlighted the need for a supportive and integrated leadership.

PRESENTATION AND DISCUSSION SUMMARIES

The workshop opened with keynote addresses outlining the current challenges faced in health care and suggesting pathways by which engineering principles might improve the way care is delivered. Sessions that followed examined how engineering disciplines engage system complexity, explored some of the impediments and failures in health care that engineering might help ameliorate, and presented case studies of successful transformations via applied systems engineering. Further sessions looked in depth at the value that could be derived from systemic change in the healthcare system, at specific types of change that would create the greatest value, and at the entities and actions that might best facilitate change.

Engineering a Learning Healthcare System

Opening the workshop and providing context for the meeting were Brent C. James, executive director of the Institute for Health Care Delivery Research at Intermountain Healthcare, and W. Dale Compton, the Lillian Gilbreth Distinguished Professor (Emeritus) of Industrial Engineering at Purdue University. In his keynote on the second day, Donald M. Berwick, then president and chief executive officer (CEO) of the Institute for Healthcare Improvement, offered an overview of some of the key factors in initiating health system change. Together, the speakers addressed the central systemic shortfalls and challenges in health care today, reflecting on the changes needed and how systems engineering might help foster a healthcare system that delivers care that we know works, and that learns from the care delivered.

Learning Opportunities for Health Care

As the first keynote speaker, James suggested that the healthcare industry is experiencing the results of a disconnect between the rapid expansion of knowledge and the traditional cultural and organizational constructs of modern medicine. This incongruity has created a system that has certain strengths, such as excellent rescue care, but also has many weaknesses, including inadequate primary and preventive care, spiraling costs, and inefficient and ineffective care delivery.

James identified several current weaknesses in the care delivery system as opportunities for improvement, including high levels of variation in services and outcomes, with often inverse associations between service intensity and outcomes; increasing rates of inappropriate care, where the risk to the patient outweighs potential benefits; unacceptable rates of care associated with adverse outcomes; inconsistent application of evidence; and significant waste within the system, leading to increased prices and limited access to care.

Although the healthcare industry continues to develop solutions at various loci in the system, James stressed the importance of additional stronger and more sustained gains that might be achieved through engineering approaches to system redesign. Opportunities include efforts to improve the protocols and predictability of care delivered, the implementation of team-based processes, structured engagement of care complexity, and active management of knowledge and learning. Perhaps most important over the long term, James said, is designing health care to be fully coordinated and interconnected as a key to the future effectiveness of American medicine.

Teaching Opportunities from Engineering

Framing the range of possible responses to the identified healthcare challenges from the engineering field, Compton discussed some of the opportunities available in making changes to a large system such as health care. He identified two particular areas where engineering can help: the organization of the delivery system and its structure. Compton suggested that appreciation of the engineering tool set can begin by clarifying several main elements, including healthcare system objectives, performance parameters, and existing control points within the system. Compton also provided relevant examples of quality and process improvement from large commercial product industries, including Ford Motor Company and Toyota, and suggested that they have relevance to current challenges facing the healthcare system. In particular, he posited that engineering principles that support continuous improvement by leveraging data, and empowering all members of the organization to communicate and participate, hold much promise for the movement toward a learning healthcare system.

In the long term, Compton said, medical and engineering professionals will need to work together much better to create common vocabulary and understanding. Specific solutions offered during his presentation included multidisciplinary involvement in research, tool development and application, and the generation and implementation of new interdisciplinary educational models for both medical and engineering professions (NAE/IOM, 2005).

Observations on Initiating Systems Change in Health Care

Citing the general areas of technique, culture, training, and economics, Berwick offered an assessment of the major challenges to the successful application of systems thinking to health care, stemming fundamentally from its basic design. That is, improvement will require fundamental changes to the system, not simply "trying harder."

Berwick outlined seven major deficiencies that must be overcome to truly wed medicine and systems knowledge: (1) a lack of emphasis on coordination and interdependence in the current practice of medicine; (2) the lack of a patient-centered approach to the care process; (3) the lack of appreciation of the power of dynamic learning and local adaptation; (4) a lack of knowledge about, or action to counteract, waste within the system; (5) the absence of a platform for interdisciplinary research and collaboration between health care and systems engineering; (6) the absence of systems thinking in the current process of healthcare providers' professional development; and (7) the lack of incentives or levers for the vast institutional rearrangement necessary to achieve the potential offered in the application of systems science to the healthcare system.

Drawing on examples, Berwick both identified the challenges and set the stage for discussion of how systems engineering principles could succeed in drawing improvement from the intersection of health care and systems thinking.

Engaging Complex Systems Through Engineering Concepts

The meeting's first panel discussion addressed how various engineering disciplines—including systems engineering, industrial engineering, operations research, human factors engineering, financial engineering, and risk analysis—deal with system complexity and how these approaches might inform and improve health care. Speakers provided examples of past successes in other industries and offered analyses about what can be learned from the contrasts.

Systems Engineering Perspectives

William B. Rouse, executive director of the Tennenbaum Institute at the Georgia Institute of Technology, provided perspectives and principles related to systems engineering approaches to complex problems, including health care. He emphasized that engineering builds on scientific findings and works to identify ways to redesign and provide for better system controls.

As a starting point, Rouse emphasized the importance of a common understanding between the healthcare and engineering vocabularies. In elaborating, he reviewed a number of engineering concepts that have applicability to health care. One class of concepts concerns the operation of a system, including *measurement*, defining and measuring the state of a system; *feedback*, comparing desired and actual outcome states of the system; and *control*, influencing system input to correct for differences between the desired and actual states. A second class of concepts concerns the creation of a system to achieve objectives of interest. The elements of this class include *analysis*, understanding input–output relationships, including uncertainties; *synthesis*, configuring input–output relationships to achieve objectives; *design*, integrating input–output relationships; *production*, creating systems that embody desired relationships; and *sustainment*, creating mechanisms to ensure the achievement of future objectives. He then went on to show how engineers use mathematical modeling to analyze the phenomena of spiraling healthcare costs caused by technological innovation, noting multiple opportunities for increased system efficiency.

Engineering Systems Analysis Tools

Operations research (OR) uses aspects of the scientific method to help frame, formulate, and solve difficult operations problems involving people and technology. Richard C. Larson, the Mitsui Professor of Engineering Systems and Civil and Environmental Engineering and director of the Center for Engineering Systems Fundamentals at the Massachusetts Institute of Technology, described the evolution of OR and provided several models of its applications in health care. Strongly systems oriented, OR has been used successfully to improve aspects of performance in healthcare settings and therefore has value and potential in developing learning healthcare systems.

Larson described how OR was used to advance cancer therapeutics through sophisticated optimization modeling and computational techniques, yielding a much safer and more reliable treatment that saved an estimated $459 million per year. He described the development of a needle exchange program in New Haven based on the application of OR modeling techniques to reduce the spread of HIV among injection drug users, leading to a 33 percent reduction in HIV/AIDS incidence. Finally, he cited his own work on the low-probability/high-consequence event of a repeat pandemic influenza on the scale of 1918, in which application of OR principles has helped to plan the application of nonpharmaceutical interventions as part of local governments' disaster planning. Larson went on to state that the most effective applications of OR to health care are likely still in the future and called for mobilization toward that goal.

Engineering Systems Design Tools

Health care can be evaluated as a service system. Indeed, the engineering of health care must recognize the fact that any service system is actually a complex integration of human-centered activities that is increasingly dependent on information technology (IT), and knowledge. As described by James M. Tien, distinguished professor and dean of the College of Engineering at the University of Miami, a service system could be considered a combination of three essential components: people, processes, and products. Services management includes managing all three toward a common end.

Tien provided an alternative systems management view of services and discussed the increasing complexity of systems, especially service systems with the attendant lifecycle design, human interface, and system integration issues. Additional elements of complexity include the increasing need for real-time, adaptive decision making within systems and the increasingly human-focused modern systems. Such a focus, Tien suggested, creates complex, customized, and personalized products and services. Methods currently used in the production of goods can be applied to improve services, such as ongoing health care, in processes that progress, for example, from supply-driven to demand-driven and from mass production to mass customization.

Engineering Systems Control Tools

In considering an approach for engineering complex healthcare systems, a patient-focused perspective is the necessary place to begin, according to Harold W. Sorenson, professor of mechanical and aerospace engineering in the Jacobs School of Engineering at the University of California, San Diego. According to Sorenson, an "integrated perspective" merges the views of management and engineering communities in navigating enterprise complexity. In health care this means marhsalling data, feedback, and control systems to improve performance in the close working relationships among all stakeholders, including healthcare administrators and practitioners, enterprise architects, and enterprise systems engineers. This notion, if successfully applied, could fundamentally change the culture, practice, and delivery of health care in the United States.

Healthcare System Complexities, Impediments, and Failures

The meeting then turned to a discussion of the inefficiencies, impediments, structural barriers, and failures within the current healthcare system that are most in need of attention and correction for progress toward a learning healthcare system to occur, with speakers offering insights on how systems engineering could address these issues.

Healthcare Culture

William W. Stead, McKesson Foundation Professor of Biomedical Informatics and Medicine and associate vice chancellor for strategy/transformation and Chief Information Officer at the Vanderbilt University Medical Center, addressed the human side of the system, one with a culture that is deep-rooted and complex and that may not always obey prescribed principles. The healthcare culture in the United States is one dominated by the current systems of education and professional survival, but it is also challenged by individual, competing forces that face discontinuous, disruptive change. In order to achieve meaningful improvement of the system and be poised to handle the continuous, disruptive change that is a fact of modern medicine, the culture will need to change to one that is outcome-driven and that values collaboration. Stead posited that opportunities for efficient and effective patient care will continue to be missed unless the healthcare culture fundamentally changes in areas such as decision-making processes, payment mechanisms, and care planning. To effect a cultural shift away from one where practitioners are instructed to trust themselves and provide care despite the system, it will be important to shift recruiting and education practices to individuals who recognize their own limits and who are comfortable with trusting the system. In moving from episodic care to patient- and population-based care, a simultaneous shift away from expert-based, mediated use of evidence to the systematic use of clinical evidence is necessary, Stead noted. He concluded by emphasizing that successful system reform will require changes in provider roles, education, decision making, financial structures, and the measurement of success on the part of every stakeholder.

Diagnostic and Treatment Technologies

The significant increase in the availability of novel diagnostic and treatment technologies has generated sustained and dramatic increases in the costs of health care. Despite the potential of new technologies to improve the quality of care and outcomes, the limited systematic integration of healthcare technologies—including IT, laboratory/radiology/imaging systems, and monitoring equipment—has led to their misuse and overuse. Using computer-aided tomography in cardiology as an example, Rita F. Redberg, director of Women's Cardiovascular Services at the University of California, San Francisco, described how the current approach to technology has resulted in use that often exceeds patient benefit. Increased collection and application of systematic data can lead to more informed decision making in the application of diagnostic and treatment technologies, Redberg suggested, and should be incorporated into practice guidelines and reimbursement policies. Additionally, a more frequent and consistent approach to reviewing evidence on the clinical benefits of new technologies might make it less likely that new practices are adopted before sufficient evidence for their effectiveness has been accumulated. Engineering integrated data collection and review into the core practices of medicine could aid in the establishment of such an approach.

Clinical Data Systems and Clinical Decision Support

In order to transform the current healthcare system into a learning healthcare system, the culture, processes, approaches to technology and the healthcare environment will all have to be transformed, said Michael D. Chase, associate medical director of quality at the Kaiser Permanente Colorado Medical Group. In particular, he noted that the U.S. healthcare system has not leveraged the available clinical data to the fullest extent possible. Data are often located in a variety of applications, cul-de-sac databases, and paper forms, which inherently limits their use. Furthermore, a lack of standardization of data models inhibits the ability of patients, clinicians, organizations, and the healthcare system to address opportunities to improve care and outcomes.

Chase described how changes could take advantage of data and health IT to develop a system of clinical decision support that is more patient-centric, takes into account process redesign, and has a team approach. He went on to describe examples of care services within Kaiser Permanente Colorado that are enabled by IT, focus on activities that improve patient outcomes, lower costs, and employ a collaborative care-giving approach. He stressed the need to take on all of the interrelated components of the healthcare system in order to achieve this level of progress on a system-wide scale.

Care Coordination and Linkage

The U.S. healthcare system has become more complex on every dimension: patient diagnosis, treatment and follow-up. Patient care is now so fragmented, disorganized, and disconnected that safety and quality depends on the ability of patients and providers to communicate and work together more effectively, said Amy L. Deutschendorf, senior director for clinical resource management at Johns Hopkins Hospital and Health System and principal of Clinical Resource Consultants, LLC. She suggested that efforts to reduce redundancies and decrease costs have challenged a healthcare system that is already marked by increased complexities, including an aging and chronically ill population, decreased lengths of stay, acute care capacity issues, convoluted payer structures and incentives, and higher consumer expectations.

To address these problems, Deutschendorf called for effective care-delivery models and new communication systems to provide the accurate, timely transfer of patient information throughout the healthcare continuum. The model she advocated focuses on the patient, fully engages all members of the healthcare team, emphasizes prevention and active care planning, and is fully integrated with the provider infrastructure. In this system, health care would go from "silo" to "systems" thinking, with stronger communication among all stakeholders, increased care based on evidence, and new approaches to staff deployment and role definitions. Additional components of this redefined system would include increased monitoring and surveillance, patient-focused care, thoughtful technology, and expedited care delivery. In closing, Deutschendorf stated that in order to achieve these major systematic changes in patient care delivery, certain healthcare "sacred cows" must be addressed—e.g., control authorities, financial rewards—and, that systems engineering principles would aid in this challenge

Administrative Business Systems

The care and administrative processes in American hospitals are still the most complex institutions in American health care, according to Ralph W. Muller, CEO of the University of Pennsylvania Health System (UPHS). These processes need to be significantly changed in order to achieve the performance improvements required of a learning healthcare system. Muller described UPHS transformation initiatives related to access to services, management and coordination of inpatient care, billing practices, data management and reporting, alignment of incentives, and change management and feedback. He described some important lessons associated with data-driven analysis and decision making for identifying opportunities and motivating change. The UPHS experience with workflow redesign and role restructuring, based in part on integrated IT, facilitated the identification of goals and improvement in performance. Muller discussed UPHS's approaches to engaging physicians, management, and staff in systems improvement initiatives as a testament to the possibility of gaining efficiency yields in an overwhelmingly complex American healthcare system through incremental changes at individual institutions.

Information Knowledge and Development

As the nation's healthcare system moves toward increasingly integrated information systems, it will be important to support information exchange and knowledge management while evaluating and improving the quality and value of healthcare practices. Eugene C. Nelson, professor in the Dartmouth Institute for Health Policy and Clinical Practice at Dartmouth Medical School and director of quality administration at Dartmouth–Hitchcock Medical Center, presented a case study, based on the Dartmouth–Hitchcock Spine Center's work, that illustrated the principles and methods of feed-forward, which builds feedback from past experiences into the future design and improvement of the system. Such an approach serves to increase the efficiency of patient care as well as to generate and manage new information about individual patients and entire patient populations.

In his presentation, Nelson outlined how the Spine Center's system focuses on the critical function of patient-reported data embedded into the process of healthcare delivery, including some of the complexities associated with developing patient-centered, feed-forward data systems. In particular, he highlighted the challenges stemming from embedding decision-support evidence into the care delivery process, and he advocated "collaboratories" in which professionally organized networks for both care and care research could develop sustainable feed-forward data systems.

Case Studies in Transformation Through Systems Engineering

Several workshop case studies illustrated the successful application of systems engineering in various circumstances and sectors.

Airline Safety

The aviation industry has successfully integrated engineering solutions that transformed safety outcomes. John J. Nance, founding member of the National Patient Safety Foundation, discussed the possibilities suggested by the aviation industry's experience. Nance summarized elements of aviation's use of engineering principles, including critical feedback systems associated with detecting and managing mechanical problems and the notion of "exquisite redundancy." The airlines built a system around the assumptions that humans are imperfect and that systems can be structured to correct—and even anticipate—human errors through training programs, procedure standardization, and variable minimization. He described the need for healthcare systems to plan for and expect failure in every aspect as well as the need for acceptance of these realities operationally and culturally. The wide scope and variety of engineering experiences adopted in aviation could be directly applicable to health care, legitimizing and inculcating known best practices, eliminating the need to reinvent every procedure, and providing operational buffers against human fallibility in order to allow for safer care delivery systems, Nance said.

Alcoa's Reorientation

Innovations designed and implemented by organizations can advance the frontiers of business operations. Earnest J. Edwards, senior vice president and controller (retired) of Alcoa, Inc., and now the vice chair of Martha Jefferson Health Service, offered what he called the five basic truths of organizational innovation: (1) high quality in tandem with low cost creates high efficiency, (2) informed decision making originates in effective systems, (3) change agents are solution-oriented, (4) strategic planning is preferred over historical reporting, and (5) vital business partners leverage their roles to make strategic decisions.

Edwards described successful applications of cycle-time reduction in the financial closing process in a leading company (Alcoa), a major government agency (the U.S. Treasury), and a community hospital (Martha Jefferson Health Service) that all achieved their goals through the application of five key strategies: (1) expecting high value, (2) effectively using information, (3) becoming solution oriented, (4) focusing on planning the future, and (5) becoming vital business partners with expanded roles in strategic decisions. In addition to streamlining financial functions, projects to reduce financial closing cycles at each of these companies provided more timely information for business decision making, served as an example of how to make major improvements to a routine process, and were a major motivating force for the staff of the organizations. Health care could benefit by adopting similar programs, he suggested.

Veterans Health Affairs

The veterans healthcare system, managed by the Veterans Health Administration in the U.S. Department of Veterans Affairs (VA), is the largest integrated healthcare system in the United States. As recently as the 1990s, the VA system was widely criticized for providing fragmented and disjointed care that was expensive, difficult to access, and insensitive to individual needs. Kenneth W. Kizer, chair of Medsphere Systems Corporation, described the radical re-engineering of VA health care that was launched in 1995, a program aimed at creating a continuum of consistent, predictable, high-quality, patient-centered care. The effort was based on specific interrelated and overlapping strategic goals: (1) create an accountable management structure and control system, (2) integrate and coordinate services across the continuum of care, (3) improve and standardize the quality of care, (4) modernize information management, and (5) align the system's finances with desired outcomes.

The effect of the reform was transformative. In recent years, the Veterans Health Administration has been hailed as providing the best health care in the United States and is held out as an exemplary model of high-quality, low-cost (i.e., high value) health care. Kizer reviewed some of the systemic changes integral to the transformation and some of the improvements in performance. Examples include decentralizing operational decision making and instituting both the computerized patient record system and the veterans equitable resource allocation methodology. He declared that relatively simple interventions can be implemented and hold promise for the reform of health care.

Ascension Health

Ascension Health is the largest not-for-profit healthcare delivery system in the United States, the largest Catholic healthcare system, and the third largest healthcare system overall (after the VA and the Hospital Corporation of America). David B. Pryor, the system's chief medical officer, detailed Ascension Health's "Call to Action," a reform effort established in October 2002 that focused on three goals: health care that works, health care that is safe, and health care that leaves no one behind.

During the presentation, Pryor focused on the steps taken to improve safety related to hospital mortality, adverse drug events, Joint Commission National Patient Safety Goals, nosocomial infections, falls and fall injuries, pressure ulcers, perinatal safety, and surgical complications, with the goal of no preventable injuries or deaths. Those steps addressed challenges in culture, infrastructure, the business case, standardization, and staff collaboration. Strategies were derived for each challenge and implemented with great success. Pryor offered several crucial factors that contributed to this success, including a clear focus with accountable goals, transparency in results reporting, addressing all challenge areas, and a deep organizational commitment across all levels of leadership with mutual accountability.

Fostering Systems Change to Drive Continuous Learning in Health Care

The IOM workshop publication *The Learning Healthcare System* (2007) identified several common characteristics of a learning healthcare organization, including a culture that emphasizes transparency and learning through continuous feedback loops, care as a seamless team process, best practices that are embedded in system design, information systems that reliably deliver evidence and capture results, and results that are captured and used as feedback to improve the level of practice and the state of the science. Each speaker addressed what feedback and performance improvement look like and how impediments can be turned into enablers.

Learning, Team, and Patient-Oriented Culture

In manufacturing, heavy industry, high-tech services, aviation, the military, and elsewhere, a small number of organizations will be innovative leaders. These innovators may use similar science and technology to meet the needs of a similar customer base, depend on the same group of suppliers, hire from the same labor pools, and be subject to the same regulations as other organizations in their fields, but they deliver far more value, often with less effort and at a lower cost. These "rabbits" gain and sustain leadership by managing their systems of work in markedly different ways.

Steven J. Spear, senior lecturer at the Massachusetts Institute of Technology and a senior fellow at the Institute for Healthcare Improvement, described several such "rabbits," including Toyota and Southwest Airlines. He pointed out that healthcare organizations can and have learned from these types of companies, with impressive improvements in efficacy, efficiency, safety, and quality of care. Spear proposed that delivering better care to more people at lower costs and with less effort is achievable by adopting elements of "clinical evidence" from other organizations. He emphasized that these transformations require an approach of process reform rather than managing individual functions and also need continuous, dynamic monitoring and management.

Knowledge Development, Access, and Use

In addition to requiring education and research agendas, knowledge management for clinical decision support (CDS) also requires a policy framework. Donald E. Detmer, then president and CEO of the American Medical Informatics Association (AMIA) and professor of medical education at the University of Virginia, asserted that we do not have the appropriate policy infrastructure to support some of these goals. Drawing from the AMIA CDS Roadmap for National Action, Detmer proposed several policy solutions. The AMIA recommends a three-pillar structure of timely availability of quality knowledge, high adoption and effective use, and continuous improvement of knowledge and methods. He noted that this roadmap was used by the U.S. Department of Health and Human Services to identify priorities for CDS development, including achieving measurable progress toward performance goals for healthcare quality improvement, exploring private–public partnerships to facilitate collaboration, and accelerating development and employment through federal programs and collaborations.

Technology Management

For health care, technology management is a growing issue that continues to require significant attention. Because a large portion of the recent growth in healthcare expenditures is a direct outcome of technology development, many look to technology as an opportunity to streamline processes and reduce costs. Stephen J. Swensen, director of quality at the Mayo Clinic and professor of radiology in the Mayo Clinic College of Medicine, presented several perspectives on the issue of technology management in U.S. health care.

Swensen outlined four primary elements of healthcare technology management. First, policies—particularly those policies that create incentives, such as payment—can be central motivators of activities and performance. The appropriateness and reliability of technology offer opportunities in terms of managing the appropriate use and ensuring the high reliability of the technologies applied. Effective diffusion of best practices and safety nets is crucial for efficient and effective technology management, as it allows for the optimization of technology use. Finally, social engineering strategies, including transparency, team-work training, horizontal infrastructure, and cross-functional team-based simulations, can contribute to moving an organization toward integrated care coordination in which decisions are made with an organizational perspective. In conclusion, Swensen noted that, in order to reach technology management goals and provide reliable patient care, the healthcare industry must foster systems changes to drive continuous learning.

Information Systems Organization and Management

Simulation can help accelerate progress. Over the past decade, numerous healthcare delivery organizations have implemented clinical information systems in order to improve the quality and safety of patient care. Recent studies have suggested that, despite considerable investment in these systems, many organizations have failed in these efforts. David C. Classen, chief medical officer of First Consulting Group and an associate professor of medicine at the University of Utah, explored current approaches to evaluating clinical information systems and detailed a new simulation tool that has been developed and used by healthcare organizations to evaluate the effectiveness of these systems in improving the safety of care. He described several strategies for evaluating the computerized physician order entry system, one of the ways that hospitals work toward safe medication management. These strategies included electronic health record (EHR) product certification as well as approaches by the National Quality Forum and the Leapfrog Group that employ simulation. Classen noted that the widespread use of simulation in these instances holds great promise for the evaluation of clinical information systems.

Capturing More Value in Health Care

During a breakout session, participants assembled in small groups to discuss the engineering approach likely to yield the greatest return in health, the amount of enhanced effectiveness and efficiency that might be anticipated, and what actions might facilitate change. The main points of their discussions were reported back to the entire group.

In response to the question of how much more value (health returned for dollars invested) could be obtained through application of systems engineering principles in health care, respondents felt that the definition of value was problematic as it depends on the stakeholder in question. In contrast, other small groups reported that based on some workshop estimates, suggesting that 50 percent of the current system resources were wasted, it was reasonable to assume that a doubling of value ought to be attainable through systematic changes, including realignment of payment incentives, health IT, and better systems integration.

When asked to identify where the greatest value could be returned, participants listed a number of different areas. Among these were health IT, for better systemic coordination and informed decision making; education reform, for the necessary cultural changes within professions and greater interdisciplinary exposure and training; realignment of incentives to promote best practices; greater emphasis on collaboration; better integration of systems; adoption of processes that lead to use and evaluation; and adoption and implementation of process technologies.

Responding to the question of which actions could do the most to facilitate the needed changes, participants elaborated on some of the areas mentioned previously. Participants noted that the approach to reform was important and should start with easy, manageable issues and progress to broader, more difficult reforms. This two-tiered approach would allow for demonstrations of the potential for improvement and would thus provide the opportunity to get greater buy-in from stakeholders. Several groups mentioned the need to encourage a more collaborative approach to the care process that would involve multidisciplinary groups. Participants mentioned the need for changes in the current culture in order to allow for more integrated care, including reforms to the models of education for healthcare providers.

Changes in the availability, implementation, and application of EHRs and health IT were discussed as ways to better communicate best practices, to allow for improved analysis of process and outcomes data that can be fed back and used to improve the system, and to create better continuity of care. In order to achieve this, however, interfaces between technology and users need to be redesigned to allow for ease of use and seamless integration into the care process. Use of data from health IT systems to model and optimize care processes was discussed as a natural application of systems engineering to health care, as was the idea of combining healthcare economics models with process engineering models to get a better grasp on measuring value. Participants also discussed the need for collaboration between process engineering and medical professional organizations and other groups concerning issues of education, nomenclature, and development of best practices and core performance measures.

Finally, several groups mentioned the need to better define value in the context of a learning healthcare system and from the perspective of all of the stakeholders involved. This would make possible the creation of processes that allow for the measurement of value and its inclusion in decision-making processes.

Next Steps: Aligning Policies with Leadership Opportunities

A concluding panel discussion on aligning policies with leadership opportunities was held with five leaders from key settings in health care reflecting on their visions for changes in practice, policy, and culture. Contributing members of the panel discussion were Denis A. Cortese of the Mayo Clinic, Paul F. Conlon of Trinity Health, Mary Jane Koren of The Commonwealth Fund, Louise L. Liang of Kaiser Permanente, and Douglas W. Lowery-North of Emory University.

Several of the themes mentioned previously were raised again and expanded upon during the question-and-answer session with the panelists. Cortese, for example, shared his experiences with the achievement of interoperable systems for radiology, pointing out that it was driven by demands from the radiology professional groups. There was also discussion of the need for consideration of interoperability on the part of manufacturers in their business models as well as the need for agreement on requirements on the part of potential IT systems users in order to allow for the emergence of a unified market.

The need for a patient-centered approach was a common theme in panelists' comments. This included the use of market segmentation strategies (e.g., mass customization) to allow for the identification and individualized targeting of different groups as well as for the consideration of patient preferences in treatment and care coordination strategies.

The need for the development of value standards that factor in outcomes, safety, and cost was discussed. Panelists suggested the development of such standards for the five most common diseases as a potential first step and emphasized the need for transparency in this and all development processes.

One of the panelists proposed a human resources–focused approach to initiating reform. It would be aimed at encouraging the training of new professionals in both health care and systems engineering, as well as collaboration across those fields, and it could incentivize participation with such strategies as debt relief for new trainees.

Finally, panelists voiced an overarching concern about potential support for the work that is needed to reengineer the healthcare system and hence the importance of reforming financial incentives throughout the system.

AREAS FOR INNOVATION AND COLLABORATIVE ACTION

Presentations and discussions during the workshop offered insights into the opportunities for Roundtable members to consider along with possible follow-up actions for ongoing multistakeholder involvement to advance the integration of engineering sciences into healthcare systems improvement. Areas mentioned as possibilities include the following:

1. *Clarify terms:* The ability of healthcare professionals to draw upon relevant and helpful engineering principles for system improvement could be facilitated by a better mutual understanding of the terminology. A collaborative effort by the IOM and the NAE could create a targeted glossary and develop potentially bridging terminology for use as appropriate.

2. *Identify best practices:* Three areas of systems orientation are particularly important to improving the efficiency and effectiveness of health care: (1) focusing the system elements more directly on the key outcome—the patient experience; (2) ensuring transparency in the performance of the system and its players and components; and (3) establishing a culture that emphasizes teamwork, consistency, and excellence. Progress could be accelerated by identifying and disseminating examples of best practices from health care and from engineering on each of these dimensions.

3. *Explore health professions education change:* In the face of a rapidly changing environment in health care—the expansion of diagnostic and treatment options, much greater knowledge available, movement beyond the point at which any one individual can personally hold all the information necessary, and IT that opens new capabilities—changes to the education of health professionals can advance caregiver skills in knowledge navigation, teamwork, patient–provider partnership, and process awareness.

4. *Advance the science of payment for value:* With cost increases in health care consistently outstripping gains in performance by most measures, progress toward counteracting this trend could be achieved with a stronger focus on ways to enhance both health and economic returns from healthcare investments. This could include work in the areas of understanding, measuring, and providing incentives for value in health care.

5. *Explore fostering the development of a science of waste assessment and engagement:* Similarly, and directly related, an exploration of the elements of inefficiency in health care, how to define and measure waste, and how to mobilize responses to eliminating waste could contribute to increasing value within healthcare systems.

6. *Support the development of a robust health IT system:* The development of a health IT system, designed with systems-related continuous improvement principles in mind, must lie at the core of an efficient, effective learning system. Beginning with challenges to EHR adoption, much work remains in order to achieve a system that allows for continuous learning; permits data sharing, including the construction of databases; employs consistent standards; and addresses privacy and security concerns. Health IT is a natural place for collaborative work between engineers and caregivers, beginning with better resolution of barriers to the achievement of such a system through the employment of both expert lenses.

REFERENCES

IOM (Institute of Medicine). 2001. *Crossing the quality chasm: A new health system for the 21st century.* Washington, DC: National Academy Press.

_____. 2007. *The learning healthcare system.* Washington, DC: The National Academies Press.

IOM Roundtable on Evidence-Based Medicine. 2005. *Roundtable on Evidence-Based Medicine charter and vision statement.* Washington, DC: The National Academies Press.

NAE (National Academy of Engineering)/IOM. 2005. *Building a better delivery system: A new engineering/health care partnership*, edited by P. P. Reid. W. D. Compton, J. H. Grossman, and G. Fanjiang. Washington, DC: The National Academies Press.

1

Engineering a Learning
Healthcare System

INTRODUCTION

As the roles and complexities of provider profiles, patient care processes, and diagnostic and treatment options grow—often in an independent and disintegrated fashion—gaps in efforts concerning patient safety, clinical outcomes, reimbursement policy, medical education, and other aspects of the functioning of the healthcare system continue to widen. Defining the future state of American health care will require a clear vision on the part of the healthcare community.

The Engineering a Learning Healthcare System: A Look at the Future workshop drew together participants from healthcare and engineering disciplines to identify challenges in health care, including effectiveness, safety, and efficiency, that might benefit from a systems engineering perspective. With the baseline assumption that reform efforts must extend beyond finance to remedy the growing complexities in health care. Participants evaluated aspects of healthcare culture and practice through examples and lessons from within and outside the healthcare sector. Workshop attendees considered approaches to taking a new look at the organization, structure, function, and delivery of services in health care while maintaining a patient-centered focus.

Presentations and discussions touched on elements from prior workshops, including Clinical Data as a Public Good and the Learning Healthcare System, in an effort to synthesize topics and take advantages of various synergies. The Engineering a Learning Healthcare System: A Look at the

Future workshop addressed multiple components central to the work of the Roundtable on Value & Science-Driven Health Care:

- Facilitate *collaborative* healthcare choices of each patient and provider.
- Ensure *innovation*, quality, safety, and value in health care.
- Foster the *transformation* of the American healthcare system into a learning health system that generates and applies evidence naturally.
- Emphasize *prevention* and *health promotion* as means to increase value.
- Instill *principles* of accountability, care coordination, expectation setting, incentive alignment, and patient-centered focus.

This chapter contains a brief summary of the workshop's three keynote addresses followed by individually authored pieces based on those presentations. The three keynote talks were a commentary by Brent C. James on "Learning Opportunities for Health Care," W. Dale Compton's discussion of "Teaching Opportunities from Engineering," and Donald M. Berwick's presentation, "Observations on Initiating Systems Change in Health Care."

Engineering a Learning Healthcare System: A Look at the Future

The first two keynote addresses together outlined the landscape of issues the workshop was designed to address and framed many of the most important questions that workshop participants would explore. The third keynote address, delivered near the end of the workshop, added further depth to the intellectual framework of the workshop and contributed additional specific suggestions for moving forward in engineering a learning healthcare system.

Reflecting the fact that the workshop was sponsored by the Institute of Medicine (IOM) Roundtable on Value & Science-Driven Health Care in cooperation with the National Academy of Engineering (NAE), the program opened with two talks that addressed, respectively, issues in health care and opportunities for addressing those issues from the realm of engineering.

The first presentation, "Learning Opportunities for Health Care" was by Brent C. James, executive director of the Institute for Health Care Delivery Research and vice president of medical research and continuing medical education at Intermountain Healthcare. Based in Salt Lake City, Intermountain Healthcare is an integrated healthcare system of hospitals, clinics, a large physician group, and a health maintenance organization/ preferred provider organization insurance plan covering more than 450,000 people. James is known internationally for his work in clinical quality improvement, patient safety, and the infrastructure that underlies successful improvement efforts, such as culture change, data systems, payment methods, and management roles.

James began by discussing the historical evolution of the modern structure of healthcare delivery. He outlined five areas where care delivery currently falls short of its theoretic potential, touched briefly on the reasons for that failure, and then reflected on emerging solutions, emerging frameworks, and challenges that create a context for work on improving health care.

The five areas of health system failure noted by James were (1) the well-documented, significant variation in practices; (2) high rates of inappropriate care; (3) unacceptable rates of preventable patient injury and death; (4) a striking inability to "do what we know works"; and (5) large amounts of waste and spiraling prices, which limit access. James suggested that we may be on the verge of a head-on collision of two factors: first, the guild nature of medicine, in which physicians, nurses, and other health professionals act as stand-alone experts, and second, what James characterized as "clinical uncertainty." The latter term refers to the era of unprecedented complexity that characterizes health care today, an era marked by a lack of valid clinical knowledge and evidence regarding the best treatments and exponentially increasing new medical knowledge, in tandem with a continued reliance on subjective judgment and the innate limitations of the expert mind when making complex decisions.

James proposed four specific areas for attention in the effort to alleviate these shortfalls: (1) addressing clinical complexity, (2) developing a more robust capacity of knowledge management in a learning system, (3) improving systems for care delivery via a team approach instead of through independent experts, and (4) designing health care as a coordinated system. In particular, he called on engineering professionals to share their knowledge and expertise with healthcare professionals in order to address these issues collaboratively.

W. Dale Compton complemented James' healthcare expertise by offering the engineering perspective. Compton, the Lillian M. Gilbreth Distinguished Professor (Emeritus) of Industrial Engineering at Purdue University, brings extensive experience in engineering research from work in academia and the private sector and has served since 2000 as Home Secretary for the NAE. He offered a variety of suggestions on how engineering can help health care transition from where it is today to the point where it might realize its full potential as a learning healthcare system.

Compton explored some of the most pressing, overarching issues, including creating change within large organizations, healthcare transformations, and integrating learning into systems change. Focusing on a case study of the Ford Motor Company, Compton outlined several principles of continuous improvement that he believes could benefit health care. Organizing a comprehensive understanding of health care's disparate parts from a systems point of view will be a critically important step. It will also be vital to have adequate data—and the capacity to mine that data for knowledge—as well as to engage participation by staff at all levels of an organization.

Communication is another key factor. Although communication has many dimensions that vary among organizations, Compton asserted that engineers and healthcare professionals have considerable work to do in creating a common understanding of problems and opportunities. A cadre consisting of both engineering and medical professionals is needed to tackle some of health care's more intractable problems, working in the near term on problem solving and in the longer term on more fundamental systems design.

Later in the workshop, a keynote address from Donald M. Berwick explored in greater depth the issues that health care faces and the ways in which solutions might be engineered. Then president and chief executive officer (CEO) of the Institute for Healthcare Improvement, Berwick was also a professor of pediatrics and healthcare policy at the Harvard Medical School and professor of health policy and management at the Harvard School of Public Health. Berwick posited that there is enormous potential benefit to health care in deepening system knowledge and basing action on that knowledge. He warned, however, that real value in healthcare reform will come only if people are willing to confront the status quo, whether in technique, culture, training, or economics. The core challenge, he suggested, is that health care needs to clarify its aims, and leadership is needed to make that happen.

The heart of Berwick's presentation discussed seven issues: (1) the need to emphasize interdependence in the healthcare system; (2) the need to make the redesign of processes more visible; (3) the need to recognize the importance and value of dynamic learning and local adaptation as scientific learning processes; (4) the question of waste, which health care must confront with knowledge and action; (5) the need for a sufficient platform for robust multidisciplinary research and development at the intersection of health care and engineering; (6) the need to enrich professional education and development in health care—for example, with more attention to teamwork and systems thinking; and (7) the reform of health care in a way that would result in a radically different, integrated systems design of the fundamental healthcare infrastructure.

Following are the full presentations of the keynote addresses that set the stage and tone for the discussions that took place throughout the remainder of the workshop.

LEARNING OPPORTUNITIES FOR HEALTH CARE

Brent C. James, M.D., M.Stat., Institute for Health Care Delivery Research, Intermountain Healthcare, Inc.

The healing professions have always been central to human society. Humanity's earliest written records refer to clinical practice. For example, the Code of Hammurabi, written almost 1,800 years BCE, addresses the legal implications of medical treatment. Artifacts from Stone Age cultures indicate the presence and importance of healers and the healing professions in preliterate times.

Until relatively recently, the healing role was limited to two basic elements: when approached by a patient suffering a health problem, a healer could give unique insight into what was happening—that is, he could explain the present; and, drawing on experience with similar cases from the past, the healer could predict the patient's potential health future. But for most of human history, healers had little to offer in the way of effective treatment. Any "healing" that occurred was mainly of a spiritual nature—a shoulder to lean on, a listening ear, and (2) compassion and understanding that could help a patient reach balance, acceptance, and closure. While no one made careful measurements of the health outcomes of early medical care at a population level, educated observers routinely opined that if one were seriously ill and sought the attentions of a typical physician, chances of survival actually declined. For many centuries, the most common approaches to treatment centered on a humoral theory of disease, which held that the human body was made up of four basic humors: black bile, yellow bile, white phlegm, and red blood. Disease was thought to arise from imbalances in the humors. Health could be restored by bringing the humors back into balance, usually by removing some of the red humor. As late as 1900, the most common physician-prescribed treatment in the United States was bloodletting. The second most common therapy was the administration of purgatives, producing chemically induced vomiting and diarrhea. Hospitals were where poor people went to die (Porter, 1997; Rosenberg, 1987; Starr, 1984).

Around the turn of the 19th century, medical practice underwent a massive transformation. Between the 1860s, during the American Civil War, and about 1910, clinical leaders introduced four important changes (Porter, 1997; Rosenberg, 1987; Starr, 1984).

First, they adopted the scientific method as the foundation for "how we know what we know" within the allopathic healing professions. Driven by the scientific method, a germ-based theory of disease rapidly replaced competing frameworks and their related treatments, such as the humoral theory. Over time, this approach greatly improved the professions' understanding of the human organism in health and disease. It also produced literally thousands of effective treatments and fundamentally changed the medical model: where before physicians could explain the present and predict the future, medical science gave them the ability to "change a patient's future."[1]

Second, clinical leaders created the modern model of clinical education. The transformation of medical education started with a report of the American Medical Association published in 1902. That report led Andrew Carnegie to commission Abner Flexner, a high school teacher, to conduct a more detailed evaluation. Flexner found that the average course of study to become a licensed physician took about 4 months. (Apparently, little effort was needed to understand the humoral theory of disease, bloodletting, and purgatives.) That training usually took place exclusively in a classroom setting, with no exposure to patients or patient care. Flexner's report, published in 1910, led to the closing of more than half of all so-called "medical schools" in the United States. A new 2-year curriculum, centered in hospitals at the patient bedside, emerged.

Third, the leaders tightened the process of professional licensing. Previously, laws regarding professional licensure had served primarily to protect the guild of medicine from external competition. Those laws took on new meaning when they rested on the foundation of medical science and effective clinical education. Clinical leaders refined the licensing laws, produced a new definition of medical professionalism, and used the resulting tools to hold the profession as a whole uniformly accountable to a much higher level of demonstrated knowledge, skills, and ethical conduct.

Finally, clinical leaders created a new organizational structure for care delivery. In 1895 physicians planning the new Johns Hopkins University Hospital divided management of the facility from the practice of medicine. A new class of health facility administrators managed staffing, supplies, and the physical plant, freeing physicians to focus exclusively on patients' clinical diagnoses and treatment.

Collectively, these changes led to dramatic gains in human health measured at a population level. A child born in the United States in 1900 had a life expectancy of 49 years. A child born 100 years later, in 2000, could expect almost 77 years of life (Cutler et al., 2006) (Figure 1-1). The years from 1900 to 1960 might be called the Public Health Era. Essentially all of the life expectancy gains achieved over those six decades came from sanitation, safe food, clean water, vaccination, and immunization. For example, the cholera epidemics that killed thousands at a time during the

---

[1] The phrase comes from Dr. James Reinertsen through a personal communication. He describes the role of the physician as (1) explain the present, (2) predict the future, and (3) change a patient's health future.

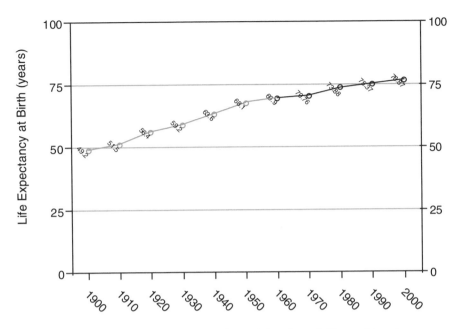

From 1900–1960: 20.7 years gained over 6 decades = 3.45 years/decade.
Since 1960: 6.97 years gained over 4 decades = 1.74 years/decade.

FIGURE 1-1 Increases in life expectancy at birth within the United States, by decade, 1900 through 2000.

latter half of the 19th century disappeared almost completely following the introduction of easily accessible clean drinking water. Typhus fever, one of the most common killers in human history, was virtually eliminated through improvements in living conditions that reduced the infestations of fleas that spread the disease. Deaths from smallpox, a true scourge, ceased with the introduction of effective vaccination programs. In 1900, somewhere between one-fifth and one-third of all children died before reaching the age of 5 years, victims of common pediatric infectious diseases—diphtheria, pertussis, measles, mumps, and polio (CDC, 1999). Widespread childhood immunization makes such deaths very rare today. During the Public Health Era, life expectancy at birth increased by an average of 3.45 years with each passing decade (as calculated by the author from the data presented in Figure 1-1).

Life expectancy gains due to advances in public health plateaued in the decade following the end of World War II. As these public health–related gains attenuated, however, a new source of health improvements emerged. For the first time in human history, physicians and nurses began to have treatment tools that could change a patient's future. Starting midcentury, disease treatment began to have a major impact on how long and how well people lived as measured at the population level. For example, since 1960 age-adjusted mortality from ischemic cardiac disease (the number one killer in modern first-world nations) has decreased by 56 percent (from 307.4 to 134.6 age-adjusted deaths/100,000 people), and since 1950 age-adjusted mortality from stroke (the number three killer in industrialized nations) has decreased by 70 percent (from 88.8 to 26.5 age-adjusted deaths/100,000 people) (CDC, 1999; Cutler et al., 2006; National Center for Health Statistics, 2000). This is remarkable progress, particularly when considered in the context of the entirety of human history. The evidence is clear: modern health professionals now routinely offer treatments that would have appeared miraculous to any previous generation.

Aim Defines the System

Given these achievements, it is worth reflecting on what is known about the factors most important in determining a person's total health—that is, how long and how well one lives. In an analysis of the actual causes of death in the United States, roughly 40 percent of total health was found to be determined by individual behavioral choices (McGinnis and Foege, 1993). The top three behavior-based challenges to health are tobacco use, obesity, and consumption of alcohol and other recreational drugs. For example, alcohol consumption is associated with about 65 percent of fatal violent crimes, 70 percent of all domestic abuse, and 60 percent of all fatal non–motor vehicle accidents (Doonon, 1998). Other behaviorally related health issues include sexually transmitted diseases, including AIDS; pregnancies among unwed teens; and suicide, accidents, and violence, particularly among young men (McGinnis et al., 2002). Healthy behaviors are closely linked with educational level, which in turn is associated with income level and health insurance coverage.[2]

One's genetic inheritance determines another 30 percent of total health. Some scientific progress has been made in understanding linkages between genes and disease, but the field is still relatively new. Some estimate that we are still 20 to 30 years away from being able to broadly offer treatments to counter genetic determinants of health.

Another 20 percent of total health relates to environmental and public health factors. These factors include clean air, safe water, and the control of epidemic infectious disease through immunization and sanitation.

---

[2] These four elements usually appear in combination and are very difficult to separate: (1) low levels of education are directly associated with (2) unhealthy behaviors, (3) low income levels, and (4) lack of health insurance.

Only 5 to 10 percent of total health—an estimated 3.5 to 7 years of lifespan—derives from the health care delivery system.

In 1977 Aaron Wildavsky published a classic essay in which he defined "the Great Equation" as the belief that "health equals health care" and that "health care means access to care." He cited statistics to show that the Great Equation is fundamentally false (Wildavsky, 1977). Such findings underscore the importance of understanding the returns achieved from our current national investment in health care.

In 2006, the United States spent about $7,100 per person on health care. For a typical family of four, healthcare expenditures far exceed the costs of owning a home. (Total national health care expenditures for a family of four totaled about $2,375 per month in 2005, while the median family home cost only $1,040 [KFF, 2006].) U.S. expenditures are high compared with those of other Organisation for Economic Co-operation and Development (OECD) countries (Peterson and Burton, 2007; Reinhardt et al., 2002). Sweden, for example, has the reputation of having the finest socialized medicine system in the world. Despite that country's spending less than half of what the United States spends on health per capita, the average Swede lives about 3 years longer than the average U.S. citizen. Likewise, although infant mortality rates have decreased very significantly worldwide over recent decades, the United States has rates roughly twice as high as those reported in Sweden.[3] Wildavsky's argument raises serious questions about whether differences in overall health at a national level can be traced back to a country's spending on health care. But even if U.S. health outcomes were equivalent to those of other developed nations, the United States still spends twice as much per person as most other modern nations. What do we get for all that extra money? Dr. W. Edwards Deming, the father of modern quality theory, regularly noted that "[a]im defines the system." Relative to health spending, what are the aims of healthcare delivery? The current national healthcare debate implicitly assumes, without examination, that the primary aim of healthcare delivery is "total health"—how long and how well we live. There are, however, two additional possible aims.

When carefully asked, most U.S. citizens say they value their relationship with a trusted medical counselor very highly. They appear to judge their health outcomes according to their opinion of that relationship, suggesting that to patients, the clinician–patient relationship may be even more

---

[3] Although these figures are often thought to represent a direct reflection of the quality of each nation's healthcare delivery system, it is important to note that the Swedish advantage disappears when risk adjustments are made for the infant mortality rate for gestational age. Each country defines preterm birth differently at a functional level, with implications for whether the infant is treated as a stillbirth or is placed in newborn ICU, with massive amounts of money invested in his/her care.

important than health outcomes. "High touch" care denotes the idea of caring, not just curing. Emeril Szilagyi captured the essence of high touch care quite accurately in his 1965 essay "In Defense of the Art of Medicine":

> A man stricken with disease today is assaulted by the same fears and finds himself searching for the same helping hand as his ancestors did five or ten thousand years ago. He has been told about the clever tools of modern medicine and somewhat vaguely, he expects that by-and-by he will profit by them, but in his hour of trial his desperate want is for someone who is personally committed to him, who has taken up his cause, and who is willing to go to trouble for him. *(Szilagyi, 1965)*[4]

High touch care leads to patient satisfaction with the healthcare delivery system. Effective primary care networks, in which people have easy access to a clinical counselor, facilitate this kind of care. Compared with other countries, the United States performs poorly in providing easy access to high touch care (Schoen et al., 2007).

Another possible aim of health care delivery is rapid response, or "rescue care." Jonsen defined the Rule of Rescue as "the imperative people feel to rescue identifiable individuals facing suffering or death" (McKie and Richardson, 2003). For the Rule of Rescue to apply, there needs to be an emotional link. There must be a name and a face so that the sufferer becomes a human being rather than a statistic (McKie and Richardson, 2003). Some commentators have pointed out that this view of care reflects a "Do something! She's dying!" reaction. They note that the interventions applied do not have to be effective—that humans feel an overwhelming need to try to help, regardless of the chance for a positive result. For example, about a year ago, six miners were underground when a coal mine in central Utah collapsed (the Crandall Mine disaster). Their plight gripped the state of Utah and the nation, as the news media shared pictures of the six men, their life stories, and interviews with their distraught friends and families. Those six men probably died in the initial collapse, but tens of millions of dollars was spent and three would-be rescuers died on the chance that the six might be alive. Other examples of the Rule of Rescue are easy to find. Indeed, the response is so powerful that in many cases, the "victim" need not be human; we respond in similar fashion to heartrending stories of animals in distress.

When examined through the lens of rapid-response rescue care, the U.S. healthcare system is the best in the world. For example, mortality rates following major trauma in the United States are about half those seen in Europe. Mortality following a heart attack in the United States is roughly

---

[4] Of particular interest, Szilagyi defined the "art of medicine" as the knowledge and skills to optimize the clinician–patient relationship.

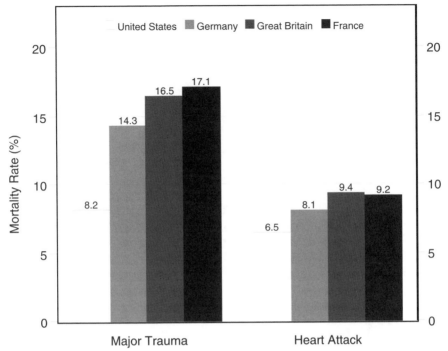

FIGURE 1-2 System performance by nation for two major examples of rescue care.
SOURCE: Based on data from OECD (2006).

a third lower than the European rates (Figure 1-2). Mortality rates for very small (less than 1,500-gram) preterm neonates in the United States are about half those observed in other developed nations (OECD, 2006). Renal dialysis rates are five times higher in the United States than in Sweden and almost twice as high as in the closest European country (Germany). Similar differences exist for other classes of high-technology, specialty-based rescue care, such as cancer treatment (Coleman et al., 2008; Verdecchia et al., 2007).

Many other countries' healthcare systems outperform the U.S. system from the perspective of total health and patient satisfaction. This advantage appears to be attributable to healthier behaviors, better public health, and easily accessible primary care. Conversely, the U.S. healthcare system performs significantly better for patients suffering from severe illness or injury, both of which require easy access to technology and subspecialists. Yet despite the massive investment it requires, rescue care is not strongly asso-

Deaths per 100,00 population

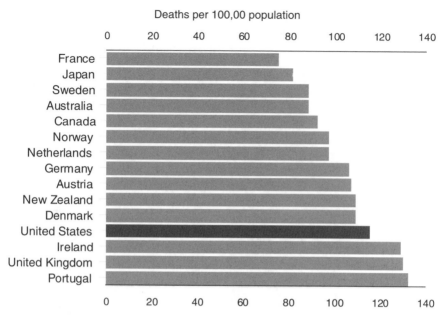

FIGURE 1-3 Mortality amenable to health care among OECD nations.
SOURCE: Based on data from OECD, 2006.

ciated with better total health at a population level. Health promotion and
disease prevention, implemented through effective primary care networks,
appear to have a greater effect on how long and how well populations
live. Figure 1-3 compares OECD nations in terms of mortality amenable
to health care. The United States fares poorly. A more recent update of
the same study places the United States dead last among 19 high-income
democracies on the same measure (Nolte and McKee, 2003).

Americans place a high value on rescue care and are willing to pay
for it. But rescue is just one of three possible aims of health care delivery,
suggesting that there are immediate opportunities to improve the quality of
health care delivered in the United States.

Opportunities for Improvement

Over the last 40 years, a broad range of health services investigations
have found that current U.S. health care delivery falls short of its theoretical
potential. The shortcomings represent significant opportunities for improvement. They fall into five broad categories.

First, care varies widely by geographic location (i.e., care received in one community is often very different from that received in another). The differences are so large that even with full access to care (health insurance), it would be impossible for all Americans to receive high-quality care. More than 40,000 articles documenting or discussing variations in care delivery have been published in peer-reviewed journals over the last 40 years. These well-documented, massive variations in practice are an important entry point for understanding how best to improve the quality of care received by all Americans.

Second, some investigators have suggested that geographic variation in quality of care might arise from inappropriate care, with a treatment's innate risk to the patient outweighing any potential clinical benefit. An evaluation of a series of major treatments performed in U.S. hospitals found that 2 to 32 percent of those treatments were clinically inappropriate. For professions that hold as their primary tenet "First, do no harm," these findings are deeply troubling. However, inappropriate care does not explain geographic variation. On average, communities with high rates of utilization show about the same proportion of inappropriate care as low-utilization communities (Chassin et al., 1998).

Third, a landmark IOM report estimated that between 44,000 and 98,000 people die each year from preventable injuries sustained as part of care delivery in U.S. hospitals (IOM, 2000). That makes American hospitals somewhere between the fourth and sixth most common cause of preventable death in the United States.

Fourth, the U.S. healthcare system is characterized by a striking inability to execute. For example, McGlynn and colleagues identified a series of treatments with strong evidence for effectiveness. The resulting list of treatments was noncontroversial; there was strong professional consensus that the treatments should routinely be provided to patients. However, such care was actually provided just 55 percent of the time (McGlynn et al., 2003). Undertreatment exists side by side with overtreatment (the second category discussed above). U.S. healthcare delivery misses by wide margins on both sides of the target of effective, beneficial care, which probably explains why inappropriate care does not account for geographic variation in care.

Fifth, by some estimates more than 45 percent of all resource expenditures in hospitals is quality-associated waste, such as recovering from preventable errors, building unusable products, providing unnecessary treatments, and simple inefficiencies (Anderson, 1991; James et al., 2006). These costs and the spiraling prices they produce limit patient access to care. They contribute to the fact that 46.6 million Americans currently lack health insurance.

Most studies documenting shortcomings in healthcare delivery have examined the U.S. healthcare system. However, similar studies in each of the above categories have been conducted in other nations, which appear to suffer from the same failings. These findings suggest that the failure of care delivery to achieve its theoretical potential arises from a deeper set of causes than simply national health policy.

Collision Between the Craft of Medicine and Clinical Uncertainty

The same body of research that documents the ways in which healthcare delivery falls short of its theoretical potential also points to a likely cause: a head-on collision of two factors inherent in current approaches to health care.

The first factor is practice based on the craft of medicine—the idea that physicians, nurses, and other health professionals should act as stand-alone experts who draw on a massive personal knowledge base gained from formal education and practice experience and who honor an ethical trust that places a patient's healthcare needs above any other end. From that foundation, each professional starts largely with raw material, then crafts a unique diagnostic and therapeutic experience customized to the needs of the individual patients who seek care or consultation. The healing professions hold that this approach guarantees the best possible result for each patient.

The second factor is what Eddy (1984) calls "clinical uncertainty." It is a direct product of the professions' decision to adopt the scientific method at the turn of the 19th century. Since then, clinical science has greatly increased understanding of the human organism in health and disease and has generated literally thousands of ways clinicians can intervene to change a patient's future. This explosion of medical knowledge has had a secondary effect: Eddy argues that "the complexity of modern medicine exceeds the capacity of the (expert) human mind." Clinical uncertainty includes four principal elements that, operating within the framework of craft-style practice, produce the opportunities for improvement catalogued in the previous section.

The first of these elements is *a lack of valid clinical knowledge about best treatment across a range of competing options.* For most conditions, modern healthcare delivery offers a range of possible treatments. A series of investigations led to the idea that clinicians have Level I, II, or III evidence (Lawrence and Mickalide, 1987) that identifies the best treatment for a particular patient in a specific circumstance only about 10 to 20 percent of the time (Ferguson, 1991; IOM, 1985; Williamson et al., 1979).[5] In 80 to 90 percent of cases, practicing clinicians can have legitimate differences of

---

[5] Level 1 is the randomized controlled trial, Level 2 is observational design, and Level 3 is expert consensus from a group of respected authorities using formal methods.

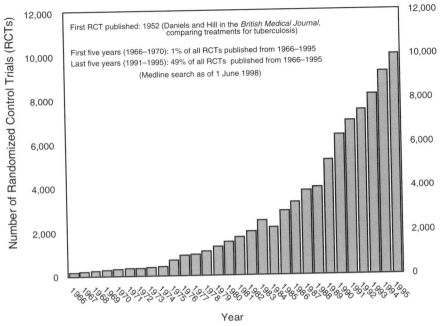

FIGURE 1-4 Rate of generation of Level 1 evidence, 1966 through 1995.
SOURCE: Chassin, 1998.

opinion about what is best, differences that are reflected in wide variation in actual practice.

The second element is *the rate of increase in new biomedical knowledge*. Figure 1-4 shows the number of randomized controlled trials (RCTs) published in the peer-reviewed medical literature each year from 1966 to 1995 (Chassin, 1998). Not only is medical knowledge increasing dramatically, but it appears that the rate of increase itself is increasing. The last year the National Library of Medicine relied primarily on manual abstraction to add new computer-searchable entries to its Medline archive of biomedical research was 2004. During that year, Medline grew by more than 11,000 references per week, representing about 40 percent of all articles published worldwide in peer-reviewed biomedical and clinical journals (National Library of Medicine, 2006). In other words, more than 27,000 articles are published each week in peer-reviewed biomedical and clinical journals. Shaneyfelt (2001) addresses the topic more directly. He reports that within 3 to 4 years of initial board certification, both generalist and subspecialist internists (cognitive physicians) begin to show "substantive declines in general medical knowledge." He estimates that to maintain current knowledge, a general internist would need to read about 20 articles a day, 365 days a year (Shaneyfelt, 2001). It is not that physicians' knowledge decreases over time; rather, the rates of continued learning possible in a busy clinical practice cannot keep pace with the generation of new knowledge. Williamson and colleagues demonstrate that it can take almost 20 years for a major new scientific finding to achieve geographically widespread adoption and links that variation to the inability of physicians in practice to stay current (Williamson et al., 1979). Variation in the deployment of new medical knowledge results directly in variation in clinical practice.

The third element is *continued reliance on subjective recall as a foundation for clinical decision making.* The expert mind reaches conclusions by breaking a problem down into subproblems, pattern matching within each subproblem, and then summarizing results back into a synthetic whole. In the case of problems that require primarily pattern matching, the expert mind performs significantly better than other competing approaches (Groopman, 2007). However, current clinical practice relies increasingly on rate estimation rather than pattern matching. For example, once a physician reaches an accurate diagnosis, the next step is offering the patient accurate information about the likely outcomes—probabilities, in the form of rates—arising from each treatment choice. The same literature that documents the expert mind's dominant performance on problems that require pattern matching also shows that the expert mind fails abysmally when asked to summarize information accurately across groups over time (rate estimation). Eddy (1992) reports that when different groups of expert physicians were asked to estimate complication rates based on subjective recall ("in my experience"), the groups typically gave responses that covered almost the full range of possible answers, and no group showed a detectable pattern of response. Eddy notes that, on any such issue, one could find a physician who honestly believed in—and was willing to testify in court to—any desired value ranging from close to 0 to almost 100 percent. Other investigators have asked practicing clinicians to estimate subjectively rates for their own performance in circumstances where measured rates were available but unknown to the physicians, and have found that respondents typically underestimated their own rates by about 20 to 50 percent (e.g., Lomas et al., 1989).

The final element is *limitations in the number of factors the expert mind can consider when making a clinical decision.* In a seminal article, Miller (1956) estimates that the expert mind can consider only five to nine factors when making a complex decision. Subsequent investigations have empirically demonstrated similar results. For example, Morris and colleagues (1994) were able to document significant variation in ventilator settings from morning to evening rounds in individual patients directly managed in an ICU by the same intensivist physician. They estimate that an intensivist needed to assess as many as 40 important physiological factors to make a treatment decision. Even after compartmentalizing the problem (breaking it into subcomponent parts, such as respiratory rate, tidal volume, and oxygen concentration), expert physicians appeared to be selecting a small subset of six to eight factors each time they saw a patient. By their own assessment, it appeared that the factor selection process was subconscious and random (Morris et al., 1994).

The vast majority of care delivery practices require that expert clinicians consider more than nine factors when making a clinical decision. Variation in how physicians subconsciously select and prioritize factors could directly contribute to geographic variation in care delivery patterns overall.

Early Solutions, Emerging Frameworks, and Refined Challenges

When the inherent complexity of modern medicine and the limitations of the human mind collide with the craft of medicine, the result is wide variation, high rates of inappropriate care, unacceptable rates of care associated with injury and death, a striking inability to apply well-established proven therapies consistently and broadly, and huge amounts of waste. However, some proven solutions have emerged. At Intermountain Healthcare, our primary vehicle is called Shared Baselines. We first identify a high-priority clinical process (in terms of health risk to each patient and volume of patients affected). We then organize a team consisting of all the health professionals associated with that specific process of care, including physicians, nurses, pharmacists, therapists, technicians, and even administrators. The team develops an evidence-based best-practice guideline. This guideline is then blended into the clinical work flow, embedded in staffing, training, supplies, physical layout, educational materials, and measurement/information flow. A physician need not remember, but can simply follow the default path to implement evidence-based best practice.

The shared-baseline approach then moves one step further. We have compelling internal evidence that it is functionally impossible, outside of a very narrow range of circumstances, to write a practice guideline that perfectly fits any patient. The people who come to us for care have had different exposures to potential toxins and pathogens in the environment. More important, they are genetically different. That means they will exhibit different responses to pathogens, different expressions of disease, and different responses to treatment. They also bring different expectations and values and have different personal resources. We therefore do not just allow, or even suggest, but rather demand that each physician adapt our shared-baseline, evidence-based best-practice guideline to the needs of each individual patient. The physician must judge what should vary and how. We use the shared baseline to track that variance. A physician will undergo just as much scrutiny for complying with a shared baseline too often, compared with his or her peers, as for complying too infrequently. In either circumstance, when physicians differ significantly from their peers working in the same practice environment, either they have something to teach or something to learn. A shared-baseline protocol is the opposite of "cookbook medicine." It is, rather, a measurement tool designed to drive peer-based learning. Over time, variation arising from professionals disappears, while variation arising from patients is retained.

Intermountain Healthcare currently has more than 50 shared-baseline protocols operating under measurement. Roughly 5 to 15 percent of a protocol's content is routinely adjusted to meet the needs of a particular patient. This approach is an example of a promising method for managing complexity. Within Lean (a recent sub-branch of quality theory), it is called mass customization. Mass customization is a tool for managing complexity. It allows a physician to focus on a handful of critical factors for each individual patient because the rest of the care delivery process is reliable through standardization and measurement.

Shared baselines have produced dramatic improvement in many care processes in Intermountain. Figure 1-5 illustrates one such instance, involving door-to-balloon inflation times for patients suffering acute myocardial infarction. Figure 1-6 shows reductions in mortality rates associated with the better execution resulting from the shared-baseline approach.

Shared baselines produce another important advantage. Beyond measurement and feedback of variation data in a peer-driven learning network, they establish a framework that directly supports the generation of scientifically valid knowledge from routine care. A shared baseline standardizes routine care. It can function like the control arm of an RCT. In fact, Intermountain has used shared-baseline protocols in just that way. We build them initially as care management tools to guarantee the best possible patient outcome at the lowest necessary cost. With consistent practice, error rates fall (better execution), costs fall, and a team can apply the scientific method to improve systematically. Technically, Intermountain is a community-based care delivery system. However, our shared-baseline protocols have led to a surge in publication of clinical results in peer-reviewed journals that rivals the publication rates of many academic medical centers. Within a typical academic setting, fewer than 5 percent of patients ever contribute to new medical science (i.e., enter some sort of trial); within an Intermountain shared baseline, that number approaches 100 percent.

Conclusion

Over the past century, modern medicine has evolved into a system that routinely performs miracles. In a very real sense, that same progress has moved us beyond our original roots. As the science has grown, the prob-

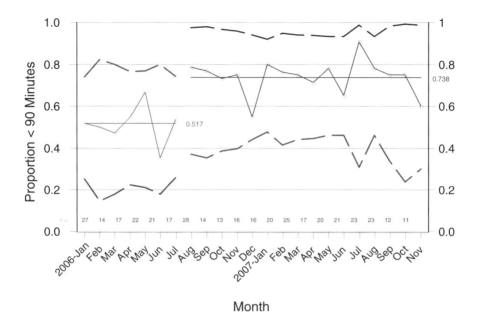

FIGURE 1-5 Proportion of all ST-segment elevated myocardial infarction patients with emergency room door to coronary angioplasty first balloon inflation time of less than 90 minutes, all Intermountain Healthcare facilities (21 hospitals), 2006 through 2007.

lem has shifted. While pattern matching is still important, an increasing portion of good clinical execution relies on assessing results across groups over time. The craft-of-medicine approach to care delivery that produced so many important results cannot address the complexity that defines modern medicine.

Engineering professionals have sought to understand and manage complex systems in many sectors and disciplines. Medical professionals could benefit from the counsel and shared learning of our engineering colleagues. As we shift from a craft-based to a profession-based practice, the idea of care delivered by a team—an organized system of care delivery, as opposed to a loose conglomeration of poorly coordinated parts—presents a number of challenges. How might engineering concepts such as system analysis, design, and control provide insight into some of the key issues facing optimal care delivery? Where can we find the best leverage for rapid, effective change? How might we better address clinical complexity? How do we build knowledge management into a learning system that lives at the heart

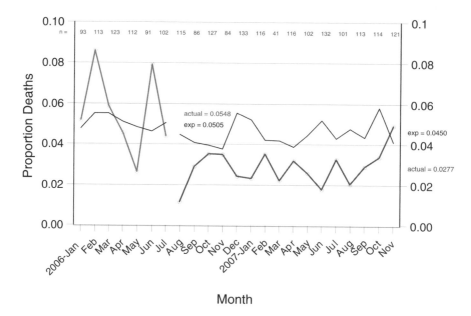

FIGURE 1-6 Mortality rates following ST-segment elevated myocardial infarction, all Intermountain Healthcare facilities (21 hospitals), 2006 through 2007.

of routine care delivery? In sum, how can we design health care as a coordinated system of production as we enter a new century?

TEACHING OPPORTUNITIES FROM
ENGINEERING: LEARNING BY EXAMPLE

W. Dale Compton, Ph.D., Purdue University

Change is difficult for large organizations, but the successful ones find ways of overcoming the challenges. This paper focuses on some of the successful approaches used by organizations and suggests that the healthcare delivery system might consider undertaking similar attempts to better serve its customers.

Any large organization faces many challenges, some organizational and others related to human behavior. Setting common objectives for a new organization is one such challenge. Ensuring the fairness of performance evaluations of individuals and groups in a changed organization is another. There are also issues concerning the fairness of the reward system. These challenges are common and contribute significantly to the silos that frequently exist in large organizations. On the human behavior side, there is a natural resistance to change. Enlisting a diverse and perhaps geographically dispersed workforce to pursue common goals can be very difficult as well.

How do organizations generally go about combating such challenges? They use various tools, they move people about, they establish cross-departmental committees, and they reorganize—even when doing so is not necessary—all in an effort to get people in different areas to work together, think along common lines, and commit to cooperation. Numerous examples demonstrate that these approaches generally do not work very well.

How can a large, diffuse, diverse organization learn to do things differently in order to go in a different direction? "Large," "diffuse," and "diverse" are emphasized because they are terms that describe the healthcare delivery system. As we think about a learning healthcare system, we must first recognize that this system has two distinct parts: the clinical part, which encompasses biologically targeted intervention processes, and the delivery part, which consists of the processes intended to support the clinical part. With this second part—the organization and structure of the delivery system—engineering can be of assistance. From an engineering perspective, we might begin by asking the following questions: What are the system objectives? What determines performance? What changes are needed or wanted? What are important points of controlling this system?

Fortunately, the overall objectives of the healthcare system are well accepted. The system must be safe, effective, timely, patient centered, efficient, and equitable. It is interesting to note that this list usually does not include cost, even though cost affects and is affected by each of these objectives and is becoming an increasingly important issue in health care.

In thinking about the steps that might prove pertinent to changing the healthcare delivery system, it is helpful to draw on experience from another industry. Although there are many differences between the operation of a large, diverse, global manufacturing company and the healthcare enterprise, some of the experiences of the former may be useful. The comparison offered here is with a member of an industry in which success is determined by the acceptance of one's products in a very competitive environment. Although there are multiple participants in the healthcare industry and although competition in that industry is less obvious and more difficult to quantify, it can be thought of as a consumer industry.

So allow me to describe a few experiences concerning how a large company faced the issue of quality in the 1970s. I joined Ford Motor Company in 1970. The first meeting of all corporate management that I attended dealt with quality. There was a great deal of consensus during that meeting. Everyone agreed that our product quality was poor, and everyone agreed that something had to be done about this situation. The meeting ended, and everyone went back to work and *continued doing the same thing they had done before,* with the result that product quality remained poor. Why?

There were no real incentives. After all, our principal competitor was just across town, and they had the same problems with product quality as Ford. So why change? Besides, everyone thought that quality cost money, and no one wanted to be the first to acknowledge having extra money.

Then, however, a crisis occurred. There was an oil embargo, and vehicle fuel efficiency became very important to the public. Big, gas-guzzling cars became unpopular. The public discovered that Japanese manufacturers offered smaller vehicles with better fuel economy and flocked to buy them. Then those customers discovered that the Japanese cars also had high quality. That was the beginning of the Japanese entry into the automotive market of the United States.

Although some commentators tried to explain the success of the Japanese as the result of their having better technology, this was not what made the Japanese cars so attractive. Rather, the Japanese products had better fuel economy because they were smaller and lighter in weight. They exhibited better quality because the Japanese had put in place procedures that kept their manufacturing processes under control. Although the Japanese had the right products for the market at the time, we must remember that when the Japanese first tried to enter the U.S. market after World War II, they were quite unsuccessful because they had poor product design and poor quality. They learned what was needed and, with the help of some key consultants, came back a few years later with superior products.

Chrysler's dire financial circumstances at the time are well known, but Ford's financial situation is less so. On one occasion, Ford was within a couple of days of running out of money. It was a grim situation. The Ford system had to change to survive. Quality had to be improved. But how?

First, it was recognized that in the short term, errors in the assembly of the vehicles could be eliminated so that customers would receive products with fewer problems, and the company would experience lower warranty costs. Members of Ford's upper management, from the CEO down, were committed to this goal and served as salespersons for the need for change. The union management was brought into the process of explaining why things needed to change and how to begin. The unions agreed with the strategy and participated actively with management in enlisting everyone in the effort.

One plant was chosen to determine how to make the necessary changes. The progress achieved in that plant in a short period of time surprised everyone. Quality improved almost immediately. Now came the task of disseminating the knowledge learned there to the entire organization. Workers from the first plant were used to teach workers in other plants. People with experience in the tasks on the line taught others how to do things better. They were the most credible teachers. For the company, quality became what was known as "Job One," the most important timing issue in the launch of a new product.

While the manufacturing system was being changed dramatically, project engineers put in place a process to improve the design of the next major Ford product. No longer would a design by the engineers simply be passed on to the manufacturing people, who would often return it to the engineers within a few weeks, saying it could not be manufactured with either the facilities in place or those planned. This process cost time and money, and ultimately led to a misunderstanding between the two groups—an example of the perils of the silo system.

Ford introduced the concept of simultaneous engineering to reduce the silo mentality among the design engineers, the development engineers, the sales force, and the so-called "parts activities" that handled warranty problems. Cooperation across boundaries became the operating mode. This new approach led to the creation of one of the most successful Ford products—the first Ford Taurus.

Of course, there are obvious differences between Ford and the healthcare system. At Ford, there was a clear management hierarchy that could set objectives. There was a single objective, *quality*. It was an objective that everyone could understand and support. Everyone in the Ford system could see why the objective was needed, how they could contribute, and how they would benefit. All involved came to understand that improving quality was not simply something they would work on for a while and then return to the old ways as soon as a couple of senior managers retired.

The Ford organization also recognized that it was necessary to adopt another important Japanese concept—*continuous improvement*. Of the many aspects of continuous improvement, four are particularly relevant to this discussion.

First, how does one tell if improvements are occurring? To begin, one must have data. Ford had large amounts of data. Its task was to create an organization that recognized the importance of letting individuals on the assembly line use those data without having to get permission from a supervisor to try new ways of doing business. Continuous improvement can work only if employees at all levels are informed, trusted, and empowered. One important result of recognition of this idea was the introduction of some key engineering tools, such as statistical process control, whereby workers control and regularly document performance against operating objectives.

The healthcare industry faces a problem that much of our industry did not face: there are large amounts of data on the clinical side of the system but not on the delivery side. As an example, I have talked with a number of representatives of ambulatory clinics and hospitals about improving patient flow in their facilities. If one can improve patient flow, one can then improve scheduling of resources and people. To accomplish good patient flow, one needs data on the arrival rate of patients at every station, that is, at every point where they stop. One needs to know the average time they spend at each station and the paths they follow. These data are normally gathered by having someone with a notepad and a stopwatch follow patients around. That is fine, but there is no assurance that these data will be representative of another time in that facility or another facility. As a result, few facilities have these data. It is not that the data cannot be collected, but the collection costs money and time. Yet without these data, it is difficult to use the engineering tools that can determine optimal flow.

A second aspect of continuous improvement focuses on participation by all involved. To quote from a recent publication, *Adapting Process-Improvement Techniques in an Academic Medical Center*, by Paul Levy, president and CEO of Beth Israel Deaconess Medical Center in Boston,

> Here is an example of ventilator-associated pneumonia (VAP), a problem relevant to anyone who has been or will be in an intensive care unit (ICU) or who will have a loved one in an ICU. A patient on a ventilator who contracts pneumonia has a 30 percent chance of dying, a pretty high rate of mortality. The good thing is that we know how to prevent many of these cases by taking five well-documented steps. . . . [I]n the months since the ICUs began working on reducing cases of VAP, performance of the five-step bundle, and the oral care, have risen to 100 percent.
>
> Note that the change was not a response to an order from CMS [Centers for Medicare & Medicaid Services]. . . . Neither the insurance companies nor patients nor even the hospital administrator insisted that these things be done. In fact it was academic physicians who read journals and other publications from around the world who instigated the changes. After several of them had read the recent literature about preventing VAP, they decided that they would change the way that ICUs cared for patients. But—and here's the key—they then had to organize the 200 people who work in the ICUs. Respiratory therapists, nurses, doctors all had to be trained to change the 'industrial' process, with no increase in staff and with basically no increase in resources. The doctors went to work and made it happen.
>
> Many of the changes were not very complex. . . . I watched the results of the changes and started posting them before they reached the 90 percent rate. At that point, the head of the group sent an e-mail to his colleagues that read something like this: 'As you may have heard, Mr. Levy has a blog on which he is now posting our success rates with ventilator-associated pneumonia prevention. Perhaps we should take this as an additional emphasis to do even better, because people out there are watching. (Levy, 2008)

The organization of the system is also a very important aspect of allowing these changes to take place. For a complex system to be manageable, the people who design it must recognize the interactions that take place among its parts, and the design must be informed by how the actions of each element of the system affect the performance of the other elements. Seeking to optimize each of the elements by itself does not guarantee the optimization of the whole. (It can be shown mathematically that this is the case except under very limited circumstances.) One must understand the details of the interactions of the various elements.

Failure to recognize this reality is not unique to any one industry. In the manufacturing industry, we often talk about profit centers, the assumption being that the company is divided into elements and each is allowed to work to optimize its own profits, with the expectation that the total profit of the company will be optimized. Where this notion becomes patently spurious is when one part of the company makes and sells products to another part of the company. Large amounts of time and effort are spent trying to arrive at the proper "transfer price" between the two parts of the company when in fact the outcome does not matter to the company as a whole. The lesson is that the silos must be broken down. This applies to all corporate objectives, not just profit.

The third aspect of continuous improvement is communication. Both engineers and healthcare professionals must work hard to create a common understanding of problems and opportunities. It is impossible to achieve continuous improvement if people are not communicating. The report *Building a Better Delivery System* (NAE/IOM, 2005), produced by a committee that the late Jerry Grossman and I co-chaired, was well over a year late being published not because of disagreements among committee members, but because we had to rewrite the report several times in an effort to ensure that both engineers and healthcare professionals would—or could—read it. The language was important. I saw similar communication difficulties at Purdue when we launched the Regenstrief Center for Healthcare Engineering. Engineers and healthcare professionals do not have a common language. Simply put, most healthcare professionals do not know what questions to ask and what to do with the answers they receive, and similarly, most engineers do not understand the constraints within which healthcare professionals work. The only experience most engineers have had with health care is being patients.

The final aspect of continuous improvement is related to the first aspect of needing good data. Not only are such data needed, but the data need to be collected, distributed, and analyzed, and this requires information technology systems. The healthcare delivery system does not yet have the sort of comprehensive information technology system it needs. Some relevant bills were recently considered in Congress. The Health Care Information Enterprise Integration Initiative—H.R. 2406—would "authorize [National Institute of Standards and Technology] to increase its effort in support of the integration of the healthcare information enterprise in the United States." A second bill, the 10,000 People Trained by 2010 Act, would authorize the National Science Foundation "to award grants to institutions of higher education to develop and offer education and training programs." The former bill would allocate $3.5 million to $3.8 million per year over 4 years for health informatics and an additional $9 million to $9.6 million per year over 4 years to establish multidisciplinary centers for informatics research on healthcare information. Although the first bill was never voted on, and the second passed in the House but was not voted on by the Senate, they represent a promising start.

In the long term, it will be necessary to create a cadre of both engineering and medical professionals who can work together. They must understand each other and be able to tackle collectively some of the difficult problems facing the healthcare industry. In particular, the NAE/IOM report *Building a Better Delivery System* recommends the creation of centers that would bring together members of the medical and engineering professions in a multidisciplinary environment where joint research would prosper, where the development of new tools would be undertaken, where the existing and new tools would be demonstrated to healthcare providers, where new joint educational tools could be created, and where assistance in implementing these tools could be provided to the healthcare community. The report calls for the establishment of 30 to 50 of these centers at a cost of about $3.5 million each (NAE/IOM, 2005). The total investment would be $100 million to $150 million per year—a modest investment compared with the approximately $500 billion currently being wasted.

A long-term refocusing of some of the educational aspects of both professions will be necessary, as well as help with problem solving in the near term. Multidisciplinary research does not mean that one discipline works on a problem while another watches or simply consents to having the first one around; there is some possibility of falling into this trap. Medical professionals are becoming more open to letting engineers into their practices, but they appear to be involved less frequent in joining the engineers in actually conducting research.

All interested parties should become actively involved in encouraging members of Congress and other officials to see the importance of investing not only in the short-term but also in long-term activities that can improve the system. Collaboration is needed to help people understand what healthcare professionals and engineers can accomplish together in the proper environment.

For a large, diverse, diffuse system to learn and change requires the involvement of all people at all levels, starting with a committed CEO. It is also necessary to have a common understanding of where the system is going, what is needed, and the tools that are available to assist in those changes, along with a recognition of the importance of creating an environment that fosters continuous improvement. The tools that engineers possess need to be brought to bear to help improve the care delivery process, and more powerful tools need to be developed. Finally, the successes achieved by individual teams need to be demonstrated to others.

It will not be easy for the healthcare delivery system to learn and change. Change can be accomplished, individually and collectively, by applying knowledge learned in other industries. Clearly a crisis is imminent in the form of safety failures, the knowledge–practice gap, waste and inefficiency, and so forth. In the short term, the tools that can be used to implement immediate changes must be identified. For the long term, it will be necessary to develop convincing arguments that research and development must receive greater funding if a stable system is to be created.

Ford learned. It changed. It survived, and it prospered. Then it went on to forget some of the important lessons it had learned. The latter must not happen to health care. Leaders in the field have a responsibility to make change occur, as well as the wherewithal to collectively make it happen; this opportunity must not be allowed to stagnate or slip away.

OBSERVATIONS ON INITIATING SYSTEMS CHANGE IN HEALTH CARE: CHALLENGES TO OVERCOME

Donald M. Berwick, M.D., M.P.P.,
Institute for Healthcare Improvement, (former)
Centers for Medicare & Medicaid Services

The potential benefit to the healthcare system of deepening system knowledge and of action based on that knowledge is enormous. The result would be equivalent to the sea change seen in health care with the entry of statistical rigor and formal experimental design in the evaluation of healthcare practices in the mid-20th century, led by pioneers such as Fred Mosteller, Tom Chalmers, Archie Cochrane, Ian Chalmers, and David Sacket. These courageous intellectual leaders changed the collective thinking about evidence, to the enormous benefit of patients. The wedding of fields that is being explored at this meeting has the same potential, and it may require equal courage. The potential for the IOM and the NAE to work together as intellectual leaders is extraordinary. Few other agents of change could carry us through the transitional barriers that this intellectual expertise is encountering.

The major challenges to instituting systems thinking in health care lie with the status quo—in technique, culture, training, and economics. It will not be possible to realize the benefits of such thinking without confronting some of those challenges, the same sort of challenges that intellectual transitions in any field encounter. The core notion behind this change in perspective is, "Every system is perfectly designed to achieve the results it gets." Therefore, the key to better performance in most complex environments is to redesign systems. Just as any car has a top speed, health care of any particular design has a characteristic safety level. The car has a top speed as a property of the car; in health care, similarly, elements such as error rates, costs, and defects are properties of the system as currently designed. That is a scientific premise: that system designs explain system performance. Some commonly espoused views fail to acknowledge performance as a characteristic of a system. These are "black box" views—unscientific views—of how things get better. Even though some of these views are today quite hegemonic in public discourse, especially the reliance on incentives to produce change, there are reasons to be skeptical of them.

A reliance on incentives, on motivation, on encouraging effort, and on markets is widespread in popular theories of healthcare change today. However, the healthcare problem is mainly one of improper designs, not an imperfect market. The great scholar of quality, W. Edwards Deming, used to say that trying harder is the worst plan. Nonetheless, most of the current dominant theories of public policy aimed at making health care perform better are "try harder plans," and consequently they are likely to fail.

Market mechanisms are particularly worrisome when applied at the level of individuals. The majority of the healthcare workforce is trying quite hard now—and mostly doing its best. The advice offered by Donald Norman in his book on human factors *The Design of Everyday Things* is, "Honor thy user" (Norman, 1988). The worst thing to do when human factors are at play is to blame the human for the factors. In pursuit of excellence, someone who understands human factors works instead to construct dikes around the frailties of human beings in order to have systems perform better than human beings do and much closer to what those humans really wish they could accomplish. There is little point in trying to mold individual behavior to achieve excellence through effort. Rather, the ownership of improvement lies squarely on the shoulders of leaders of systems rather than those of individuals within the workforce.

This paper examines seven challenges. One challenge that is not included in this list because it is so basic is the challenge of setting aims. Deming used to say that without an aim, there is no system. A variation on this saying with a more positive tone is, "Aim creates a system." One of the serious barriers to wedding engineering, sciences, and health care lies outside these fields; it is the absence of aim. A country that cannot make a clear decision that its health care will be safe, or efficient, or effective, or patient centered, or timely, or equitable will not achieve those aims. This is not a technical problem. It is a political problem, a problem of leadership.

Without aim there is no system, and without it all of our explorations of systems thinking will be fruitless.

Beyond the need to set aims, at least seven challenges to the wedding of medicine and systems knowledge can be identified. The first is *the difficulty of getting people to emphasize interdependence in their thinking.* Romantic views of professionalism emphasize personal responsibility, hierarchy, specialization, independence, and professional autonomy. Such views are evident everywhere in health care. Take, for example, architecture. In hospitals there are "doctors' conference rooms" and "nurses' conference rooms" and even "patient bathrooms" and "staff bathrooms." There are discipline-specific spaces. The fragmentation is also evident in training: schools are separate, and the experiences offered to young people to develop their self-images are separate. Separateness, not interdependence, is emphasized in the preparation of professionals.

The separateness is further evident in the framings of professional ethics. Each discipline has its own statement of its ethics, and this statement is nowhere unified with another. There is no common, shared description of the ethical center of health care that applies to everybody, from a physician to a radiology technician to a manager. Physicians have the Hippocratic oath, nurses take pledges, and therapists take pledges, but they do not take the same pledges together.

Fragmentation is evident in the lack of financial compensation for coordinating mechanisms. It is a habit of payment systems to pay for interactions but not for coordination, as evidenced by the institutional boundaries that exist. I am engaged in a great debate right now in one of the committees on which I serve concerning whether hospitals' mortality rates should include deaths that occur beyond the hospital walls. Is it fair to characterize a hospital mortality rate within 30 days of discharge? Hospitals are saying, "No, we are not responsible for what happens once a patient has left our building." That attitude represents fragmentation and a failure to understand, let alone embrace, interdependence.

Failure is evident in chronic care hand-offs, and it is embedded in the language used. The word "discharge," for example, is a peculiar one. It implies that there is an "admission" and then a "discharge," as if the patient were a type of effluent. The word suggests the patient is no longer a responsibility, and it is a symptom of a lack of sensitivity to interdependence. Proper systems in health care will place interdependence and its management at the top of the hierarchy of professional concerns. That is not the current culture.

The second challenge is *the need to increase the visibility of care processes, from the viewpoint of patients.* Paul Batalden once said that health care lacks catwalks. It is extremely difficult to see processes of care. It is not easy to "hover" above the work, to see the workflow, because of the way space and time are divided. When processes *are* seen, they are not always seen accurately because they are seen from the supply side, not the patient side. The work is described as it is performed, not as patients and their loved ones experience it. The immediate effect is very toxic—patients are expected to adjust to processes instead of having processes molded to their needs, even at the level of the individual. This is a vicious cycle: the more that patients are forced into processes that do not fit them as individuals, the more their expectations will be construed as unreasonable and their capacities seen as constrained.

Possibilities derive only from the redesign of processes, not from the reinforcement of current processes. The first step is to make the processes visible from the viewpoint of the people served. I have recently been studying, to my enormous benefit, with Amory Lovins, founder of the Rocky Mountain Institute and one of the world's leading scholars in the fields of energy and the environment. In 1976 Lovins proposed a focus on what he called *end use efficiency* as the hallmark of proper energy design and policy. A concern with end use efficiency is exactly what is needed in health care, as opposed to centralized efficiency, which is not going to meet the needs of patients.

Currently, there are few mechanisms for the coordination and commitment necessary to make processes visible. Taichi Ohno, the creative genius behind the Toyota Production System, offered an important observation. He wrote, "When waste is at a minimum, every customer can be seen as an individual." Not being focused on process, the healthcare system operates with exactly the opposite premise, assuming that trying to meet the needs of the individual drives costs up. It does not. Rather, when done properly, it drives costs down.

The third challenge is *the need to recognize the importance of nonlinearities and the value of dynamic learning and of local adaptation as scientific learning progresses.* The nonlinear nature of system dynamics in health care, as in any nonlinear system, weakens the learning power of many formal and classical methods of evaluation and inquiry. Some formal methods of inquiry tend to be insensitive to contacts, mechanisms, and recurring and meaningful stratification. Those methods also weaken the contribution of local knowledge because they are trying to protect against bias.

Health care today lacks habits and norms of inquiry that capitalize on processes and knowledge growth in a nonlinear context. That is actually the side effect of a major intellectual achievement in health care: the establishment of a hierarchy of scientific evidence as a basis for evaluating clinical practices. That hierarchy places RCTs at the top—where they surely belong when considered relative to other forms of inquiry. However, RCTs usually do not belong at the top of the hierarchy of learning processes when nonlinear complex systems are involved. Most sound learning in complex systems occurs in local and individual settings. Currently, there are no powerful ways to harvest the knowledge accumulating through innovation in local settings in health care.

There is a chasm between, on the one hand, pragmatic engineering sciences (which are very sensitive to nonlinearities) and local learning and system improvement methods and, on the other hand, the current hegemonic hierarchies of evaluation of clinical procedures. Journals have not opened their review processes and pages to the former kind of knowledge. The RCT continues to be placed at the pinnacle of methodologies even in those settings where it simply cannot provide the information needed. I recently received an extremely discouraging e-mail from a very discouraged leader of improvement, a quite senior physician at a major medical center, who forwarded to me the instruction that he had received from his chief of medicine ordering that "no further Plan-Do-Study-Act cycles will be permitted in this department." The chasm between formal trials and local improvement is enormous, and the cost to knowledge growth is very high.

The fourth challenge has to do with *attention to waste—knowledge of and action on waste in health care.* One early benefit of proper system views is knowledge concerning waste, including the degree of waste and its different forms. Waste is often the manifestation of system failure and illiteracy. In the nonsystemic view, being mired in that waste can even feel productive. What might otherwise be seen as waste feels like necessary activity. One who attacks waste, even if the attempt is to avoid suboptimization, can appear to be ill-motivated and sinister. For example, the following can feel extremely risky and assaultive in a fragmented system: (1) using someone else's laboratory findings instead of repeating them, (2) eliminating inventories that buffer against poor flow, (3) automating processes, and (4) using capital fully. It is wasteful when the neurosurgery operating room is never touched by the orthopods and when the orthopods never allow the neurosurgeons to use their room. From the viewpoint of waste, this is poor management of capital, yet many would regard such "ring fencing" as absolutely necessary to achieving excellence in the current system.

The forms of waste in health care are just as vast as they are in other industries: rework, scrap, inventory, queues, motion, unused space and equipment, idle capital, excess information, records of no value, loss of ideas, and, most of all, demotivating of the workforce through insult and indignity. The economics of health care today are in some sense founded on waste. Waste means jobs; it means profit; it means income; it means familiar habit and comfort. Surely, waste levels exceed 30 percent in the healthcare industry; that is 30 percent of the $2.6 trillion spent. In fact, waste may exceed 60 percent, but that would be more difficult to prove. Indeed, if formal value chain analysis were used, the figure might prove to be even higher. Despite the opportunity, it should be noted that there is no formal research agenda in health care in the nation that is intended to discover and identify waste in its myriad forms.

The fifth challenge is *the missing platform for multidisciplinary research and development in the intersection of systems sciences and health care.* My career benefited enormously from leaders at Harvard—Howard Hiatt the first among them—who built a platform for the intersection of quantitative analysis methods and healthcare delivery. That platform was the foundation of my own career. With Hiatt and others, I studied a variety of sciences not usually associated with health care, and that study was made easier because there was a platform that linked one part of my brain, performing quantitative analysis, to the other part of my brain, learning to be a doctor. The intersections for the collaborative efforts being explored at this workshop are insufficient. That is, the most valuable potential forms of collaborative research and development among engineering sciences, system sciences, and health care are not yet dignified.

Of interest, the barrier is dyadic. It is symptomatic of the history of the distance between the fields that engineers feel unwelcome, unfamiliar, and intimidated in the healthcare setting. They become silent, as all people tend to do when they are awed in the cathedral of health care. Healthcare leaders tend not to be aware of the engineering disciplines or to be suspicious of their applicability. Although this wall is being broken down slowly, much remains to be done. Bridge building here will be expensive and it will take time, but it will pay off. The recent examples of, say, Steven Spears' work in health care or Eugene Litvak's work are already paying off handsomely in settings where the participants are wise enough to seek these experts' counsel.

As the IOM and others forge these intersections (I love the idea of a master of sciences and engineering degree in health systems), the days when industrial engineers were very common in healthcare settings should be remembered. Somehow that situation never grew into the truly fertile interaction it might have become. The question of what stalled it should be addressed. The idea of more physician-engineers is intriguing. There are physician-information technologists, physician-bioscientists, and molecular biologists who are physicians; now there need to be more engineers who are physicians, people like Kate Sylvester, who is a leader of such syntheses in the United Kingdom.

The sixth challenge has to do with *the implications of systems thinking for professional development.* Today there are *no* requirements for physicians and nurses for training in safety science and safety practices. Medical schools are just starting to incorporate these subjects into their curriculums. No physician is emerging from training today who has not heard of Osler or Watson and Crick or the Krebs Cycle, yet thousands of physicians graduate every year who have never heard of James Reason or W. Edwards Deming or Karl Weick—or even Robert Brooke or Jack Wennberg, who are right here within the field. Nor have most of the teachers heard of these luminaries, which is probably the reason the students do not hear about them. The preparation of professionals today dismisses systems sciences through its silence. Moreover, the siloing of professional preparation itself deemphasizes the role of interdependency. I trained for 9 years in medicine before I was a fully qualified physician. In that training, I spent not a single day of study self-consciously with students of nursing, even though we would then spend our professional lives together locked in interdependency.

The seventh challenge is the greatest in some sense: *institutional redesign, or the institutional rearrangements, will be needed if systems sciences are to be fully exploited.* If process literacy, process knowledge, and investment in process redesign were increased, the institutions created to preserve the current fragments would become visibly inadequate, and the spaces between them would appear larger and larger. The waste incurred through fragmentation would be obvious. Systems knowledge inevitably leads to the desire for integrated design. It is not at all clear that upon emerging from that exploration, there would be a need for hospitals or offices or insurers or professions in anything close to their current forms.

Some caution against this kind of grandiose thinking about redesign, but it may be that the science would lead there, that system redesign—not political or financing rearrangement—would be the true manifestation of what should be called healthcare reform. It would be *care* reform, not financing reform or insurance reform or coverage reform, and yet little, if any, of that kind of change is being discussed in the current political debate.

It is doubtful that the political or social will to go there yet exists. If it did, the issues being faced in health care, such as financing, coverage, and costs, would melt away, or at least begin to do so. Furthermore, hospitals would look profoundly different. Indeed, a measure of whether health care had become truly system-minded would be whether hospitals, at last, would seek to be empty, not full. Instead, virtually every hospital board of trustees is holding virtually every executive in virtually every hospital in America accountable for making sure that occupancy levels are trending up, not down. This tells us that "success" has been defined incorrectly from the viewpoint of the true social need for health and gives some idea of the level of institutional rearrangement that would be needed if a truly rational system design were chosen.

The discussion encouraged by this workshop, about a merging of engineering, sciences, and health care, does make sense. It makes a great deal more sense than the status quo. Systems thinking and knowledge are manifest already in many areas of human endeavor other than health care, and someday they will be seen as too promising to continue to be ignored by the healthcare enterprise.

REFERENCES

CDC (Centers for Disease Control and Prevention). 1999a. Decline in deaths from heart disease and stroke—United States, 1900-1999. *JAMA* 282(8):724–726.

CDC. 1999b. Vaccines dramatically reduced disease in the 20th century. *Morbidity and Mortality Weekly Report* 48(12):21.

Chassin, M. R. 1998. Is health care ready for six sigma quality? *Milbank Quarterly* 76(4):565–591.

Coleman, M. P., M. Quaresma, F. Berrino, J. M. Lutz, R. De Angelis, R. Capocaccia, P. Baili, B. Rachet, G. Gatta, T. Hakulinen, A. Micheli, M. Sant, H. K. Weir, J. M. Elwood, H. Tsukuma, S. Koifman, G. A. Silva, S. Francisci, M. Santaquilani, A. Verdecchia, H. H. Storm, J. L. Young, and the CONCORD Working Group. 2008. Cancer survival in 5 continents: A world-wide population-based study (CONCORD). *Lancet Oncology* 9(8):730–756.

Cutler, D. M., A. B. Rosen, and S. Vijan. 2006. The value of medical spending in the United States, 1960–2000. *New England Journal of Medicine* 355(9):920–927.

Doonon, M. 1998. *Issue brief: Will alcohol be the next tobacco?* Boston: The Massachusetts Health Policy Forum.

Eddy, D. M. 1984. Variations in physician practice: The role of uncertainty. *Health Affairs* 3:74.

Eddy, D. M. 1992. *A manual for assessing health practices and designing practice policies: The explicit approach.* Philadelphia, PA: The American College of Physicians.

Ferguson, J. H. 1991. Forward. Research on the delivery of medical care using hospital firms. Proceedings of a workshop, April 30 and May 1, 1990, Bethesda, MD. *Medical Care* 29(7 Suppl.):JS1–JS2.

Groopman, J. 2007. *How doctors think.* Boston, MA: Houghton Mifflin.

IOM (Institute of Medicine). 1985. *Assessing medical technologies.* Washington, DC: National Academy Press.

IOM. 2000. *To err is human: Building a safer health system.* Washington, DC: National Academy Press.

KFF (Kaiser Family Foundation). 2006. *Wall Street Journal* (February 22). (2005 data.)

Lawrence, R. S., and A. D. Mickalide. 1987. Preventive services in clinical practice: Designing the periodic health examination. *JAMA* 257:2205–2207.

Levy, P. 2008. Adapting process-improvement techniques in an academic medical center. *The Bridge* 38(1):6–9.

Lomas, J., G. M. Anderson, K. Domnick-Pierre, E. Vayda, M. W. Enkin, and W. J. Hannah. 1989. Do practice guidelines guide practice? *New England Journal of Medicine* 321:1306–1311.

McGinnis, J. M., and W. H. Foege. 1993. Actual causes of death in the United States. *JAMA* 270(18):2207–2212.

McGinnis, J. M., P. Williams-Russo, and J. R. Knickman. 2002. The case for more active policy attention to health promotion. *Health Affairs* 21(2):78–93.

McGlynn, E. A., S. M. Asch, J. Adams, J. Keesey, J. Hicks, A. DeCristofaro, and E. A. Kerr. 2003. The quality of health care delivered to adults in the United States. *New England Journal of Medicine* 348(26):2635–2645.

McKie, J., and J. Richardson. 2003. The rule of rescue. *Social Science & Medicine* 56(12):2407–2419.

Miller, G. A. 1956. The magic number seven, plus or minus two: Some limits on our capacity for processing information. *Psychological Review* 63(2):81–97.

Morris, A. H., C. J. Wallace, R. L. Menlove, T. P. Clemmer, J. F. Orme, L. K. Weaver, N. C. Dean, F. Thomas, T. D. East, N. L. Pace, M. R. Suchyta, E. Beck, M. Bombino, D. F. Sittig, S. Böhm, B. Hoffmann, H. Becks, S. Butler, J. Pearl, and B. Rasmusson. 1994. Randomized clinical trial of pressure-controlled inverse ratio ventilation and extracorporeal CO^2 removal for adult respiratory distress syndrome. *American Journal of Respiratory and Critical Care Medicine* 149:295–305.

NAE (National Academy of Engineering)/IOM. 2005. *Building a better delivery system*. Washington, DC: The National Academies Press.

National Center for Health Statistics. 2000. *Health, United States, 2000 with adolescent health chartbook*. DHHS Publication No. (PHS) 2000-1232-1. Hyattsville, MD: U.S. Department of Health and Human Services, Centers for Disease Control and Prevention, p. 7.

National Library of Medicine. 2006. *Fact sheet MEDLINE*. http://www.nlm.nih.gov/pubs/factsheets/medline.html (accessed April 22, 2010).

Nolte, E., and M. McKee. 2003. Measuring the health of nations: Analysis of mortality amenable to health care. *British Medical Journal* 327(7424):1129–1133.

Norman, D. 1988. *The design of everyday things*. New York: Currency Doubleday.

OECD (Organisation for Economic Co-operation and Development). 2006. *OECD health data—OECD website*. http://www.oecd.org/dataoecd/29/52/36960035.pdf (accessed June 22, 2010).

Peterson, C. L., and R. Burton. 2007. *U.S. healthcare spending: Comparison with other OECD countries*. Congressional Research Service Report for Congress, September 17, order code RL34715.

Porter, R. 1997. *The greatest benefit to mankind: A medical history of humanity*. New York: W. W. Norton.

Reinhardt, U. W., P. S. Hussey, and G. F. Anderson. 2002. Cross-national comparisons of health systems using OECD data, 1999. *Health Affairs* 21(3):169–181.

Rosenberg, C. E. 1987. *The care of strangers: The rise of the American hospital system*. New York: Basic Books.

Schoen, C., R. Osborn, M. M. Doty, M. Bishop, J. Peugh, and N. Murukutla. 2007. Toward higher-performance health systems: Adults health care experiences in 7 countries, 2007. *Health Affairs* 26(6):w717–w734.

Shaneyfelt, T. M. 2001. Building bridges to quality. *JAMA* 286(20):2600–2601.

Starr, P. 1984. *The social transformation of American medicine*. New York: Basic Books (The Perseus Books Group).

Szilagyi, D. E. 1965. In defense of the art of medicine. *Archives of Surgery* 91:707–711.

Verdecchia, A., S. Francisci, H. Brenner, G. Gatta, A. Micheli, L. Mangone, I. Kunkler, and the EUROCARE-4 Working Group. 2007. Recent cancer survival in Europe: A 2000–02 period analysis of EUROCARE-4 data. *Lancet Oncology* 8(9):784–796.

Wildavsky, A. 1977. Doing better and feeling worse: The political pathology of health policy. In J. H. Knowles, ed., *Doing better and feeling worse: Health in the United States* (pp. 105–123). New York: W. W. Norton & Co.

Williamson, J., P. Goldschmidt, and I. Jillson. 1979. *Medical practice information demonstration project: Final report*. Office of the Assistant Secretary of Health, DHEW, Contract #282–77–0068GS. Baltimore, MD: Policy Research Inc.

2

Engaging Complex Systems
Through Engineering Concepts

INTRODUCTION

Along with the increasing interest and concern for the problems sur-
rounding health care in the United States has come an increasing awareness of the implications of the healthcare system's complexity. In seeking
to engage engineering sciences for insight and strategies for healthcare
improvement, it was important to frame the workshop presentations and
discussions with a common foundation in and understanding of engineering concepts. The engineering disciplines presented as possible opportunity
areas for improving healthcare delivery and management included systems
engineering, industrial engineering, operations research, human factors
engineering, financial engineering, and risk analysis.

William B. Rouse, executive director of The Tennenbaum Institute at
Georgia Institute of Technology, described the fundamental perspectives by
which systems engineering approaches complex problems. With a particular
focus on the nature of prediction, control, and design, Rouse presented a
model that shed light on the roots of spiraling healthcare costs and then
suggested some likely effects of alternative approaches to controlling costs.
Offering a list of standard options from the systems engineering toolbox
that might be applied to build processes for controlling costs, as well as
some new options described in a Commonwealth Fund report (Schoen et
al., 2008), Rouse provided practical insights into how engineers might approach a representative set of issues in health care.

Richard C. Larson, Mitsui Professor of Engineering Systems and Civil
and Environmental Engineering and director of the Center for Engineering

63

Systems Fundamentals at the Massachusetts Institute of Technology, introduced some principles of operations research (OR), a systems-oriented approach that draws on the principles of the scientific method to help frame, formulate, and solve difficult problems involving people and technology. Larson offered examples of the application of OR to health care, including work that used sophisticated optimization modeling and computational techniques to advance cancer therapeutics. He said that the techniques of OR have much to offer to the reengineering of systems and processes in health care. He further suggested that the applications of OR and engineering systems with the greatest potential to transform health care have not yet been identified and that further attention is needed to determine opportunities for future progress.

Discussing the engineering of systems design tools, James M. Tien, distinguished professor and dean of the College of Engineering at the University of Miami, observed that health care is a complex, integrated collection of human-centered activities that is increasingly dependent on information technology and knowledge. In particular, he explained, health care is a service system. By definition a service system combines three essential components—people, processes, and products—and Tien suggested that managing services means, in effect, managing an integrated and adaptive set of people, processes, and products. He outlined an alternative systems management view of services, discussing the increasing complexity of systems; the increasing need for real-time, adaptive decision making within these systems; and the reality that modern systems are becoming increasingly more human centered. One result is that products and services are becoming both more complex and more personalized or customized. Tien suggested that the methodologies he discussed can be applied to help improve basic services in health care.

Essential methodologies of systems engineering were also the focus of a paper by Harold W. Sorenson, professor of mechanical and aerospace engineering in the Jacobs School of Engineering at the University of California, San Diego. Sorenson discussed the principles of an "integrated perspective" for managing complex systems. He outlined the questions that typically apply in engineering complex enterprises, and he described typical approaches that a systems engineer might use to articulate the nature of a problem and to design an appropriate architecture to address it. He provided an overview of how systems engineers think about managing complexity, developing solutions, and assessing those solutions. For health care, Sorenson suggested, such an approach could allow a rapid enhancement of capabilities, the development of better working relationships among stakeholders, and the identification of new and more effective ways to deliver patient care—with the potential to lead ultimately to significant changes in healthcare culture, practice, and delivery.

CAN WE AFFORD TECHNOLOGICAL
INNOVATION IN HEALTH CARE?

*William B. Rouse, Ph.D., The Tennenbaum Institute,
Georgia Institute of Technology*

The enormous cost of U.S. health care is often cited as a key national challenge (CBO, 2008). Health care is consuming an increasingly large portion of the nation's gross domestic product (GDP). At the same time, there are concerns that the quality of health care in the United States lags behind that of other countries (IOM, 2000, 2001). It is clear that substantial improvements in the delivery of healthcare value are needed, and, it is argued, these improvements should be achievable through value-based competition (Porter and Teisberg, 2006). Of course, it should be kept in mind that our healthcare system did not become the way it is overnight (Stevens et al., 2006).

A recent report published by the Congressional Budget Office (CBO) attributes 50 percent of the cost growth in health care over the past four decades to technological innovation (CBO, 2008). Science and engineering research has yielded a steady stream of innovations for detection, diagnosis, and treatment, whose use in many cases has grown by 10 to 15 percent per year. Compounding such growth over 40 years results in a very large level of use. In many domains, such as personal electronics or cellular telephones, such growth would be seen as an enormous success. However, the third-party payers of most healthcare bills see this growth as a threat to the viability of the healthcare system.

This paper approaches this threat as an engineering problem rather than as a problem of medical science. First, it outlines the engineering approach and contrasts that approach with science. It then explores the CBO's conclusions a bit more deeply. It proposes three models for controlling the costs of health care so that the growth of these costs tracks the growth in GDP, providing insight into the magnitude of the efficiency gains needed to accomplish this goal. The paper concludes with a discussion of possible ways to achieve these gains.

Engineering Approach

Determination of the best way to control healthcare costs should be approached as an engineering problem rather than as a medical science problem. The potential of engineering to enhance health care has, of late, received increasing attention (NAE/IOM, 2005). This potential can be understood in terms of the following levels of understanding of any phenomenon:

- *Describe* past observations.
- *Classify* past observations.
- *Predict* future observations.
- *Control* future observations.
- *Design* future observations.

Science progresses from describing and classifying past observations to predicting future observations. If these predictions turn out to be accurate, science concludes that the theory or model employed has credence. If not, the theory or model needs revision. The goal is to create valid knowledge.

Engineering builds on scientific knowledge, particularly in using models to predict. However, engineers usually are not content just to predict. They also want to control the state of the system of interest or, if they can, to design or redesign the system to facilitate better control. In some cases, this penchant for design and control has enormous societal implications (McPhee, 1990).

Predict

Taken simplistically, there are two basic approaches to prediction. One is extrapolation. Equations are fit to data collected under particular conditions. These equations are then used to project the outcomes for similar conditions. Statistical models, such as those used in medicine for randomized controlled trials (RCTs), are examples of equation fitting. To the extent that the conditions of the trials adequately reflect the eventual conditions of use, we can be reasonably confident that similar outcomes will be attained when a treatment moves from trials to clinical use.

RCTs work well, although slowly and expensively, when there are large populations that can be observed under controllable conditions. However, this approach cannot be employed for the study of large-scale systems such as health care. There simply are not enough healthcare systems to achieve statistical significance in a study of the large, systemic changes likely to be needed to control costs and enhance quality to the extent outlined earlier.

Engineering approaches to solving large-scale problems typically rely on models as a basis for prediction. These models are formulated from "first principles" drawn from a range of scientific domains. These principles, usually stated as fairly simple mathematical relationships, become elements of much larger mathematical and computational models that are used to predict the outcomes of different approaches to the design and control of complex systems. Engineering approaches are illustrated later in this paper.

Control

Engineering the control of a system involves measurement, feedback, and compensation to achieve system objectives. Measurement is used to ascertain the state of the system. This, of course, requires defining system state variables, their units of measure, and how such measurements can be made. Feedback involves comparing predicted and actual system states in order to correct errors. Such feedback results in a "control loop." Compensation concerns adding dynamic elements to the control loop in order to counteract delays and lags in system response.

Design

Engineering design involves problem analysis, solution synthesis, production of an artifact that embodies the solution, and then sustainment of the system in its use. Analysis involves understanding input–output relationships, including uncertainties, and then creating models, as discussed above. Synthesis is a matter of designing input–output relationships to achieve system objectives. Production involves the various actions—fabrication, construction, programming, and so forth—necessary to create systems that embody the desired relationships. Finally, sustainment concerns creating mechanisms that ensure that system objectives will be met in the future.

Summary

Engineering approaches to prediction, control, and design have much to offer health care with respect to making systemic improvements by decreasing costs and increasing quality. The remainder of this paper provides an illustration of how engineering might help in meeting the challenges faced by health care.

Healthcare Illustration

As discussed earlier, the past four decades have seen enormous increases in healthcare costs. Specifically, real healthcare costs tripled as a percentage of GDP in the period from 1965 to 2005, with half of this growth due to technological innovation (CBO, 2008). The magnitude of these increases has led some to conclude that the healthcare system is "running on empty" (Peterson, 2005). There appears to be virtually unanimous agreement that the system must change significantly.

Figure 2-1 summarizes the overall phenomenon discussed in the CBO report. Technological inventions become market innovations as they increase in effectiveness and the associated risks decrease. The result is in-

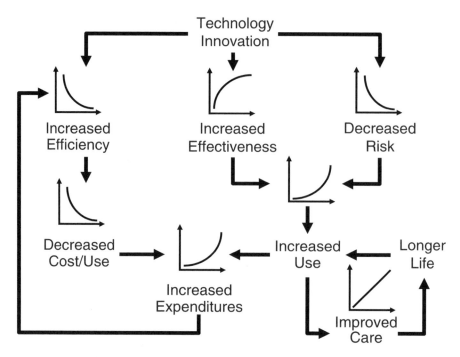

FIGURE 2-1 The dynamics of escalating healthcare costs.

creased use, which in turn leads to increased expenditures. In parallel, increased efficiency through production learning (discussed further below) leads to decreased cost per use, although not enough to keep pace with the product's growing use in health care. Finally, increased use yields improved care, which leads to longer lives and increased chances of again employing the technology of interest.

The concern in this illustrative example is how to control the phenomenon depicted in Figure 2-1. In typical engineering fashion, we approach this control problem with a series of models, beginning with a very simple model and then elaborating as the limits of each model become clear.

Model 1: Growth

The first model considers what efficiencies are needed to counteract the growth in Figure 2-1. We start with a simple equation:

(1)   Cost $(1 - \alpha)$ Use $(1 + \beta)$ = Total $(1 + \delta)$,

where α is the annual rate of cost reduction, β is the annual rate of usage growth, and δ is the annual allowable total growth. A bit of algebra shows that the annual rate of cost reduction required is given by the following:

$$(2) \qquad \alpha = (\beta - \delta)/(\beta + 1).$$

Table 2-1 shows the cost reductions needed for five of the technologies discussed in the CBO report, assuming zero allowable growth. These are rather significant decreases. However, these decreases are more instructive than definitive because of the simplicity of the model. In particular, the model is quite limited in that it provides no mechanism for achieving cost reductions and does not differentiate between the various elements of the healthcare delivery process. Thus we need to elaborate on model 1.

Model 2: Learning

The second model considers production learning, a well-understood concept in industrial engineering (Hancock and Bayha, 1992). Quite simply, as one produces more of an item, one gets better at it, and unit costs decrease. In some industries, such as the semiconductor industry, these decreases are a primary source of profit margins. Many manufacturing industries employ production learning curves to predict costs and hence profits. The basic learning equation is given by

$$(3) \qquad \text{Cost } (t = T) = \text{Cost } (t = 0) \text{ No. Uses } (t = T)^{-\text{Rate}}.$$

This learning phenomenon is usually discussed in terms of "percent curves." For example, a 70 percent curve means that after each doubling of the number of units produced, unit costs drop to 70 percent of what they were after the previous doubling. Table 2-2 provides a few examples of the rates required in equation (3) to achieve different percent curves.

TABLE 2-1 Cost Reductions Needed to Accommodate Growth

Treatment	Annual Rate of Usage Growth (%)	Minimum Annual Rate of Cost Reduction (%)
Angiography	10	9
Angioplasty	15	13
Dialysis	12	11
Hip replacement	10	9
Knee replacement	11	10

TABLE 2-2 Production Learning Parameters

Percentage Cost Per Use for Each Doubling of Uses	Rate for Learning Model
70	0.515
80	0.322
90	0.152

Most learning curves fall in the 70 to 90 percent range. This range reflects the experiences of many industries, including producers of airplanes, automobiles, and electronics. Curves below 70 percent are rare. As the results given below will show, controlling healthcare costs may require achieving significantly below 70 percent—a significant challenge.

Figure 2-2 shows learning curves for the three learning rates in Table 2-2, assuming a 10 percent annual rate of growth in usage. Note that the initial conditions were 100 uses at $100 per use, yielding an initial total expenditure of $10,000. Figure 2-3 shows the growth of total expenditures, again assuming a 10 percent annual growth in usage.

Table 2-3 shows the overall results for annual growth rates of 5 and 10 percent, assuming a 70 percent learning curve. Unit costs have dropped significantly, but the growth in usage has overwhelmed these efficiencies. Overall, this model exhibits impressive cost reductions from production learning, but it does not indicate where or how this learning happens. Furthermore, the model does not reflect the process whereby health care is delivered.

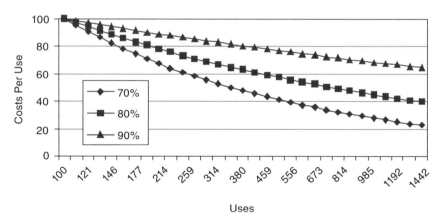

FIGURE 2-2 Learning curves for the three learning rates from Table 2-2.

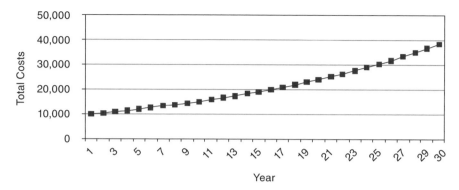

FIGURE 2-3 Expenditure growth at 10 percent annual growth in use.

TABLE 2-3 Impacts of Production Learning

Rate (%)	Results at 30 Years		
	No. of Uses	Cost/Use ($)	Total Expenditures ($)
5	412	48	19,874
10	1,586	24	38,256

Model 3: Process

The third model explicitly considers the process by which healthcare service is provided. As shown in Figure 2-4, this process includes multiple stages and differentiates labor from technology. A rich experience base allows us to define the learning rates for technology. For present purposes we, somewhat optimistically, set the technology learning rate at 70 percent. The question then is, What labor learning rate is needed to control the growth in costs to an acceptable level? This model is given by the following equations:

(4)   Cost (t) = Cost of Labor (t) + Cost of Technology (t),
(5)   CTOT (t) = CPUL (t) NU (t) + CPUT (t) NU (t),
(6)   CPUL (t) = CPUL (1) NU (t)$^{-Rate}_L$,
(7)   CPUT (t) = CPUT (1) NU (t)$^{-Rate}_T$, and
(8)   NU (t) = NU(1) (1+β) $^{t-1}$.

where CTOT, CPUL, and CPUT denote total costs, labor cost per unit, and technology cost per unit, respectively, while NU denotes number of units.

Figure 2-5 shows the efficiency required to control increases in health-

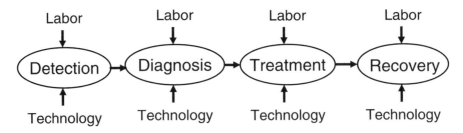

FIGURE 2-4 Service delivery process model.

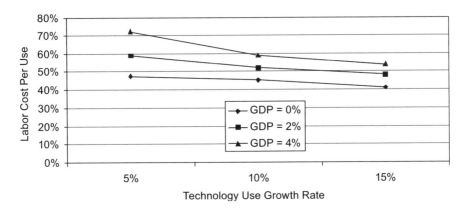

FIGURE 2-5 Required efficiency (% cost per use per doubling) for healthcare costs to track gross domestic product (GDP).

care costs to the point that they track increases in the GDP. The best case is for 4 percent GDP growth and 5 percent usage growth, which requires a learning curve of greater than 70 percent for labor. This magnitude of learning is imaginable. The worst case is for 0 percent GDP growth and 15 percent usage growth, which would require a learning curve of greater than 40 percent. This level of learning has never been achieved in any domain.

Implications

The implications of the results of these three models are quite clear. To limit the growth in total healthcare spending to the growth in GDP, some combination of the following three things is needed:

- Limit the growth of technology use.
- Limit the cost of technology use.
- Decrease the cost of labor associated with technology use.

Overall, the savings due to learning are the key to affordability. Achieving these savings will, however, be a significant challenge since learning rates of less than 70 percent are difficult to achieve.

Sources of Learning

In industries in which production learning curves have long been used, the sources of learning include labor efficiency, changes in personnel mix, standardization, specialization, method improvements, better use of equipment, changes in the resource mix, product and service redesign, and shared best practices. The Commonwealth Fund recently published recommendations for "bending the curve" (Schoen et al., 2008). Based on extensive economic analyses, the following are recommended as ways to reduce healthcare costs:

- Producing and using better information
  - Promoting health information technology
  - Center for medical effectiveness and healthcare decision making
  - Patient shared decision making
- Promoting health and disease prevention
  - Public health: reducing tobacco use
  - Public health: reducing obesity
  - Positive incentives for health
- Aligning incentives with quality and efficiency
  - Hospital pay-for-performance
  - Episode-of-care payment
  - Strengthening of primary care and care coordination
  - Limit on federal tax exemptions for premium contributions
- Correcting price signals in the healthcare market
  - Resetting of benchmark rates for Medicare advantage plans
  - Competitive bidding
  - Negotiated prescription drug prices
  - All-payer provider payment methods and rates
  - Limit on payment rate updates in high-cost areas

The report *Bending the Curve* provides projections of the savings that could be realized by adopting these recommendations (Schoen et al., 2008).

Conclusions

This paper has illustrated an engineering approach to addressing the complex problem of escalating healthcare costs. Ironically, it has done so in the context of an engineering phenomenon, namely, the successful technology innovation that has led to growing markets and increased revenues. The problem in health care is that increasing revenues to innovators translate into increasing costs to payers. Such growth is viewed more favorably when individuals pay rather than when third parties pay.

It may be possible to devise market-based mechanisms to control the growth in demand. De facto rationing is also likely, although we do not like to talk about the use of this mechanism. The other primary mechanism, which was the main focus of this paper, is increasing system efficiency to lower supply costs and hence prices. Such efficiency is needed to ensure the affordability of technology innovations. Although the required improvements are substantial, the estimates of their magnitude provided here offer some guidance concerning how aggressive efficiency initiatives need to be.

In searching for efficiencies of this magnitude, it will be important to focus on the whole system (Rouse, 2008). Consider the architecture of healthcare delivery shown in Figure 2-6. The efficiencies that can be gained

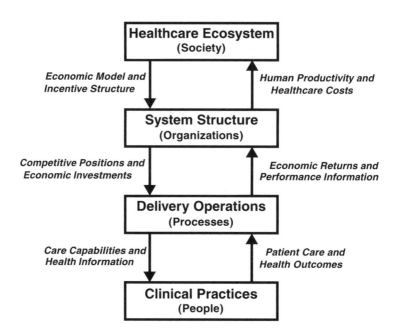

FIGURE 2-6 The architecture of healthcare delivery.

at the lowest level (clinical practices) are limited by the nature of the next level (delivery operations). For example, functionally organized practices are much less efficient than delivery that is organized around processes.

Similarly, the efficiencies that can be gained in operations are limited by the level above (system structure). Functional operations are driven by organizations structured around specialties, such as radiology. In addition, efficiencies in the system structure are limited by the healthcare ecosystem in which organizations operate. The experiences of other countries provide ample evidence of this.

The fee-for-service model central to U.S. health care ensures that provider income is linked to activities rather than to outcomes. The focus on disease and restoration of health rather than on wellness and productivity ensures that healthcare expenditures will be viewed as costs rather than investments. Recasting of "the problem" in terms of outcomes characterized by wellness and productivity may enable the identification and pursuit of efficiencies that cannot be imagined within our current frame of reference.

OPERATIONS RESEARCH FOR THE OPERATING ROOM AND MUCH MORE!

Richard C. Larson, Ph.D., Massachusetts Institute of Technology

The intent of this paper is to introduce the principles of OR to professionals in the healthcare community, with the goal of demystifying the OR approach by giving examples of its use in health care and elsewhere. As originally defined by OR cofounder Philip M. Morse, OR uses all aspects of the scientific method to help frame, formulate, and solve difficult operations problems involving people and technology. OR is a strong "systems-oriented" approach for use in developing learning healthcare systems.

Morse, a physicist at Massachusetts Institute of Technology (MIT), was the founder of OR in the United States in the late 1930s and early 1940s. Other physicists founded OR in Great Britain. According to the seminal book *Methods of Operations Research*, OR is an applied science that uses all known scientific techniques as tools to solve a specific problem (Morse and Kimball, 1951). It uses mathematics but is not a branch of mathematics, although the dominant mode in the OR field has become more mathematical. One of the ways in which OR can be most valuable is by offering an alternative and more insightful definition of the problem at hand.

At MIT I am at the junction of traditional OR and an emergent field called engineering systems. The way engineering systems are approached at MIT is to look at complex systems problems and put them in a box, framing them in such a way that it is possible to include all of their complexities—complexities that typically include issues from traditional engineering as well as management issues and issues from the social sciences. To the extent feasible, the full complexity that exists at the intersection of those three disciplines is embraced. The healthcare system, however it is defined, has many such problems. From an OR perspective, what kinds of interventions are required?

Going back to Morse's definition, OR requires multidisciplinary teams, not teams representing just one area or specialty. It also requires the development of an intimate knowledge of the operations in question, as well as a willingness and ability to invent new models and methods. Finally, we cannot simply pontificate from ivied buildings—we must get our boots on the ground.

OR of the 1940s and 1950s, in effect, evolved into the engineering systems of today. Those systems can bring many relevant applications to bear on health care. A special issue of OR's flagship journal, *Operations Research*, was recently devoted entirely to such considerations. Similarly, a recent book, *Operations Research in Healthcare: Handbook of Methods and Applications* (Brandeau et al., 2004), has some 40 or 50 chapters devoted to different applications of OR in the healthcare sector.

There are many success stories that may not be widely known outside of the OR field, but these are success stories within the broader definition of the healthcare system. For example, Ed Kaplan, who happens to be a member of both the National Academy of Engineering and the Institute of Medicine, won the Edelman Prize in 1992 for his New Haven Health Department Study on clean-needle exchange (Kaplan and Heimer, 1992). As is now widely known, heroin addicts often share needles; if anyone in a group of addicts has an HIV infection, the probability of infecting the others is rather high. Kaplan applied fundamental OR probabilistic modeling techniques—some actually developed from the study of wildlife—to this problem. The equations were not elaborate, but the lateral thinking was very impressive. Kaplan's results predicted a substantial reduction in the HIV/AIDS progression that occurred through the use of dirty needles if the government sponsored clean-needle exchanges. The city of New Haven adopted the approach, and studies suggest that the program reduced HIV/AIDS incidence by 33 percent. This is an example of OR on the ground. Kaplan went into the field, talked with people who were involved in the system at all levels, and then applied some basic mathematical modeling techniques.

More recently, Marco Zaider from Memorial Sloan-Kettering Cancer Center and Eva K. Lee from the Georgia Institute of Technology School of Industrial and Systems Engineering and Health Systems Institute used OR to advance cancer therapeutics. Their team devised sophisticated optimization modeling and computational techniques to implement an intraoperative 3-dimensional treatment planning system for brachytherapy (the placement of radioactive "seeds" inside a cancerous tumor) that offers a much safer and more reliable treatment. The system eliminates preoperation simulation and postimplant imaging, leading to savings of an estimated $459 million per year on the treatment of prostate cancer alone. Quality of life is improved through the use of treatment plans that deliver less radiation to healthy structures, which results in a drastic reduction (45 to 60 percent) in complications. This was a major application of OR at Georgia Tech, which also is well known for applying OR optimization techniques to airline crew and flight scheduling. More recently still, Kaplan and his colleague Larry Wein have received national acclaim for their OR-based ideas, presented in papers and in congressional testimony, on how best to respond to bioterrorism and its associated health risks.

The city of Stockholm was a 2008 finalist for the Edelman Prize for the project "Operations Research Improves Quality and Efficiency in Social Care and Home Help." The program led to an annual savings of €20 million to €30 million ($30 million to $45 million) and improvement in the quality of home care provided to patients.

The Larson research group at MIT has used OR to assess a low-probability/high-consequence event: the possibility of a return of pandemic influenza of the magnitude of that seen in 1918 to 1919. The so-called Spanish flu, this pandemic had its genesis in Kansas and eventually killed roughly 50 million people worldwide (although the precise death count will never be known). Depending on how Bayesian one is, the probability of such a recurrence in any given year may be anywhere from 1 to 5 percent. If we are not prepared for such a pandemic worldwide, it has the potential to kill more people than a full nuclear exchange between two nuclear powers. There will be no way to cordon off boundaries. If such a pandemic strikes anywhere in the world, it will reach the United States with high probability. So it is a possibility well worth studying.

Basically, as with any respiratory infectious disease, the Spanish flu spread from person to person through face-to-face contact or by people touching contaminated objects. Today, states have responsibility for influenza prevention, with each state expected to prepare its own pandemic influenza plan. These plans were read and discussed at MIT, with 12 states being represented. One need only imagine 50 Hurricane Katrinas all happening at the same time, with each state left to cope on its own and with no expectation of federal aid. The goal of the Larson research group is to apply OR thinking, lateral thinking, and some creative thinking to determine the best ways to apply nonpharmaceutical interventions (NPIs) should an influenza pandemic occur. There is strong evidence that NPIs can greatly reduce the probability of infection should such a pandemic strike. Possible NPIs include various forms of social distancing, such as closing schools, which could be government mandated; personal choice, such as deciding to telecommute or altering one's shopping patterns; and hygienic behavioral changes, which can be something as simple, but important, as intensive hand washing.

Another object of study—again using probability models of OR—is one of the most popular and fundamental parameters in epidemiology: R_0, which is defined as the mean number of new infections generated by a typical newly infected person in a fully susceptible population. If R_0 is something like 2, for instance, a person who becomes infected with the disease will, before being isolated from the rest of the population, infect two more people on average. These two will cause the infection of four people, who will cause the infection of eight, and so on, doubling each generation. If the R_0 is greater than 1, the number of infections will increase exponentially; if the R_0 is less then 1, there will be a geometric decay in the number of infections.

The problem is that many in the medical community treat R_0 as a constant of nature. They will say in a paper: consider an infectious respiratory disease where R_0 equals 2.6003724, and we will work from there. Recent evidence suggests strongly that R_0 can be decomposed into behavioral components, as is suggested in the following equation:

$$R_0 = p\lambda.$$

That is, R_0 equals p times λ, where λ is the frequency of daily contacts, and p is the probability of transmitting the infection, given contact. Seen this way, it is clear that the transmission parameter can be changed. Recent research has indicated that about 15 percent of the population has 4 or fewer face-to-face contacts per day. Another 15 percent of the population has 100 or more face-to-face contacts per day. Most of us have a value of λ that is between these extremes. The other parameter, p, represents the probability of giving the infection to someone—say, if I am infected and I shake your hand, what is the probability of giving it to you? Both λ and p are somewhat controllable by us, by our family members, and by our coworkers, and therefore we can influence R_0. This was done in 2003 when severe acute respiratory syndrome struck Hong Kong and elsewhere, as members of the population drastically changed their behaviors.

There are many roads forward. Paul O'Neill's article in *OR/MS Today*, "Why the U.S. Healthcare System Is So Sick and What OR Can Do To Cure It" (O'Neill, 2007), should be required reading for us all. Although additional research concerning how OR can improve the healthcare system is available, more is needed. Most notably, studies that connect OR and the social sciences (e.g., understanding how physicians and patients view uncertainty in healthcare delivery) could greatly expand the applicability of OR to healthcare improvement. Every day physicians and healthcare providers must make decisions based on many confounding factors. Doing so requires the calculation of conditional probabilities, something that is very difficult for most of us, not just physicians. Most people, including physicians, appear not to understand probability and risk as well as they should. A nice short read on the subject can be found in the book *Complications: A Surgeon's Notes on an Imperfect Science* (Gawande, 2002).

Going forward, it is likely that the most transformative applications of OR and engineering systems to health care have not yet been identified, but we do need feet on the ground, and we cannot pontificate from our offices. One of the key issues can be summed up this way: Imagine that you or a loved one is in a hospital receiving treatment. In the spirit of Harry Truman, you might ask, "Where does the buck stop?" That is, who is in charge? What single individual assumes responsibility? Too often, decisions appear to be the responsibility of a committee, with the result that important decisions fall between the cracks.

ON DESIGNING AN INTEGRATED AND ADAPTIVE HEALTHCARE SYSTEM

James M. Tien, Ph.D., College of Engineering, University of Miami, and Pascal J. Goldschmidt, M.D., Miller School of Medicine, University of Miami

Introduction

Health care can be considered a service system. In general, services are carried out with knowledge-intensive agents or components that work together as providers and consumers to create or coproduce value. Indeed, anyone performing the engineering design of a healthcare system must recognize that the system is a complex integration of human-centered activities that is increasingly dependent on information technology and knowledge. Like any service system, health care can be considered a combination or recombination of three essential components: people (characterized by behaviors, values, knowledge, etc.), processes (characterized by collaboration, customization, etc.), and products (characterized by software, hardware, infrastructures, etc.). Thus, a healthcare system is an integrated and adaptive set of people, processes, and products. It is, in essence, a system of systems whose objectives are to enhance its efficiency (leading to greater interdependency) and increase its effectiveness (leading to improved health). Integration occurs over the physical, temporal, organizational, and functional dimensions, while adaptation occurs over the monitoring, feedback, cybernetics, and learning dimensions. In sum, service systems such as health care are indeed complex, especially because of the uncertainties associated with their human-centered aspects. Moreover, the system complexities can be dealt with only through methods that enhance system integration and adaptation. The purpose of this paper, then, is to highlight the critical importance of integration and adaptation when designing, operating, or refining a complex service system such as health care.

On Services

Before discussing a healthcare service system as an integrated system, an adaptive system, and a complex system, it is helpful to start by defining services and discussing their uniqueness, especially in contrast to goods. Some concluding insights are provided later.

As detailed by Tien and Berg (1995, 2003, 2006, 2007), the importance of the services sector cannot be overstated. This sector employs a large and growing percentage of workers in the industrialized nations. As reflected in Table 2-4, the services sector in the United States includes a number of large industries and accounts for 82.1 percent of total jobs, while the other 4 economic sectors (manufacturing, agriculture, construction, and mining), which together can be considered the physical "goods" sector, employ the remaining 17.9 percent. Health care, which employs 10.8 percent of the U.S. workforce, is, of course, one of the largest industries

TABLE 2-4 U.S. Employment, by Industry/Sector, 2006

Industries	Employment (M)	Percentage
Trade, transportation, and utilities	26.1	19.0
Professional and business	17.2	12.6
Health care	14.8	10.8
Leisure and hospitality	13.0	9.5
Education	13.0	9.5
Government (except education)	11.7	8.5
Finance, insurance, and real estate	8.3	6.1
Information and telecommunication	3.1	2.2
Other	5.4	3.9
Services Sector	**112.6**	**82.1**
Manufacturing	14.3	10.3
Construction	7.5	5.5
Agriculture	2.2	1.6
Mining	0.7	0.5
Goods Sector	**24.7**	**17.9**
Total	137.3	100.0

SOURCE: Bureau of Labor Statistics, 2006.

in the services sector. Yet, as Tien and Berg (2006) point out, engineering research and education do not reflect this distribution, as the majority of research is still manufacturing or hardware oriented, and degree programs are still offered mainly in those traditional disciplines that were established in the early 1900s. On the other hand, medical research and education are somewhat more sensitive to the services need of health care; for example, evidence-based protocols are becoming more prevalent in the practice of medicine. Nevertheless, Hipel and colleagues (2007) maintain that services research and education deserve more attention and support now that the computer chip, information technology, the Internet, and the "flattening of the world" (Friedman, 2005) have all combined to make services—and services innovation—the new engine for global economic growth.

What constitutes the services sector? It can be considered "to include all economic activities whose output is not a physical product or construction, is generally consumed at the time it is produced and provides added value in forms (such as convenience, amusement, timeliness, comfort or health) that are essentially intangible" (Quinn et al., 1987). Implicit in this definition is the recognition that services production and delivery are so integrated that they can be considered a single, combined stage in the services value chain, whereas the goods sector has a value chain that includes supplier, manufacturer, assembler, retailer, and customer. Alternatively, services can be viewed as knowledge-intensive agents or components that work together as providers and consumers to create or coproduce value (Maglio et al., 2006).

Unfortunately, the U.S. healthcare system is a good example of a people-intensive service system that is in disarray. It is the most expensive healthcare system in the world, yet it is among the least effective of any developed country; a minority of the population receives excellent care, while an equal minority receives inadequate care (NAE/IOM, 2005). This situation is not due to a lack of well-trained health professionals or to a lack of innovative technologies; rather, it exists because the U.S. healthcare system consists of a fragmented group of mainly small, independent providers driven by insurance companies focused on costs. Clearly it is, at best, a nonsystem (Rouse, 2008). The natural conclusion to draw is that an integrated and adaptive healthcare system must be designed and implemented, one that will involve the participation and support of a large number of stakeholders (consumers, doctors, hospitals, insurance companies, and so on). For example, patients will need to take increased responsibility for their own health care in terms of access to and use of validated information.

The remainder of this section focuses on three overarching influences. First, the emergence of electronic services is totally dependent on information technology; examples include financial services, banking, airline reservation systems, and consumer goods marketing. As discussed by Tien and Berg (2003) and detailed in Table 2-5, e-service enterprises interact or "coproduce" with their customers in a digital medium (including e-mail and the Internet), as contrasted with the physical environment within which traditional or bricks-and-mortar service enterprises interact with their customers. Similarly, in contrast to traditional services delivered by low-wage earners, e-services typically employ high-wage earners and are more demanding in their requirements for self-service, transaction speed, and computation. With regard to data input that can be processed to produce information that, in turn, can be used to help make informed service decisions, it should be noted that both sets of services rely on multiple data sources; however, traditional services typically require homogeneous (mainly quantitative) data input, while e-services increasingly require nonhomogeneous (i.e., both quantitative and qualitative) data input. Paradoxically, the traditional service enterprises have been driven by data, although data availability and accuracy have been limited (especially before the pervasive use of the Universal Product Code and the more recent deployment of radio frequency location and identification [RFLID] tags). Likewise, the emerging e-service enterprises have been driven by information (i.e., processed data), although information availability and accuracy have been limited as a result of the current data rich, information poor (DRIP) conundrum (Tien, 2003).

Consequently, while traditional services—such as traditional manu-

TABLE 2-5 Comparison of Traditional and Electronic Services

| Issue | Service Enterprises | |
	Traditional	Electronic
Coproduction medium	Physical	Electronic
Labor requirement	High	Low
Wage level	Low	High
Self-service requirement	Low	High
Transaction speed requirement	Low	High
Computation requirement	Medium	High
Data sources	Multiple homogeneous	Multiple nonhomogeneous
Driver	Data driven	Information driven
Data availability/accuracy	Poor	Rich
Information availability/accuracy	Poor	Poor
Economic consideration	Economies of scale	Economies of expertise
Service objective	Standardized	Personalized
Service focus	Mass production	Mass customization
Decision time frame	Predetermined	Real time

facturing—are based on economies of scale and a standardized approach, e-services—such as electronic manufacturing—emphasize economies of expertise or knowledge and an adaptive approach. Another critical distinction between traditional and electronic services is that although all services require decisions to be made, decisions made in traditional services are typically based on predetermined decision rules, while e-services require real-time, adaptive decision making. It is for this reason that Tien (2003) advanced a decision informatics paradigm, one that relies on both information and decision technologies from a real-time perspective. High-speed Internet access, low-cost computing, wireless networks, electronic sensors, and ever-smarter software are the tools necessary for building a global services economy. Thus e-commerce, a sophisticated and integrated service system, combines product selection (i.e., selection of goods or services), order taking, payment processing, order fulfillment, and delivery scheduling into a seamless system, all provided by distinct service providers; in this regard, an electronic service system can be considered to be a system of different systems.

The second influence on services is their relationship to manufacturing. The interdependencies, similarities, and complementarities of services and manufacturing are significant. Indeed, many recent innovations in manufacturing are relevant to the service industries. Concepts and processes can, for the most part, be recast in terms that are relevant to services. These concepts and processes include cycle time, total quality management, quality circles, six-sigma design for assembly, design for manufacturability, design for recycling, small-batch production, concurrent engineering, just-in-time manufacturing, rapid prototyping, flexible manufacturing, agile manufacturing, distributed manufacturing, and environmentally sound manufacturing. Thus, many of the engineering and management concepts and processes employed in manufacturing can also be used to deal with problems and issues arising in the services sector.

Nonetheless, there are considerable differences between goods and services. Tien and Berg (2003) provide a comparison of the two sectors. The goods sector requires material as input, is physical in nature, involves the customer at the design stage, and employs mainly quantitative measures to assess its performance. By contrast, the services sector requires information as input, is virtual in nature, involves the customer at both the production and delivery stages, and employs mainly qualitative measures to assess its performance. Of course, even when there are similarities, it is critical that the coproducing nature of services be taken into consideration. For example, physical parameters, statistics of production, and quality can be quantified more precisely in the case of manufacturing; because a services operation depends on an interaction between the recipient and the process

TABLE 2-6 Services Vs. Manufactured Goods

Focus	Services	Goods
Production	Coproduced	Preproduced
Variability	Heterogeneous	Identical
Physicality	Intangible	Tangible
Product	Perishable	"Inventoryable"
Objective	Personalizable	Reliable
Satisfaction	Expectation related	Utility related
Life cycle	Reusable	Recyclable
OVERALL	CHIPPER	PITIRUR

of producing and delivering, the characterization is necessarily more subjective and different.

A more insightful approach to understanding and advancing services research is to consider explicitly the differences between services and manufactured goods. As shown in Table 2-6, services are, by definition, coproduced, they are quite variable or heterogeneous in their production and delivery, they are physically intangible and perishable if not consumed either as they are being produced or by a certain time (e.g., before a flight's departure), they are focused on being "personalizable," they are expectation related in terms of customer satisfaction, and they are reusable in their entirety. On the other hand, manufactured goods are preproduced, quite identical or standardized in their production and use, physically tangible, "inventoryable" if not consumed, focused on being reliable, utility related in terms of customer satisfaction, and recyclable with regard to their parts. In mnemonic terms and referring to Table 2-6, services can be considered to be "chipper," while manufactured goods are a "pitirur."

Although the comparison of services and manufacturing highlights some obvious methodological differences, it is interesting to note that, while physical manufactured assets depreciate with use and time, virtual service assets are generally reusable and may in fact increase in value with repeated use and over time. The latter assets are predominantly processes and associated human resources that build on the skill and knowledge base accumulated through repeated interactions with the service receiver, who is involved in the coproduction of the service. Thus, for example, a surgeon should improve over time, especially if the same type of surgery is repeated. Indeed, clinical productivity increases for the average physician from the dawn of a career to almost end of a career, with a slight slowing toward the end. Likewise, while most U.S. physicians practice at a financial loss during the first few years of their career, they progressively improve their financial standing.

In services, automation-driven software algorithms have transformed human resource–laden, coproducing service systems into algorithm-laden, self-producing services. Thus, extensive manpower would be required to coproduce the services manually if automation were not available. Although automation has certainly improved productivity and decreased costs for some services (e.g., telecommunications and Internet commerce), it has not yet had a similar effect on other labor-intensive services, such as health care. With new multimedia and broadband technologies, however, some hospitals are personalizing their treatment of patients, including by sharing patients' electronic records. As a result, patients can take increased responsibility for their own health care.

A third critical influence on services is the computation-driven move toward mass customization. *Customization* implies meeting the needs of a customer market that is partitioned into an appropriate number of segments, each with similar needs (e.g., Amazon.com targets its marketing of a new book to an entire market segment if several members of the segment act to acquire the book). *Mass customization* implies meeting the needs of a segmented customer market, with each segment being a single individual (e.g., a tailor who laser scans an individual's upper torso and then delivers a uniquely fitted jacket). *Real-time mass customization* implies meeting the needs of an individualized customer market on a real-time basis (e.g., a tailor who laser scans an individual's upper torso and then delivers a uniquely fitted jacket within a reasonable period, while the individual is waiting).

It is interesting to note that, with regard to customization and relative to the late 1700s, the United States is in some respects going "back to the future"; that is, advanced technologies are not only empowering the individual but also allowing for individualized or customized goods and services. For example, e-education reflects a return to individual-centered learning (Tien, 2000), much like the home schooling of a previous century. Moreover, when mass customization occurs, it is difficult to say whether a service or a good is being delivered; that is, a uniquely fitted jacket can be considered to be a coproduced service/good or "servgood." The implication of real-time mass customization, then, is that the resultant coproduced servgood must be carried out locally, although the intelligence underpinning the coproduction could be residing at a distant server and delivered like a utility. Thus, while most manufacturing jobs have already been relocated overseas (with only 10.3 percent of all U.S. employees still involved in manufacturing), and while service jobs (82.1 percent of all U.S. jobs) are beginning to be relocated overseas, real-time mass customization should help stem if not reverse the job outflow trend. In this regard, real-time mass customization should be viewed as a matter of national priority.

Clearly, health care needs to transition from being a traditional (although high-wage) to an electronic-based service industry, relying on digital media for such activities as real-time access to patient data. (Some digitally based medical approaches need further assessment and improvement. Although robotic surgery is quite helpful in the repair of small nerves and blood vessels, for example, its overall efficacy is still under debate. Nevertheless, as robotic surgery is further refined, it will undoubtedly become a standard technique.) Additionally, health care must adopt some of the methods that have made manufacturing efficient (e.g., reduced cycle time and improved quality) while focusing on service effectiveness (e.g., maintaining a high standard of coproduction and meeting consumer expectations). Most important, health care must be adaptive and customize treatments to the needs of patients, with treatments ranging from evidence-based protocols to servgood or personalized therapies.

On Integration

As indicated earlier, a service system such as health care is actually an integration or combination of three essential components—people, processes, and products. The people in a service system can be grouped into those demanding services (consumers, users, patients, buyers, organizations, etc.) and those supplying the services (suppliers, providers, clinicians, servers, sellers, organizations, etc.). Similarly, processes can be procedural (standardized, evolving, decision focused, network oriented, etc.) or algorithmic (data mining, decision modeling, systems engineering, etc.) in structure, or sometimes both. And products can be physical (facilities, sensors, information technologies, etc.) or virtual (e-commerce, simulations, e-collaboration, etc.) in form.

Given the coproducing nature of services, it is obvious that people make up the most critical element of a service system. In turn, because people are so unpredictable in their values, behaviors, attitudes, expectations, and knowledge, they invariably increase the complexity of a service system. Moreover, the multistakeholder—and related multiobjective—nature of such systems serves only to intensify the complexity level and may ultimately result in the system's being indefinable, if not unmanageable. Human performance, social networks, and interpersonal interactions combine to further aggravate the situation. People-oriented, decision-focused methods are considered in a later section.

Processes that underpin system integration include standards, procedures, protocols, and algorithms. By combining or integrating service processes, one could, for example, enhance a "one-stop shopping" approach, a highly desirable situation for the consumer or customer. Integration of financial services has resulted in giant banks (e.g., Citigroup), integration of home-building goods and services has resulted in super stores (e.g., Home Depot), and integration of software services has resulted in complex software packages (e.g., Microsoft Office). Integration also enhances system efficiency, if not effectiveness. For example, the RFLID tag—a computer chip with a transmitter—serves to integrate the supply chain.

Service-related products can be grouped into two categories. First are those physical products or goods (e.g., cars, aircraft, satellites, computers) that, as indicated earlier, enable the delivery of effective and high-quality services (e.g., road travel, air travel, global positioning, electronic services). Second are more virtual products or services, including e-commerce.

More important, and as detailed in Table 2-7, service system integration can occur over many different dimensions, including physical, temporal, organizational, and functional. Physical integration can be defined by the degree of systems collocation in the natural (e.g., closed, open, hybrid), constructed (e.g., goods, structures, systems), or virtual (e.g., services, simulation, e-commerce) environment. An urban center's infrastructures (e.g., emergency services, health services, financial services) are examples

TABLE 2-7 System Integration: Dimensions

Dimension	Definition	Characteristics	Elements
Physical	Degree of systems collocation	Natural	Closed; open; hybrid
		Constructed	Goods; structures; systems
		Virtual	Services; simulation; e-commerce
Temporal	Degree of systems cotiming	Strategic	Analytical; procedural; political
		Tactical	Simulation; distribution; allocation
		Operational	Cognition; visualization; expectation
Organizational	Degree of systems comanagement	Resources	People; processes; products
		Economics	Supply; demand; revenue
		Management	Centralized; decentralized; distributed
Functional	Degree of systems cofunctioning	Input	Location; allocation; reallocation
		Process	Informatics; feedback; control
		Output	Efficiency; effectiveness

of a constructed environment. Over time, and with advances in information technology and in response to the need for improved efficiency and effectiveness, these infrastructures have become increasingly automated and interlinked, or interdependent. In fact, because the information technology revolution has changed the way business is transacted, the government is operated, and national defense is conducted, President George W. Bush (2001) singled it out as the most critical infrastructure to protect following the terrorist attacks of September 11. Thus, while the United States is considered a superpower because of its military strength and economic prowess, nontraditional attacks on its interdependent and cyber-underpinned infrastructures could significantly harm both the nation's military power and its economy. Clearly, infrastructures, especially the information infrastructure, are among the nation's weakest links; they are vulnerable to various attacks, from willful acts of sabotage to invasions of privacy. Recent technological advances toward imbuing infrastructures with "intelligence" make it increasingly feasible to address the safety and security issues, allowing for the continuous monitoring and real-time control of critical infrastructures.

Temporal integration can be defined by the degree of systems cotiming from a strategic (e.g., analytical, procedural, political), tactical (e.g., simulation, distribution, allocation), and operational (e.g., cognition, visualization, expectation) perspective. Expectation, for example, is a critical temporal issue in the delivery of services. More specifically, because services are to a large extent subject to customer satisfaction and because—as Tien and Cahn (1981) postulated and validated—"satisfaction is a function of expectation," service performance or satisfaction can be enhanced through the effective management of expectation. With respect to health care, however, it may be difficult, if not impossible, to manage a patient's expectation under certain emergency or competitive situations.

Organizational integration can be defined as the degree of systems comanagement of resources (e.g., people, processes, products), economics (e.g., supply, demand, revenue), and management (e.g., centralized, decentralized, distributed). With regard to management integration, Tien and colleagues (2004) provide a consistent approach to considering the management of both goods and services—first by defining a value chain and then by showing how it can be partitioned into supply and demand chains, which in turn can be appropriately managed. Of course, the key purpose of the management of supply and demand chains is to smooth out the peaks and valleys commonly seen in many supply and demand patterns. Moreover, real-time mass customization occurs when supply and demand chains are simultaneously managed. The shift in focus from mass production to mass customization (whereby a service is produced and delivered in response to a customer's stated or imputed needs) is intended to provide superior value to customers by meeting their unique needs. It is in this area of customization—where customer involvement is not only at the goods design stage but also at the manufacturing or coproduction stage—that services and manufacturing are merging in concept (Tien and Berg, 2006), resulting in the above-mentioned servgood.

Functional integration can be defined as the degree of systems co-functioning with respect to input (e.g., location, allocation, reallocation), process (e.g., informatics, feedback, control), and output (e.g., efficiency, effectiveness). From an output perspective, for example, it is obvious that a system should act to enhance efficiency and effectiveness, the twin pillars of productivity. However, it should be noted that manufactured goods are primarily a result of an efficient supply chain, while services are primarily a result of an effective demand chain.

Again, health care—as a service system—must be integrated with regard to people, processes, and products, as well as over the physical, temporal, organizational, and functional dimensions. Designing an efficient and effective healthcare system will not be easy; socialistic systems like Sweden's cost too much, while capitalistic systems like those in the United States both have high cost and are unfair. New design approaches are required. The information technology revolution has permitted the analysis element of system design to be carried out largely by computers; it allows a simulated and collaborative redesign process to occur until a satisfactory design that meets specified performance (e.g., morbidity, mortality, cost) criteria is achieved. The resulting integrated healthcare system will be a comprehensive, interoperable system of systems.

On Adaptation

Because a service system is, by definition, a coproducing system, it must be adaptive. Adaptation is a uniquely human characteristic, based on a combination of three essential components: decision making, decision informatics, and human interface. (Indeed, designing a healthcare system is essentially an exercise in making decisions or choices about the system's characteristics or attributes.) Figure 2-7 provides a framework for decision making. To begin, it is helpful to clarify the difference between data and information, especially from a decision-making perspective. Data represent basic transactions captured during operations, while information represents processed data (e.g., derivations, groupings, patterns). Clearly, except for simple operational decisions, decision making at the tactical or higher levels requires, at a minimum, appropriate information or processed data. Figure 2-7 also identifies knowledge as processed information (together with experiences, beliefs, values, cultures, etc.) and wisdom as processed knowledge (together with insights, theories, etc.). Thus, strategic decisions

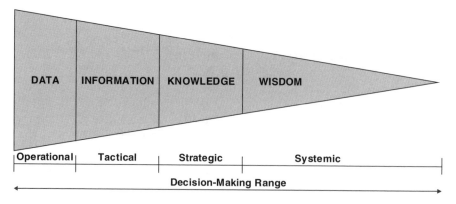

FIGURE 2-7 System adaptation: decision-making framework.

can be made with knowledge, while systemic decisions can be made with wisdom. Unfortunately, for the most part the literature does not distinguish between data and information. Economists claim that because of the astounding growth in information—really, data—technology, the United States and other developed countries are now part of a global "knowledge economy." Although electronic data technology has transformed large-scale information systems from being the "glue" that holds the various units of an organization together to being the strategic asset that provides the organization with its competitive advantage, the United States is far from having reached the level of a knowledge economy. In terms of a continuum of data, information, knowledge, and wisdom, the United States—as well as other advanced economies—is, at best, at the beginning of a DRIP conundrum, as identified earlier.

The fact remains that data—both quantitative and qualitative—need to be fused and analyzed effectively and efficiently to provide the information needed for informed or intelligent decision making with regard to the design, production, and delivery of goods and services, including health care. As depicted in Figure 2-8, the nature of the necessary real-time decision (regarding the production or delivery of a service) determines, where appropriate and from a systems engineering perspective, the data to be collected (possibly, from multiple, nonhomogeneous sources) and the real-time fusion and analysis to be undertaken to obtain the needed information for input to the modeling effort. The modeling effort, in turn, provides the knowledge needed to identify and support the required decision in a timely manner. Clearly, methods must be developed that can fuse and analyze a steady stream of nonhomogeneous (i.e., quantitative and qualitative) data, and this is especially true for health care, where quantitative data

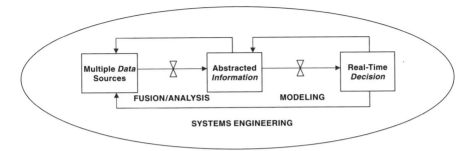

FIGURE 2-8 System adaptation: a decision informatics paradigm.

from monitoring devices must be complemented with patients' qualitative assessments before clinicians can recommend appropriate treatment. The feedback loops in Figure 2-8 are within the context of systems engineering; they serve to refine the analysis and modeling steps.

Continuing with the decision informatics paradigm in Figure 2-8, it should be noted that decision modeling includes the information-based modeling and analysis of alternative decision scenarios. They include OR, decision science, computer science, and industrial engineering. At present, decision-modeling methods suffer from two shortcomings. First, most of the available methods—especially optimization—are applicable only in a steady-state environment, whereas in the real world all systems are in transition. (Note that steady state, like average, is an analytical concept that allows for a tractable, if not always manageable, analysis.) Second, most of the available methods are unable to cope with changing circumstances. We need methods that are adaptive so decisions can be made in real time, as is required in most healthcare situations. Thus, non-steady-state and adaptive decision methods are required. More important, real-time decision modeling requires more than simply speeding up the models and solution algorithms; like real-time data fusion and analysis, it also requires additional research and development.

The systems engineering methods implicit in Figure 2-8 concern the integration of people, processes, and products from a systems perspective; they include electrical engineering, human–machine systems, system performance, and system biology. Again, the real-time nature of coproducing services—especially human-centered services that are computationally intensive and intelligence oriented—requires a real-time systems engineering approach. Ethnography, a branch of anthropology that can help identify a consumer's unmet needs, is being used to identify breakthrough products and service innovations. Another critical aspect of systems engineering is system performance, which provides an essential framework for assessing the decisions made in terms of such issues as satisfaction, convenience, privacy, security, equity, quality, productivity, safety, and reliability. Similarly, undertaking systems engineering within a real-time environment will require additional thought and research.

The human interface is another essential element of an adaptive service system; it is actually a critical tool in systems engineering. Such interfaces include the interactions between and among humans and software agents, machines, subsystems, and systems of systems. The discipline of human factors deals with many of these interactions. However, another critical interface arises from the interaction of humans with data and information. In developing appropriate human–information interfaces, one must pay careful attention to a number of factors. First, human–information interfaces are a part of any decision support model; they determine the manner in which the model output or information is provided to the decision maker. Cognition represents the point of interface between the human and the information presented. The presentation must enhance the cognitive process of mental visualization and must be capable of creating images from complex multidimensional data, including structured and unstructured text documents, measurements, images, and video. Second, constructing and communicating a mental image common to a team of, say, clinicians and nurses could facilitate collaboration and could lead to more effective decision making at all levels, from operational to tactical to strategic. Nevertheless, cognitive facilitation is especially necessary in operational settings that are under high stress. Third, cognitive modeling and decision making must combine machine learning technology with a priori knowledge in a probabilistic data-mining framework to develop models of, say, a nurse's tasks, goals, and objectives. These user-behavior models must be designed to adapt to an individual decision maker in order to promote better understanding of the needs and actions of the individual, including adversarial behaviors and intents.

More important and as detailed in Table 2-8, service system adaptation can occur in the monitoring, feedback, cybernetics, and learning dimensions. Monitoring adaptation can be defined by the degree of sensed actions with regard to data collection (e.g., sensors, agents, swarms), data analysis (e.g., structuring, processing, mining), and information abstraction (e.g., derivations, groupings, patterns). Data are acquired by sensors, which can be in the form of humans, robotic networks, aerial images, radio frequency signals, and other measures and signatures. When working with patients, for example, sensors that monitor the patients' vital signs are essential, as are verbal inputs from the patients themselves. More recently, data warehouses have been proliferating, and data mining techniques have been gaining popularity. However, regardless of how large a data warehouse is and how sophisticated a data mining technique is, problems can occur if

TABLE 2-8 System Adaptation: Dimensions

Dimension	Definition	Characteristics	Elements
Monitoring	Degree of sensed actions	Data collection	Sensors; agents; swarms
		Data analysis	Structuring; processing; mining
		Information abstraction	Derivations; groupings; patterns
Feedback	Degree of expected actions	Standardized	Prestructured; preplanned
		Procedural	Policies; standard operating procedures
		Algorithmic	Optimized; Bayesian
Cybernetic	Degree of reactive actions	Deterministic	Known states; deterministic actions
		Dynamic	Known state distributions; dynamic actions
		Adaptive	Unknown states; adaptive actions
Learning	Degree of unstructured actions	Cognition	Recognition based; behavioral
		Evidence	Information based; genetic
		Improvisation	Experience based; evolutionary

the data do not possess the desirable attributes of measurability, availability, consistency, validity, reliability, stability, accuracy, independence, robustness, and completeness.

Moreover, in most situations, data alone are useless unless access to and analysis of the data occur in real time. When developing real-time, adaptive data processors, one must consider several critical issues. First, as shown in Figure 2-8, these data processors must be able to combine (i.e., fuse and analyze) streaming data from sensors and other appropriate input from knowledge bases (including output from tactical and strategic databases) in order to generate information that can serve as input to operational decision support models or provide the basis for making informed decisions. Second, as also shown in Figure 2-8, the types of data collected and the ways in which the data are processed must depend on what decision is to be made; these dependencies highlight the difficulty of developing effective and adaptive data processors or data miners. Furthermore, once a decision has been made, it may constrain subsequent decisions, which in turn may change future data requirements and information needs. Third, inasmuch as the data processors must function in real time and be able to adapt to an ongoing stream of data, genetic algorithms, which have equations that can mutate repeatedly in an evolutionary manner until a solution emerges that best fits the observed data, are becoming the tools of choice in this area.

Feedback adaptation can be defined by the degree of expected actions based on standardized (e.g., prestructured, preplanned), procedural (e.g., policies, standard operating procedures), and algorithmic (e.g., optimized, Bayesian) approaches. In general, different models underpin these approaches. As an example, Kaplan and colleagues (2002) developed a set of complex models to demonstrate that the best prevention approach to a smallpox attack would be to undertake immediate and widespread vaccination. Unfortunately, models, including simulations, that deal with multiple systems are still relatively immature and require additional research and development. Such system of systems models are quite complex and require a multidisciplinary approach.

Cybernetic adaptation can be defined by the degree of reactive actions that can be deterministic (i.e., known states, deterministic actions), dynamic (e.g., known state distributions, dynamic actions), or adaptive (e.g., unknown states, adaptive actions). Cybernetics is derived from the Greek word "kybernetics," which refers to a steersman or governor. Within a system, cybernetics is concerned with feedback (through evaluation of performance relative to stated objectives) and control (through communication, self-regulation, adaptation, optimization, and management). Thus, cybernetic adaptation refers to actions that are undertaken based on an assessment of the feedback signals, with the corrective steps taken to modify the system so as to achieve the desired system objectives. A system is defined by state variables that are known in a deterministic manner (resulting in deterministic feedback or cybernetic actions), that are known in a probabilistic or distributional manner (resulting in dynamic feedback or cybernetic actions), or that are unknown (resulting in adaptive feedback or cybernetic actions). For example, autopilots—which are programmed to deal with deterministic and dynamic situations—can, for the most part, take off, fly, and land a plane, yet two human pilots are usually in the plane as well in case an unknown state occurs and the adaptive judgment of a human is required. Clearly, a trained human—such as a clinician or surgeon—remains the most adaptive controller, although machines are becoming more "intelligent" through adaptive learning algorithms.

System control is perhaps the most critical challenge facing system of systems designers. Because of the difficulty, if not impossibility, of developing a comprehensive solid-on-solid (SoS) model, either analytically or through simulation, SoS control remains an open problem and is, of course, uniquely challenging for each application domain. Moreover, real-time control of interdependent systems—which is required in nearly all application domains—poses an especially difficult problem. The cooperative control of an SoS assumes that it can be characterized by a set of interconnected systems or agents with a common goal. Classical techniques of control design, optimization, and estimation could be used to create parallel architectures for, as an example, coordinating numerous sensors. However, many issues that involve real-time cooperative control have not been addressed, even in non-SoS structures. For example, one issue concerns the control of an SoS in the presence of communication delays to and among the SoS subsystems.

Finally, learning adaptation can be defined by the degree of unstructured actions based on cognition (e.g., recognition based, behavioral), evidence (e.g., information based, genetic), and improvisation (e.g., experience based, evolutionary). Learning adaptation is mainly about real-time decision making at the operational level. In such a situation and as indicated earlier, the issue is not simply how to speed up steady-state models and their solution algorithms; indeed, steady-state models become irrelevant in real-time environments. Instead, learning adaptation concerns reasoning under both uncertainty and severe time constraints. In developing operational decision support models, one must recognize several critical issues. First, in addition to defining what data to collect and how they should be fused and analyzed, decisions will drive what kind of models or simulations are needed. These operational models are, in turn, based on abstracted information and output from tactical and strategic decision support models. The models must capture changing behaviors and conditions and be responsive within the changing environment, usually through the use of Bayesian networks. Second, most adaptive models are closely aligned with evolutionary models, also known as genetic algorithms, so they function in a manner similar to biological evolution or natural selection. In recent years, computationally intensive evolutionary algorithms have been used to develop sophisticated, real-time pricing schemes to minimize traffic congestion (Sussman, 2008), to enhance autonomous operations in unmanned aircraft, and to determine sniper locations in modern warfare (e.g., in Iraq). Third, computational improvisation is another operational modeling approach that can be employed when one cannot predict and plan for every possible contingency. (Indeed, much of what happened on September 11 was improvised, based on the ingenuity of the responders.) Improvisation involves learning by reexamining and reorganizing past knowledge in time to meet the requirements of an unexpected situation; it may be conceptualized as a search-and-assembly problem that is influenced by such factors as the time available for planning, the prevailing risk, and the constraints imposed by prior decisions (Mendonca and Wallace, 2004).

Again, health care as a service system must be adaptive with regard to decision making, decision informatics, and human interfaces, as well as with regard to the monitoring, feedback, cybernetics, and learning dimensions. At all levels of healthcare decision making, a spectrum of possible methods can be used, ranging from adaptive—instead of randomized—medical trials to autonomous control and from virtual-touch tools to genetic algorithms, all of which are able to cope with imprecision, uncertainties, and partial truth (Zadeh, 1996). Moreover, the methods can be used to process information, take changing conditions into account, and learn from the environment; thus, they are adaptive and, to a large extent, responsive to a data stream of real-time input. In a fully integrated and adaptive system of systems, each system must be able to communicate and interact with the entire SoS, with no compatibility issues.

On Complexities

Service systems are indeed complex, requiring both integrative and adaptive approaches to deal with their complexity. There are a number of ways to characterize the complexity of a system (Rouse, 2007), especially a service system. Table 2-9 lists seven system stages that characterize the complexity of a healthcare service system and for which integrative and adaptive methods are required to mitigate, if not handle, the complexity.

The first stage, the system's purpose, is difficult to define given the many stakeholders (patients, clinicians, insurers, etc.) involved, the multiple objectives (wellness care, emergency care, acute care, etc.) of each stakeholder, and the overarching business model (revenues, expenditures, endowments, etc.). Combining these divergent viewpoints into a consistent and viable purpose is an almost impossible task. The second stage, the system's boundary, is, at best, ill defined and shifting; the spatial (offices, clinics, hospitals, etc.), temporal (schedules, activities, resources, etc.), and interdependent (infrastructures, supply chains, demand chains, etc.) relationships are difficult to determine. Third, the system's design must be robust (to ensure reliability, quality, integrity, etc.), efficient (to minimize cost, inventory, waste, etc.), and effective (to maximize usefulness, satisfaction, pervasiveness, etc.). Fourth, the system's development must be based on models (gedanken experiments, simulations, networks, etc.), scalability (multiscale, multilevel, multitemporal, etc.), and sustainability (over time, space, culture, etc.). Fifth, the system's deployment must be with minimal risk (measured by morbidity, comorbidity, mortality, etc.), uncertainty (unexpected attitudes, behaviors, performances, etc.), and unintended consequences (delays, bad side effects, deteriorating vital signs, etc.). Sixth, the system's operation

TABLE 2-9 Complex Service Systems: Healthcare Considerations

System Stages	Healthcare System Considerations	Critical Methods	
		Integrative	Adaptive
1. Purpose	Stakeholders; triaging; business model	✓	✓
2. Boundary	Spatial; temporal; interdependent	✓	✓
3. Design	Robust; efficient; effective	✓	✓
4. Development	Models; scalability; sustainability	✓	✓
5. Deployment	Risk; uncertainty; unintended consequences	✓	✓
6. Operation	Flexible; safe; secure	✓	✓
7. Life cycle	Predictable; controllable; evolutionary	✓	✓

must be flexible (agile, transparent, redundant, etc.), safe (with minimal natural accidents, human failures, unforeseen disruptions, etc.), and secure (with minimal system viruses, system crashes, privacy intrusions, etc.). Seventh, the system's life cycle must be predictable (with regard to inputs, processes, outcomes, etc.), controllable (with appropriate sensors, feedback, cybernetics, etc.), and evolutionary (with learning capabilities, timely recoveries, intelligent growth, etc.).

Although Table 2-10 shows only a simple two-by-two, supply-vs.-demand matrix (Tien et al., 2004), it provides important insight into supply chain management (SCM, which can occur when demand is fixed and supply is flexible and therefore manageable), demand chain management (DCM, which can occur when supply is fixed and demand is flexible and therefore manageable), and real-time customized management (RTCM, which can occur when both demand and supply are flexible, thereby allowing for real-time mass customization).

Table 2-10 identifies example SCM, DCM, and RTCM methods. The literature offers abundant SCM findings (especially concerning manufacturing), only recently has focused on DCM methods (especially with regard to revenue management), and is devoid of RTCM considerations, except for a recent contribution by Yasar (2005). Yasar combines two SCM methods (capacity rationing and capacity extending) and two DCM methods (demand bumping and demand recapturing) to deal with the real-time customized management of, as examples, either a goods problem concerned with the rationing of equipment to produce classes of goods or a services

TABLE 2-10 Complex Service Systems: Integration/Adaptation Research

	Demand	
Supply	Fixed	Flexible
Fixed	Unable to Manage	Demand Chain Management
	Price established (at point where fixed demand matches fixed supply)	Product revenue management Dynamic pricing Target marketing Expectation management Auctions
Flexible	Supply Chain Management	Real-Time Customized Management
	Inventory control Production scheduling Distribution planning Capacity revenue management Reverse auctions	Customized bundling Customized revenue management Customized pricing Customized modularization Customized coproduction systems

problem concerned with the rationing of consultants to coproduce classes of services. More important, Yasar shows that the combined, simultaneous real-time management of the two SCM and two DCM methods yields a significantly more profitable outcome than the tandem application of these two sets of methods. Moreover, real-time management requires a more sophisticated solution approach than the traditional steady-state approach.

It is in this fourth, RTCM quadrant of Table 2-10 that system integration (as reflected in the SCM methods) and system adaptation (as reflected in the DCM methods) are combined and dealt with simultaneously. Thus, a combined integration/adaptation research effort is synonymous with an RTCM activity, which can occur when both demand and supply are flexible and thereby allow for real-time mass customization. This fourth quadrant also highlights the complexity involved in designing a service system that is at once both integrated and adaptive. Clearly, health care is an example of such a complex system.

On Insights

A number of insights can be gleaned from an integrated and adaptive view of healthcare services. First, electronic medical records are the glue that should keep the healthcare system integrated and adaptive. Unfortunately, most medical records—including patient data, drug prescriptions, laboratory diagnostics, clinician reports, and body scans—are still in manual folders and as a consequence are difficult to access, fuse, and analyze.

Recently Microsoft and Google launched, respectively, HealthVault and Health for use by consumers to store and manage their personal medical data online. Although patients have a legal right to obtain their medical records from doctors, hospitals, and testing laboratories, doing so is a tedious and overwhelming process because the records are usually not in electronic form. Nevertheless, sharing such electronic records with new medical providers and third-party services will make it easier to coordinate care, spot adverse drug interactions, allow for medication reminders, and track vital signs. At the same time, however, personal data residing on Microsoft or Google servers raise significant privacy concerns. At present, the Health Insurance Portability and Accountability Act (HIPAA) only requires doctors, hospitals, and third-party payers not to release information without a patient's consent. Of course, HIPAA requirements could be broadened, and new rules could be enacted that would give consumers stronger protection and legal recourse if their records were leaked or improperly shared for purposes other than those intended.

Second, because real-time healthcare decisions must be made in an accelerated and coproduced manner, the human service provider (e.g., clinician) will increasingly become a bottleneck; he or she must be supported by a smart robot or software agent. For example, anyone could make use of a smart alter ego or agent that could analyze, and perhaps fuse, all existing and incoming e-mails, phone calls, Web pages, news clips, drug prescriptions, and stock quotes and then assign each item a priority based on the individual's preferences and observed behaviors. Such a smart agent should be able to analyze a text message, judge the sender–recipient relationships by examining an organizational chart, and recall the urgency of the recipient's responses to previous messages from the same sender. The agent might add information gathered by watching the user via a video camera or by scrutinizing his or her calendar. Most likely, such a smart agent would be based on a Bayesian statistical model—capable of evaluating hundreds of user-related factors linked by probabilities, causes, and effects in a vast web of contingent outcomes—that could infer the likelihood that a given decision on the software's part would lead to the user's desired outcome. The ultimate goal is to judge when the user can safely be interrupted, with what kind of message, and via which device. In time, smart agents representing both providers and consumers will be the service coproducers; they will employ decision informatics techniques to accomplish their tasks. It should be noted that such smart agents may never be appropriate for certain situations, especially, for example, when nuanced patient behavior is critical or when a catastrophic surgical consequence is a possibility. Obviously, these situations require direct patient–doctor interaction or coproduction, perhaps assisted by smart agents that can help in the identification of alternative diagnoses and treatments.

Third, perhaps the best example of an integrated and adaptive service system is the evolving Web 2.0. It is built, centered on, and run by users. In other words, it is a social network for the integration—including collaboration and communication—of activities (eBay, Amazon.com, Wikipedia, Twitter, MySpace, Friendster, LinkedIn, Plaxo, Facebook, etc.), entertainment (Ning, Bebo, Second Life, World of Warcraft, etc.), and searches (Google, Yahoo, MSN.com, etc.). Unfortunately, the integrated Web, while a somewhat successful e-commerce platform, is unable to interpret, manipulate, or make sense of its content. On the other hand, with the encoding of Web pages in a semantic Web format, the evolving Web will make it possible for the above-mentioned smart or decision informatics–supported agents to undertake semantic analysis of user intent and Web content, to understand and filter their meaning, and to respond adaptively in light of user needs. The semantic Web, then, would be an ideal complex service system for which integration and adaptation would constitute the basis for its functionality. Several obstacles must be overcome before full functionality is reached, however. For example, semantic standards or ontologies—such as the Web Ontology Language—must be established to maintain compatible and interoperable formats; healthcare and financial services companies are now developing their own ontologies. Indeed, a healthcare SoS also needs a common ontology to allow new system components to be integrated appropriately into the SoS without a major effort so as to achieve higher capabilities and performance than would be possible with the components as stand-alone systems. Of course, the healthcare ontology must be transdisciplinary—beyond a single discipline—in scope.

Fourth, modern systems of systems are becoming increasingly more human centered, if not human focused, with products and services becoming more personalized or customized. Certainly coproduction of services implies the existence of a human customer, if not a human service provider. The implication is profound: a multidisciplinary approach must be employed for, say, health care, and it must include techniques from the social sciences (sociology, psychology, and philosophy) and management (organization, economics, and finance). As a consequence, researchers must expand their systems (i.e., holistic oriented), human (i.e., decision oriented), and cybernetic (i.e., adaptive oriented) methods to include and be integrated with those techniques that are beyond science and engineering. For example, higher patient satisfaction can be achieved not only by improving service quality, but also by lowering patient expectations. In essence, as stated by Hipel and colleagues (2007), systems, human, and cybernetics is an integrative, adaptive, and multidisciplinary approach to creative problem solving that takes into account stakeholders' value systems and satisfies important societal, environmental, economic, and other criteria to enhance the decision-making process in designing, implementing, operating, and maintaining a system or SoS so as to meet societal needs in a fair, ethical, and sustainable manner throughout the system's life cycle.

Fifth, although this paper has focused primarily on designing an integrated and adaptive healthcare system (by employing a systems engineering approach), it should be noted that a number of other engineering approaches can be applied to health care and related biological issues. Grossman (2008) identifies several disruptive engineering innovations that could change the way health care is organized, paid for, and delivered, including precision diagnostics and therapies (i.e., evidence-based medicine), advances in information and communication technologies (i.e., personal health records), and new business models (i.e., overcoming the cottage-industry structure and the dysfunctional reimbursement and regulatory framework). Indeed, as identified in Table 2-11, every engineering discipline or technology has some potential applications to biology; a number of such "technobiology" examples—developed by applying technology-based techniques to biological problems—are cited and briefly described in the table. These examples highlight the technological focus. On the other hand, "biotechnology" is about applying biology-based techniques to technological problems; such techniques include neural networks, genetic algorithms, and systems biology.

Sixth, perhaps the most critical U.S. healthcare issue is the universal access of patients to health care. Payers—particularly private insurance companies—have nearly eliminated access of at-risk individuals to healthcare providers by not allowing these individuals to enroll in their insurance programs. (At the extreme, only very healthy and relatively young individuals are able to purchase private insurance.) Thus, a huge access problem is created for the uninsured, whose solution is to go to the emergency room, where treatment must be provided at no cost, when the illness is already severe and costly to treat. A vicious subsidization cycle ensues in which individual insurance premiums skyrocket, mainly to pay for the care of individuals who are at risk and unable to obtain insurance or who cannot afford an insurance premium. The application of systems engineering—a technobiology approach—to the U.S. healthcare system is required to equilibrate the insurance imbalance and make the system efficient and effective.

Seventh, a final insight concerns the customization or personalization of medical treatment through advances in genetics, proteomics, and metabolomics. Most common illnesses will eventually be preventable; the challenge is to know which prevention effort will be most effective for a given individual. Using markers of risk (e.g., gene variants, blood levels of a protein moiety) may allow for the targeting or personalization of preventive measures in a highly cost-effective way. In this way, humans can be sheltered from chronic illnesses and remain fully functional until an advanced age,

TABLE 2-11 Technobiology Examples

Discipline	Examples	Scope
Biomedical	1. PillCam	1. Can capture 50,000 images of possible gastrointestinal diseases
	2. Nerve stimulation	2. Neurostimulator to treat migraine headaches, chronic back and leg pain, etc.
	3. Induced hypothermia	3. Lowering of body temperature to 91.5 degrees to achieve faster healing and to stem harmful chemical reactions that occur when flow of oxygen is restored following cardiac arrest
Chemical	1. Tissues	1. Regenerative medicine: engineering stem cells to create skin, muscle, bone, cartilage, fat, blood vessel, nerve, heart, liver, bladder, kidney, etc.
	2. Diagnostic	2. Test that identifies gene variations that can predict Lou Gehrig's disease, Parkinson's, Alzheimer's, etc.
	3. Microcyn	3. Electronically charged, super1-oxidized, water-based solution that attacks proteins in infectious agents of a wound, reducing need for antibiotics
Electrical	1. Bioimaging: VCT XT (low dose) computed tomography	1. A 70 percent lower-radiation, 3-dimensional, high-resolution image that can be manipulated
	2. Robotic	2. Automated assistance in surgery, walking, moving, etc.
	3. Bioinformatics	3. Large-scale analysis of data for biological purposes, including drug discovery, patient treatment, etc.
Environmental	1. Sunshine vitamin	1. Sunlight spurs body's production of vitamin D, which may reduce instances of cancer, autoimmune disease, high blood pressure, heart disease, and diabetes
	2. Hearing pill	2. Naturally occurring substance called N-acetylcysteine helps prevent hearing loss due to loud noise by helping the body promote reduced conformation of glutathione

TABLE 2-11 Continued

Discipline	Examples	Scope
Industrial	1. Evidence-based protocols, including false discovery rate	1. Data mining and analysis of past treatments can point to effective protocols, including minimization of false positives linking diseases and DNA genes
	2. Adaptive clinical trials	2. Design and success criteria adjusted as clinical results are obtained
	3. E-care	3. Integrated digital records
	4. Concierge care	4. VIP/premium services
	5. Preventive care	5. Biomarkers/diagnostic tools allow for predictive care
	6. Personalized care	6. Genomics-based adaptive, customized care
Material	1. Nanoparticle medicine	1. Focuses cancer treatment by targeting special nanoparticles that attach to cancerous cells
	2. Drug delivery	2. New drug delivery material with timed release
Mechanical	1. Haptics	1. Sensing and manipulation of objects and environments through touch
	2. Exoskeleton	2. An external anatomical feature that supports and protects a person's body
	3. Prosthetic	3. An orthopedic device that can help a mobility-impaired individual
	4. Artificial disk	4. Replaces damaged or diseased neck disks, resulting in less pain, less swelling, and fewer complications
	5. Asthma mitigation	5. Alair System employs radio-frequency energy to warm the airway and keep muscles from constricting in asthma patients

beyond which survival is genetically limited. Thus, health care is indeed a service, one that can be personalized and that can enhance the quality—and length—of an individual's life.

ENGAGING COMPLEX SYSTEMS THROUGH ENGINEERING CONCEPTS: A METHODOLOGY FOR ENGINEERING COMPLEX SYSTEMS

Harold W. Sorenson, Ph.D., Jacobs School of Engineering, University of California, San Diego

Introduction

This paper is intended to give senior healthcare leaders examples from other business sectors of problems and emerging approaches to finding solutions that may be applicable to health care and may make it possible to realize the goal of developing a learning healthcare system. In general terms, these approaches have been developed to allow complex enterprises to respond better to the challenges of globally distributed operations in a highly dynamic, event-driven environment.

The ubiquitous presence of the World Wide Web has created an environment in which entities are bonded through the exchange of information. The businesses and national security organizations that have been able to operate successfully in this information-bonded environment have demonstrated outcomes and advantages that are evident to everyone. An *integrated perspective* that merges the views of the business and engineering communities is increasingly recognized as one of the cornerstones of a successful approach to dealing with enterprise complexity. The result can be new and more effective ways to deliver health care through the rapid fielding of enhanced capabilities based on a close working relationship among all stakeholders, including healthcare administrators and practitioners, enterprise architects, and enterprise systems engineers. Consequently, the culture, practice, and delivery of patient care can change in fundamentally important ways.

Working from a perspective focused on feedback control systems and their fundamental importance in a wide variety of engineering applications, this paper reviews principles of control and their importance in the synthesis of complex enterprise systems. As with any engineering system development, consideration of the devices that must be controlled dominates the design. For example, the control of room temperature results from measuring temperature and comparing it with the desired setting. The controller regulates the operation of the heater to achieve the desired condition. An engineering model combining the environment and the heaters is fundamental to the design of the control system and its ability to maintain temperature and comfort. As the following discussion argues, the emerging methodology for engineering complex systems has conceptual similarities, but it involves people and organizations as well as technology, which presents a much more challenging problem.

Context for the Discussion

The issues motivating this workshop's discussions can be thought of in terms of an emerging paradigm that has seen increasing use in the commercial and business worlds and, to some extent, within the Department of Defense. Looking carefully at these motivating issues, we see that if we look at health care as a complex adaptive system, we can approach it with a variety of improvement strategies that many companies are currently using to help them compete in their marketplace.

Reordering and abbreviating the issues that motivate the overall workshop discussion, we can derive a related list of eight issues that motivate the discussion in this paper:

1. Focus on the patient for learning healthcare systems.
2. Improve value and eliminate capability deficiencies.
3. Apply complex adaptive systems theory to health care.
4. Make extensive data more widely available and useful.
5. Enable knowledge to be an enterprise asset.
6. Apply system and process developments to health care.
7. Recognize the dynamics of the healthcare environment.
8. Change culture, practice, and delivery.

The goal of this paper is to explore these issues, identify potential approaches, and discuss possible strategies for their engagement. In this context, focusing on the patient is exactly the right place to start for a learning healthcare system. The methodology discussed starts there, with patients as the key stakeholders. Overall, the approaches discussed are driven by the need to improve value or eliminate deficiencies in capabilities; this becomes a focus driven by the stakeholder community, which says, in essence, this is what we want to be able to do better.

One central consideration for health care is the need to make data more widely available and useful. As with many types of organizations, health care suffers from a prevalence of stovepipes, silos, and other organizational conventions that prevent data from being widely accessible to the broader community. By transforming data and information into knowledge, enterprises gain an asset that can be used to address current deficiencies in healthcare delivery directly and to allow more benefits to be delivered to the patient. In summary, knowledge must become an enterprise asset. This paper examines an emerging methodology for system and process development and suggests that such development has utility in the healthcare environment. If this methodology is successfully applied, the changes that result can have the effect of altering the culture of healthcare delivery, with concomitant changes in the practice and delivery of care.

General Approach

When we approach the problem of engineering complex enterprise systems, we typically start by asking a series of interrelated questions. How do we think about the problem? How do we manage the complexity? How do we approach the problem's solution? How do we develop the problem's solution? How do we assess the proposed solution? What is the effect of the development? Each of these questions is discussed briefly in the sections that follow, with a particular emphasis on the first three.

How Do We Think About the Problem?

Any enterprise, whether a healthcare or business or defense enterprise, involves a large number of people with a variety of responsibilities and jobs. To carry out these responsibilities and jobs, these stakeholders work using prescribed processes to accomplish desired functions and outcomes. And in performing this work, they use a variety of information and data. In most enterprises, the reality is that any given user is familiar with only a limited number of processes and data sources. Too often this implies that the function being performed has more limited utility than would be the case if the workers' knowledge of processes and data were broader and more encompassing. Because of the stovepipe or silo characteristics embedded in virtually every organization, a given user in an enterprise is unfamiliar with all the other useful components of the system and has no way to learn them in a natural way.

How do we bring order to such a system? How do we manage this environment in such a way that the users can actually use the data, the processes, and the functions that exist elsewhere in the enterprise? In much of his writing, Russell Ackoff (a seminal thinker in systems science at the Wharton School) emphasizes the need to break away from reductionist thinking in managing complex enterprises. He goes to the heart of the question in his book *On Purposeful Systems*, written with Frederick Edmund Emery (Ackoff and Emery, 1972), when he writes, "To manage a system effectively, you might focus on the interactions of the parts rather than their behavior taken separately." Indeed, the issue is all about interactions, interfaces, and the way information is shared and distributed.

A long-time collaborator with Ackoff, Jamshid Gharajedaghi, outlines the basics of systems thinking in his book *Systems Thinking: Managing Chaos and Complexity* (Gharajedaghi, 1999). Such thinking starts, he suggests, with an operational definition of a "systems methodology" that involves three interdependent variables: structure, function, and process. Those variables, together with the environment, define the whole. For present purposes, we can think of structure as defining the components and their relationships and constraints—synonymous with input, means, and effects. Similarly, function defines the outcome, which is synonymous with output, and process defines the sequence of activities required to produce the outcome—how the function is performed. A core assumption is that the development process is necessarily iterative.

As a quick example of the interdependency of function, structure, and process, consider the heart. The function of a heart is to pump. It circulates blood. Its structure can be defined in terms of its chambers, valves, and arteries. The process is basically defined in terms of alternating cycles of contraction and expansion. The environment is the body in which the heart operates. The body in turn operates in a larger environment, which certainly affects the functioning of the heart. Clearly, the variables are interdependent and cannot be separated in considering the heart as a system.

Figure 2-9 provides background on the evolution of systems thinking. A product of the competitive world in which we live, systems thinking began with the ideas of Henry Ford regarding mass production. His model posited that people and parts are interchangeable, a way of thinking that

SHIFT OF PARADIGM ► ▼	Mindless System	Uniminded System	Multiminded System
	Machine Model	Biological Model	Social Model Purposeful Society Organization Members
Analytical Approach Independent Variables	Interchangeability of Parts and Labor Henry Ford's Mass Production System	Diversity and Growth Alfred Sloan's Divisional Structure	Participative Management Self-organizing Systems Social systems are information-bonded Tavistock Institute's Socio-Tech Model
Systems Approach Interdependent Variables	Joint Optimization Ford's Whiz Kids Operations Research	Flexibility and Control Ohno's Lean Production Cybernetics Model	Redesign Ackoff's Interactive Management Choice

FIGURE 2-9 Evolution of systems thinking.

led to people and parts being treated as independent variables. The analytical result was to look at each part by itself. As people first experimented with mass production, they learned that the factors they regarded as being independent actually were not, but rather were *interdependent*. This interdependence led to a systems approach, which can be said to be the roots of operations research. The analytical problem became a search for optimal solutions that would enable an organization to do things better. An oft-cited example of the acceptance of the OR approach is the scenario involving the "whiz kids" at Ford Motor Company around 1960.

Ford started with the motto that one could have any color Ford one wanted as long as it was black. As mass production gained in popularity, it became apparent that everybody could institute mass production techniques; as a result, the first adapters of mass production, such as Ford, would lose their competitive edge. Alfred Sloan started General Motors (GM) with the idea that diversity would lead to growth. Buyers of GM products could get cars with different colors and in different varieties. To manage the resulting interdependencies, Sloan introduced a reductionist approach that was reflected in the divisional structures of the company. Organizational structures were broken down and reduced to the point where the company considered marketing to be separate from human resources, which was separate from sales, and so forth. That led to the divisional structure that is still taught in management schools today. This is much more of a biological model than Ford's mass production model. It is a biological model because there is a brain (i.e., the chief executive officer) in charge who tells his or her arms (i.e., the divisional structure) what to do. The divisions implemented the strategy from the corporate office to develop diverse products and to stimulate corporate growth and profit.

This business model evolved to another stage with the concept of lean production, developed by Ohno at Toyota. Lean production is based on a cybernetics model in which one measures the production process and feeds that information back into decisions about inventory and production to gain efficiencies and reduce costs. This is essentially the state of the practice in most organizational theory today.

The past decade, however, thanks in large part to the power of the Web, has seen the rise of participative management. The person in charge no longer has the sole word. Based on personal experience working at high levels in companies, I can say that collaboration and participation provide the essential mechanisms to manage large, complex enterprises effectively. Top-down direction is increasingly complemented by bottom-up involvement in the decision-making process. A fundamental characteristic of this new, productive environment is its social nature. The power of these social networks is a primary source of the complex adaptive systems we are starting to recognize and address.

Social systems are information bonded, in contrast to the systems of the past, which were energy bonded. Consider the car. It has an engine, and when the car is started, the gas in the engine explodes, and the energy from that explosion is transferred through the camshaft to the driveshaft, to the axle, and to the wheels. Everything is connected by various forms of energy transfer. Most electric power grid systems operate the same way, with the electrical energy being transferred in ways that allow us to do what we want. Energy-bonded systems are created by well-known systems engineering processes that are based on well-developed requirements. In essence, it is the statement of requirements that separates project management from corporate management. In the case of a technology, its usefulness is the primary developmental concern, but enterprise systems must be concerned with organizational interactions and with the people involved in them. Learning healthcare systems can be described as being information bonded and operating through social networks.

The social model basically says that if one is purposeful and seeks to reach some kind of enterprise objective, one should take a holistic view that includes society, the organization, and, finally, the various members of that society or organization who may be involved in what one is trying to do. This holistic set of concerns leads to a totally different approach from the traditional systems engineering, which is reductionist in nature. Now, instead of analyzing things, one designs, one tries out, one builds, one fields, and one learns. The development proceeds in an iterative fashion, with new capabilities appearing on a time scale of days or a few weeks. Collaboration among stakeholders and managers becomes the necessary development interaction style. Often no single person is in charge in the sense of having tight control over the development plan. Flexibility and adaptation are central to the process and the participative management style.

To make an important point, let me introduce a little engineering jargon. Entropy is the measure of randomness in the universe. According to the Second Law of Thermodynamics, total entropy in a closed system increases over time. However, open-living systems display an opposite tendency; they move toward order, thus generating negative entropy. Emergent behaviors are a result. The Internet is a good example. Think of all the behaviors that have emerged from the use of the Internet. I am sure the creators of the Internet had no idea of the sorts of behaviors that would arise and garner so much interest, such as the information-sharing power of Google, the online auctions of eBay, and communication sites such as MySpace. These emergent behaviors are the key to understanding the potential for changing the culture, practice, and delivery of health care.

How Do We Manage the Complexity?

Data and information must be at the heart of any discussion of information-bonded systems. Consequently, the methodology being described here starts with a consideration of the mechanisms for making data and information available across an enterprise in ways that are effectively transparent to the system user. In this approach, sources and generators of data and information *publish* to a *registry* that is used to make potential users aware of the existence of the data and information and that has pointers defining how the data are found and retrieved. The users, generally, *subscribe* to the types of data and information they are interested in accessing. The mechanism for accomplishing this publish/subscribe operation is referred to as a *service registry*. The registry is important because it guarantees that data will not be warehoused. Ownership and responsibility for the data remain with those who generate them, and once the registry has been established, the methodology says that information is retrieved, processed, integrated, and managed to achieve a purpose. If new information is generated, it is registered for future users of the results. The pointers are provided so that subscribers can quickly get the information needed to solve a problem or answer a question. Alternatively, Web standards allow the discovery of information that supplements the subscriber information that is registered. For example, Google provides a search engine people use regularly in their daily lives. Standards that have already been developed for the Web are fundamental to the development of the mechanisms used to define interfaces and govern the exchange of data and information. The processes for dealing with data and information form the basis of the methodology.

Enterprises must adapt and respond in a timely and effective manner to a variety of planned and unplanned events. To deal with this ever-present situation, it is important that there be a seamless interoperation of disparate organizational entities, often in unplanned and complex ways. The rapidly changing environment has led to a search for *solution invariants* that might provide stability for the creation and evolution of the system that supports information interoperation (referred to here as the enterprise knowledge system [EKS]). The current approach for managing enterprise complexity, which is continuing to evolve and mature, is based on three interdependent variables: structure, function, and process. The structure, which we refer to as an *architecture*, provides a blueprint for evolving the EKS. It defines the components or actions of the system and their functional interconnections. The architecture is also used to capture the constraints on the system (e.g., quality of service, security and privacy rules, regulatory constraints such as HIPAA). The structural description does not involve detail on the implementation of the components, communications, or constraints. Instead, it should be developed relatively quickly and should provide a documented basis for the implementation and evolution of the EKS itself. As with the design of a building, the architecture provides a reference that changes less often than the implementation and permits a framework within which processes and functions are allowed to change to accomplish the objectives of the business.

How Do We Approach the Problem's Solution?

Deriving and defining the architecture is the key step of the development process for complex, adaptive systems. Fundamental to the design process is the concept of separation of concerns. Generally, the first step in separating concerns is to assume that the architecture is defined as consisting of *layers* or *tiers*. Each layer communicates with its adjoining layer through well-defined interfaces. An activity in one layer cannot interact directly with any internal feature of any other layer. This structure allows changes to be made within a layer without disturbing other layers as long as the interface descriptions remain unchanged (i.e., concerns are separated). A fundamentally important layer is the presentation layer. Users interact with the system using a *portal*, sometimes referred to as the human–system interface. For our architecture construct, users, through the portal, have access to the service registry and the elements of the system they are interested in using. Users can ask questions and, essentially, tell the system what they are trying to do. Everyone should be familiar with the function of a portal through Web interactions. For example, the AOL browser serves as a portal to the global community and its services.

Behind the registry is an infrastructure that allows the complexity of the networked system, such as the Web, to be hidden and transparent to the user. Through this *common information infrastructure* (CII), information that addresses the needs of a user is routed to appropriate functions, applications, processes, and services. An architectural style that is gaining wide acceptance is *service-oriented architecture* (SOA). In this style, the CII is generally referred to as the *enterprise service bus*.

A very simple model of architecture has users who can access the system through various kinds of hardware devices and *communities of interest* that are defined through having a common interest or mission that requires a variety of business applications or services. Underpinning this architecture is the CII. In this simple model of an enterprise architecture, it is important to recognize that a network simplifies the system connections of many users and their applications. A set of N users can communicate directly with one another without being connected in a point-to-point fashion. The latter mode of communication would generate an enormously complicated requirement because the number of point-to-point connections for N users is proportional to the square of the number of users. With a networked system, the number of connections is simply N. Each user connects to the network, and the network accomplishes the point-to-point connectivity.

Returning to the SOA, the term *service* denotes a broad set of useful artifacts that enable users to accomplish their tasks. A service can be an application that may be useful for people across the enterprise, it can be data sources or databases that have widespread utility, or it can be computational tools that support implementations invisible to the user. In essence, a service is a reusable artifact that simplifies the development and implementation of, and facilitates the introduction of, new processes and functions that broaden the existing system capability. The SOA model is based on the differing needs and roles of service consumers and providers. The consumers interact with the system through a presentation layer. The business processes must be precisely defined and are used to derive essential services. The composition of the services produces the desired process. Required services are located via the service registry, wherever they may be located physically. The registry is used to inform the service provider of the request for the service, and the enterprise service bus executes and allows the execution of the desired business process.

In summary, one starts by asking, "What are we going to do in our business?" In the present case we might ask, "How are we going to deliver health care?" One then defines the processes that describe a healthcare function. From these processes and from the actors using the system, services are defined and added to the service registry. As described, the architecture of the system is layered, and an emphasis in the system development is on the interfaces between layers. One can change a business process without changing the service or presentation layer except in the details of that process. The value of managing the complexity of the EKS through the use of layered, or N-tiered, architectures then starts to make sense.

How Do We Develop the Problem's Solution?

Having defined a framework for managing the complexity, it is logical to ask, "How do we develop the problem solution?" First, one identifies a function or mission that is to be provided by the healthcare delivery system. Then one identifies the people, or actors, who should be involved in using, describing, architecting, and implementing the desired capability. This group of people constitutes a *community of interest,* and the members are referred to as *stakeholders*. The future users of the system are requested to answer the question, "As an actor, how am I going to use this system?" The answers are called *use cases,* which become the basis for discussions between the architect and the users as the architecture is developed. The architect guides the discussion but must always be sensitive to the needs of the user community. For the healthcare delivery community, the use cases should focus on the needs of and the services desired by and delivered to each patient. They are key actors for this system development.

The manner in which the architect translates the use case information into the structure of the desired system is not addressed here, but the architecture must provide guidance to the engineers who implement the system. The architect implements governance procedures that enable the implementation to be measured against the requirements of the architecture. A key part of the governance process is continuing interaction among the stakeholders, architects, and implementers. This interaction drives the iterative development of the system and must serve to put in place useful capabilities, often in small increments, on a frequent basis. The implementation approach is referred to as *agile development.* Practice has revealed a desirable phenomenon that often emerges from providing new capabilities in small, easily understood increments. Because the users can live with and use the capability, a fan club develops that facilitates the adoption of the capability across a broader community. This is one example of a desirable emergent behavior that can appear when one is working within a highly complex environment. These behaviors are observed to change cultures in a natural manner that comes from bottom-up participation, not from the top down.

How Do We Assess the Proposed Solution?

Early in this paper, I mentioned the importance of feedback control and its great utility in virtually all systems and their useful operation. There has been no discussion of the role of feedback control in this methodology, but there was an implicit reference in the previous paragraph. In essence, it is through various types of feedback that we address the question, "How do we assess the proposed solution?"

The development of complex systems such as healthcare delivery advances because of feedback and communication among all the participants. The architect serves as the feedback controller during the development of the architecture. Because the systems being developed are inherently complex, it is often difficult for the architect to determine whether the logic and behaviors dictated by the architecture will achieve the goals of the stakeholders. Systems of the type discussed here are event driven. Using theory and methods drawn from discrete-event dynamic systems, the architect can develop models of the capability being developed that can be used to assess the adequacy of the logical architecture and the behavior of the processes implemented by the architecture. These architectural models do not involve the actual implementation of any capabilities. They can be applied before time and resources are expended to actually build the system. In fact, they are useful in saving later development costs and delays in situations where fundamental problems are discovered late in the process. Finally, the architect serves as the controller in the governance policies that are imposed on the implementers. As useful capabilities are presented to the user community, the architect again assesses the reactions of the users to identify desirable modifications, additions, and improvements.

As a capability moves into daily use, however, the architect must have planned for the possibility of behaviors arising either from events outside the community of interest or from unplanned events occurring within the system that can adversely affect the system's usefulness. To anticipate the effects of complex events on the desired system, the architect must introduce mechanisms for measuring the internal message traffic. Sometimes referred to as business activity monitoring, these measurements are used to provide feedback that allows the earlier identification, recognition, and correction of anomalous behaviors. Thus, feedback control becomes essential in the long-term operation and performance of the system.

What Is the Effect of the Development?

In closing, we consider the question, "What is the effect of the development?" This paper has asserted that it is possible to build an environment that will lead to the rapid fielding of enhanced and new capabilities. This result can be achieved only through close working relationships among all stakeholders, including patients, healthcare administrators and practitioners, and enterprise architects and engineers. Not only can there be planned developments that provide more effective ways of delivering health care, but unexpected and useful emergent behaviors can appear. As a result, the culture, practice, and delivery of patient care will change fundamentally in important and beneficial ways. This change will be driven from the bottom up by the participants while being guided by the leadership of the healthcare community.

REFERENCES

Ackoff, R., and F. E. Emery. 1972. *On purposeful systems.* Chicago, IL: Aldine-Atherton.
Brandeau, M. L., F. Sainfort, and W. Pierskalla (Eds.). 2004. *Operations research and health care. A handbook of methods and applications.* New York: Springer.
Bush, G. W. 2001 (October 16). *Executive order on critical infrastructure protection.* Washington, DC: The White House.
CBO (Congressional Business Office). 2008. *Technological change and the growth of health care spending.* Pub. No. 2764. Washington, DC: CBO.
Friedman, T. L. 2005. *The world is flat: A brief history of the twenty-first century.* New York: Farrar, Strauss & Giroux.
Gawande, A. 2002. *Complications: A surgeon's notes on an imperfect science.* New York: Metropolitan Books.

Gharajedaghi, J. 1999. *Systems thinking managing chaos and complexity: A platform for designing business architecture.* Boston, MA: Butterworth–Heinemann.

Grossman, J. H. 2008. Disruptive innovation in health care: Challenges for engineering. *The Bridge* 38(1):10–16.

Hancock, W. M., and F. H. Bayha. 1992. The learning curve. In G. Salvendy (Ed.), *Handbook of industrial engineering*, 2nd ed. (pp. 1685-1698). New York: Wiley.

Hipel, K. W., M. M. Jamshidi, J. M. Tien, and C. C. White. 2007. The future of systems, man and cybernetics: Application domains and research methods. *IEEE Transactions on Systems, Man, and Cybernetics Part C* 30(2):213–218.

IOM (Institute of Medicine). 2000. *To err is human: Building a safer health system.* Washington, DC: National Academy Press.

_____. 2001. *Crossing the quality chasm: A new health system for the 21st century.* Washington, DC: National Academy Press.

Kaplan, E. H., and R. J. Heimer. 1992. HIV prevalence among intravenous drug users: Model-based estimates from New Haven's legal needle exchange. *Acquired Immune Deficiency Syndrome* 5(2):163–169.

Kaplan, E. H., D. L. Craft, and L. M. Wein. 2002. Emergency response to a smallpox attack: The case for mass vaccination. *Proceedings of the National Academy of Sciences* 99(16):10935–10940.

Maglio, P., S. Srinivasan, J. Kreulen, and J. Spohrer. 2006. Service systems, service scientists, SSME, and innovation. *Communications of the Association for Computing Machinery* 49(7):81–85.

McPhee, J. 1990. *The control of nature.* New York: Farrar, Straus and Giroux.

Mendonca, D., and W. A. Wallace. 2004. Studying organizationally-situated improvisation in response to extreme events. *International Journal of Mass Emergencies and Disasters* 22(2):5–29.

Morse, P. M., and G. E. Kimball. 1951. *Methods of Operations Research.* Cambridge: Technology Press of Massachusetts Institute of Technology.

NAE (National Academy of Engineering)/IOM. 2005. *Building a better delivery system: A new engineering/health care partnership.* Washington, DC: The National Academies Press.

O'Neill, P. 2007. Why the U.S. healthcare system is so sick and what OR can do to cure it. *OR/MS Today* 34(6). www.lionhrtpub.com/orms/orms-12-07/frhealthcare.html (accessed May 28, 2010).

Peterson, P. G. 2005. *Running on empty.* New York: Picador.

Porter, M. E., and E. O. Teisberg. 2006. *Redefining health care: Creating value-based competition on results.* Boston, MA: Harvard Business School Press.

Quinn, J. B., J. J. Baruch, and P. C. Paquette. 1987. Technology in services. *Scientific American* 257(6):50–58.

Rouse, W. B. 2007. Complex engineered, organizational and natural systems. *Wiley Inter-Science Online: Systems Engineering* 10(3):260–271.

_____. 2008. Health care as a complex adaptive system: Implications for design and management. *The Bridge* 38(1):17–25.

Schoen, C., S. Guterman, A. Shih, J. Lau, S. Kasimow, A. Gauthier, and K. Davis. 2008. *Bending the curve: Options for achieving savings and improving value in U.S. health spending.* New York: The Commonwealth Fund.

Stevens, R. A., C. E. Rosenberg, and L. R. Burns. (Eds.) 2006. *History and health policy in the United States.* New Brunswick, NJ: Rutgers University Press.

Sussman, J. M. 2008. Intelligent transportation systems in a real-time, customer-oriented society. *The Bridge* 38(2):13–19.

Tien, J. M. 2000. Individual-centered education: An any one, any time, any where approach to engineering education. *IEEE Transactions on Systems, Man, and Cybernetics Part C: Special Issue on Systems Engineering Education* 30(2):213–218.

_____. 2003. Towards a decision informatics paradigm: A real-time, information-based approach to decision making. *IEEE Transactions on Systems, Man, and Cybernetics, Special Issue, Part C* 33(1):102–113.

Tien, J. M., and D. Berg. 1995. Systems engineering in the growing service economy. *IEEE Transactions on Systems, Man, and Cybernetics Part C* 25(5):321–326.

_____. 2003. A case for service systems engineering. *Journal of Systems Science and Systems Engineering* 12(1):13–38.

_____. 2006. On services research and education. *Journal of Systems Science and Systems Engineering* 15(3):257–283.

_____. 2007. A calculus for services innovation. *Journal of Systems Science and Systems Engineering* 16(2):129–165.

Tien, J. M., and M. F. Cahn. 1981. *An evaluation of the Wilmington Management of Demand Program*. Washington, DC: National Institute of Justice.

Tien, J. M., A. Krishnamurthy, and A. Yasar. 2004. Towards real-time customized management of supply and demand chains. *Journal of Systems Science and Systems Engineering* 13(3):257–278.

Yasar, A. 2005. *Real-time and simultaneous management of supply and demand chains*. Ph.D. thesis. Troy, NY: Rensselaer Polytechnic Institute.

Zadeh, L. A. 1996. The evolution of systems analysis and control: A personal perspective. *IEEE Control Systems Magazine* 16(3):95–98.

3

Healthcare System Complexities, Impediments, and Failures

INTRODUCTION

The extent to which health care for Americans is timely, efficient, and appropriate for a given individual is determined by the characteristics of the delivery system. Moving to a learning healthcare system will require the identification of specific areas where system complexities slow or inhibit progress and the development of solutions geared toward overcoming impediments and failures.

Workshop discussions considered a number of process inefficiencies, structural barriers, and system failures that are significant impediments to quality and that preclude the delivery of highly effective, highly efficient, evidence-based health care. In the second workshop session, the focus turned to the areas of underperformance that may need the most attention and correction from an engineering perspective. Presenters in this session examined select obstacles inherent in multiple healthcare system components and certain flawed processes that particularly affect the generation and application of evidence. One goal of the session was to frame suggested ideas for how systems engineering might address some of health care's most troublesome shortfalls.

This chapter begins with an overview of the healthcare culture. In his presentation William W. Stead, chief information officer of Vanderbilt University Medical Center, described the current healthcare environment as being characterized by competition, misaligned incentives, and inherent distrust among stakeholders. Throughout health care, Stead sees competing cultures at loggerheads—as exemplified by the tensions among consumers who want high service and low out-of-pocket costs, payers who want to select risk and limit cost, and purchasers who want more value at the lowest cost. Looking to a future that will be defined by individualized medicine, Stead suggested that tomorrow's opportunities may not be fully realized without fundamental changes in the healthcare culture. Education for health professionals is only one area that needs reform. Another requirement will be to move from the business of managing episodes of care to the business of caring for patients and populations. He added that similar fundamental reforms will need to be engineered into the business models of virtually every healthcare stakeholder—in payment mechanisms, and, notably, in the role of the individuals in managing their own care.

Speaking from her perspective as a cardiologist and health policy analyst, Rita F. Redberg, director of Women's Cardiovascular Services at the University of California, San Francisco, noted that a marked proliferation in new diagnostic and treatment technologies has resulted in a precipitous increase in healthcare costs. Moreover, limited integration in the design of systems for health information technology (HIT) and technologies such as imaging systems has allowed their misuse and overuse, thus impeding their ability to improve healthcare quality. Redberg surveyed the current landscape of diagnostic and treatment technologies available for heart disease and offered suggestions for systemically evaluating and using these technologies in ways that improve care and reduce costs. She proposed that more systematic data collection and the development of more prospective registries would lead to better-informed decisions in health care.

Addressing a concern that was raised throughout the workshop about the need for more robust data collection and mining capacities, Michael D. Chase, associate medical director of quality, Kaiser Permanente Colorado, asserted that the U.S. healthcare system has not fully leveraged clinical data to improve health outcomes. Impediments to full use of the data include limited data access, a problem that is exacerbated by inadequate adoption of electronic health records (EHRs) and lack of data standards. As health care has become more complex, the lag in the sophistication of data applications in evidence generation has become more acute. Engineering principles, Chase suggested, could help those in charge of health care manage various complex processes and increase the use of data for clinical decision support. Chase offered examples and suggestions concerning how key delivery systems could be better integrated into healthcare systems in order to address critical areas in health care. For example, Chase proposed a patient-centered, population health–based view grounded in the principle of getting the right information to the right member of the healthcare team—including the patient—at the right time during the workflow or decision-making process. Chase presented a model that takes a broad look at decision support opportunities across a continuum of patient needs, available healthcare professionals, tools and systems, and an extended time line for patient care.

Amy L. Deutschendorf, senior director for clinical resource management at Johns Hopkins Hospital and Health System and principal of Clinical Resource Consultants, also observed that there has been an escalation in system and patient complexities throughout the current healthcare environment. The crush of information, a plethora of new technologies, increased regulatory oversight, an aging population, and heightened consumer awareness and expectations have all contributed to the disorganization, fragmentation, and discontinuity of patient care. Consequently, she argued, effective care coordination and linkage have become even more important. Deutschendorf spoke of the need for processes that ensure patient-centered alignment of care. One application is a care delivery process with communication models and systems that can ensure the accurate and timely transfer of patient information throughout the healthcare continuum. Deutschendorf suggested a number of other changes, including more clarification, definition, and distinctions between acute patient care and ambulatory care; better management of consumer expectations; and increased communication and collaboration between caregiving team members. Because models of care need to be based more firmly on evidence, she proposed that rigorous research be conducted to determine which care delivery models can yield appropriate safety outcomes and the highest possible quality outcomes.

Speaking from his perspective as chief executive officer (CEO) of the University of Pennsylvania Health System (UPHS), Ralph W. Muller discussed areas of successful transformation in administration and business systems at his institution. He highlighted projects on patient registration, billing, and revenue cycle management, and he discussed how each was transformed in order to be more effective. He also described a project that examined how UPHS inpatient and outpatient operations were improved through a combination of systems analysis, reporting systems, incentive alignment, and continuous change management. In discussing lessons learned in several areas of day-to-day practice—as well as from significant, documented results—Muller illustrated how engineering-specific interventions can change systems of care. In recounting examples of reform at UPHS, Muller also highlighted elements of a methodology for conceptualizing change in the face of entrenched health cultures. He offered specific lessons learned about using data and analysis to identify opportunities and motivate change, redesign workflows and restructure roles, integrate information technology, establish goals and monitor performance, and create meaningful incentives.

The final speaker in the second session, Eugene C. Nelson of the Dartmouth–Hitchcock Medical Center, said that we will need a healthcare system information environment that provides critical knowledge that can be used to effectively manage individuals over time, evaluate and improve the quality and value of clinical practice, and facilitate basic translational and outcomes research. Nelson described a successful transformative activity at the Dartmouth–Hitchcock Spine Center that designed, tested, and refined patient-centered "feed-forward" and "feedback" data systems, which are built into the flow of healthcare delivery in order to support patient care and generate information and knowledge concerning entire patient populations. Nelson detailed the issues and concerns that motivated the project, discussed the challenges of designing the systems, and described their positive impacts on system effectiveness and patient satisfaction. He also outlined a promising approach for creating sustainable feed-forward data systems based on the formation of "collaboratories," or professionally organized networks for advancing health care and healthcare research.

HEALTHCARE CULTURE IN THE UNITED STATES

William W. Stead, M.D., Vanderbilt University Medical Center

This paper begins with three observations about the culture of health care in the United States. First, that culture is centered on individual expert health professionals; their behaviors reflect the way they are selected, the way they are educated, and what it takes to survive in their work environment. These cultural roots of the health professions must be addressed if change in health care is to be realized. Second, the culture of health care in this country is one of a clash among competing forces. Stakeholders work against each other to obtain advantage for themselves at the expense of others. If we are to achieve meaningful improvement, this competitive clash needs to be transformed into a competition to work together to achieve the right results for the patient. Third, today's health care faces discontinuous, disruptive change. The way health professionals make decisions will not scale up to handle the data load that is resulting from biological discoveries in genomics, proteomics, and other areas. This last observation is good news. As the health professions and other stakeholders realize that they cannot escape disruptive change, we will have a once-in-a-century chance to test better approaches to health care. Building on these observations, this paper contrasts the current healthcare culture with a future culture in which care is delivered through systems approaches.

The Culture of the Health Professions

The culture of the health professions is rooted in their education. In the first phase of that education, the scientific basis of health and disease and the scientific method are taught. The goal is for each professional to have a current fact base and to know the method by which facts are discovered. This phase of education is preparation to act on what is known, interpret new literature, and learn from practice. By way of analogy, at the end of this phase, students have learned how the car works and how it is built, but they have no idea how to plot a path from point A to point B. In the second phase of education, students learn practice through an apprenticeship model in which they are mentored by a variety of individual experts. To continue the analogy, in this phase students learn the many ways to use the car to get from point A to point B and which ways work best. The third phase of education extends throughout the career as learning continues through practice and reading. If something unusual is seen in a patient or something new is tried on the chance that it might work, case reports are written to share observations. When the effects of alternative approaches are sought, a trial is conducted and the results written up. However, learning remains individual. Each health professional seeks to be the best expert at caring for the cases he or she sees.

The culture of the health professions is influenced by the way decisions are made. The reasoning of health professionals, because they are experts, takes place through the recognition of patterns. A person with fever, cough, infiltrate on a chest X-ray, and an elevated white count is suspected of having pneumonia, while a low white count causes concern that the immune system is overwhelmed. These conclusions are based on the entire picture, in much the same way that a constellation in the night sky is recognized. There is no systematic processing of data and calculation of combinatorial probabilities as is done by a novice in a learning situation. In addition, the data used to make decisions are imprecise. Many measurements used in clinical practice are correlative measures, not direct measurements of the substance itself. For example, nephrologists used to measure serum creatinine, an indicator of renal function, by the light absorption of a compound formed by the adduct formation between creatinine and the picrate ion. Other compounds were absorbed at the measured frequency, causing falsely elevated measures. At a time when the sensitivity of the test was ±0.3, the threshold for treating transplant patients for rejection was a change of 0.3. In other words, physicians erred on the side of treatment with a toxic drug because treatment had to be started early to save the transplant. That kind of reasoning was used regularly, in the face of uncertainty, in life and death situations, under an oath that says "do no harm."

The culture of the health professions has also been shaped by the exponential increase in biomedical knowledge and technology. This overload is handled through specialization and subspecialization. In the process, some are learning more and more about less and less, while the rest are learning less and less about more and more. The workflow requires large amounts of multitasking, is interruption driven, and is nontransparent. There is no chance to sit and reflect. Compensation models reward piecework, procedures, and technology. Health professionals do their best to deliver exceptional care despite the "system." Time is the most limited resource.

The combination of these internal roots and external pressures has led the culture of the health professions to become one in which circumstances that conflict with quality health care are accepted. Variability in practice is accepted as well. The best experts are sought out and expected to disagree. What other industry would report success if there were a shift in performance on a recommended practice from 60 to 80 percent of cases? If 5 practices need to be followed for each patient with a condition, and each is performed correctly 80 percent of the time, the probability that all 5 will be done correctly for a given patient is just 33 percent. The health professions' culture accepts process improvement targets that are far lower than necessary to have the desired effect on clinical outcomes.

Autonomy is a goal of training. Challenges from those lower in the hierarchy are not acceptable. The conditions under which health professionals function lead to increased self-confidence and cynicism (Gray et al., 1996). The fragmentation in care results in less of a sense of responsibility. Although everyone knows the healthcare system is broken, each individual believes his or her own practice is quite good. Data showing the variability in practice are met with surprise. By and large, health professionals are passionate about doing the right thing and are attempting to provide care for patients despite the system. Most of the time, they do a good job. The trouble is that most of the time is insufficient to avoid the quality problems that are ubiquitous in health care.

The Clash Among Competing Forces

The culture of the health professions is just one of many cultural challenges to achieving better health care. The healthcare system in the United States is a clash among competing forces; it is not a system. Health professionals, for example, focus on payment for services and autonomy. Care facilities seek high-margin services and low supply costs. Suppliers focus on intellectual property protection and volume. Meanwhile, consumers seek accessible services and low out-of-pocket costs. Payers pursue the right to select risk and limit cost. Purchasers want more value at the lowest cost.

As Porter and Teisberg (2006) point out, the different stakeholders compete in a zero-sum game. The only way a payer can reduce costs for a purchaser, such as an employer, is to negotiate with the provider to take less or force the consumer to receive less. Because employers are working outside of the direct care process instead of improving that process, they add administrative overhead. As the other stakeholders respond, the increase in overhead is compounded, and the system becomes more expensive and less workable for the patient.

This clash among stakeholders raises several cultural barriers to quality health care. Incentives are not aligned. Providers are paid more if they overuse resources and if they provide poor care leading to rework. They are paid less if they provide such good care that other care is not necessary. They are paid more for technical and episodic tasks and little for cognitive, coordinative work. Healthcare CEOs have limited power given the autonomy of health professionals and the competition among hospitals for physicians.

The stakeholders distrust each other. Although individuals trust their own physicians, they do not trust the "system" (Norris, 2007). They are the ball in the healthcare ping-pong match. They are forced to change health plans regularly as employers and government seek to control costs. A Medicare beneficiary sees a median of two primary care providers and five specialists per year, and Medicare beneficiaries with multiple chronic diseases see up to 16 health professionals (Pham, 2007).

The culture of health care accepts waste. In his keynote address, Brent C. James outlined the data. Administrative overhead in U.S. health care may be as high as 40 percent. Thirty percent of the care provided may be unnecessary; as much as 70 percent may be preventable. Given the rapidly escalating cost of health care, tension exists over the cost of new technology, which has accounted for half of that increase in recent decades. Can we afford ever better technology? Does the increased cost of health care hurt the economic competitiveness of the country by increasing the cost of everything we do?

Finally, the culture accepts poor outcomes on a population basis. In the United States, 109 deaths per 100,000 patients each year are attributable to health care, as compared with 65 in France (Nolte and McKee, 2008). Yet France's per capita healthcare spending is about half that of the United States.

Toward a New Healthcare Culture

Even if today's health care provided acceptable quality and access at an affordable cost, the healthcare culture would face disruptive, discontinuous change because of the inevitable demise of expert-based practice (IOM, 2009a). Cognitive research shows that a human can handle from five to nine facts in a single decision (Miller, 1956). Even with today's clinical descriptions of phenotype, the number of facts bearing on a decision already can exceed this capacity, contributing to the overuse, underuse, and misuse of medical care. The additional data from structural genetics will probably push us into the range of ten facts per decision. Full data on a person's

functional expression may create a ten-fold increase in the facts per decision, and data on proteins may add a second ten-fold increase. Imagine a
primary care provider trying to cope with such a massive amount of data in
a 15-minute encounter. Clearly a new paradigm for clinical decision making
will be necessary. This inescapable change will create a once-in-a-century
chance to rethink roles—and therefore culture—in health care.

Table 3-1 contrasts the current culture with a possible future culture in
which systems approaches to health and health care are used to deliver the
desired results every time. In the current culture of a clash among forces,
people attempt to fix the nonsystem by layering fix on top of fix from the
outside. Each fix adds complexity and cost without changing the fundamentals of care delivery. The goal should be a future culture in which the
system is continuously refined from the inside out. In this culture, people
are recruited and educated to know their limits, to trust the system and their
teammates, and to expect perfect collective performance or correction with
each failure. Care is coordinated around populations, and the care delivered is right for the individual through systematic use of evidence (IOM,
2009b). Each individual is a data point in a population database. Providers
are taught to practice in multidisciplinary, high-performance teams, using
simulation to perfect their skills and outcomes to guide course corrections
(IOM, 2007). Coordinated care is paid for and, on the basis of the value,
delivered.

In the process of shifting toward this vision or other possible futures,
health professionals must strive to preserve the best of the current culture.
Most people engaged in health care are passionate about what they are do-

TABLE 3-1 Comparison of Current and Possible Future Healthcare
Cultures

Current Culture	Future Culture
• Layer fix on fix from outside	• Improve from the inside out
• Trust oneself; provide care despite the system	• Know one's limits; trust the system and one's team
• Care safe for the masses	• Right care for the individual
• Manage episodes of care	• Care for populations and the patient as a whole
• Expert-mediated use of evidence	• Systematic use of evidence
• Each patient is an experiment with n = 1	• Each patient is a data point in a population
• Learn in disciplinary silos	• Learn in teams
• Learn by applying science through practice	• Learn from simulation and outcomes
• Pay for piece work and process steps	• Pay for coordination and outcomes

ing and about being in health care. Every day, in every hospital or clinic, there are people who go far out of their way to help their patients, despite the ecology in which they work. That passion must be preserved. At the same time, changes must be made to roles, education, decision-making processes, payment structures, and the way success is measured—in short, to the professional and business models of every stakeholder in the system.

DIAGNOSTIC AND TREATMENT TECHNOLOGIES

Rita F. Redberg, M.D., M.Sc., University of California, San Francisco

A marked proliferation of new diagnostic and treatment technologies has resulted in a precipitous increase in the costs of health care. Moreover, despite the potential of these technologies to improve the quality of health care, the limited integration in system design for such technologies as HIT; laboratory, radiology, and imaging systems; and monitoring and surgical equipment has allowed their misuse and overuse. This paper surveys the current landscape of diagnostic and treatment technologies available for treatment of heart disease and examines how they might be evaluated and employed more systematically to improve care and reduce costs.

In the late 1970s, John Eisenberg and Sankey Williams at the University of Pennsylvania were studying the behavior of the house staff with the goal of changing their routine daily lab test ordering for inpatients. However, Eisenberg and Williams's daily reminders to the house staff to order only those tests that would affect patient management were not successful in reducing the number of daily lab tests ordered. It was difficult to be criticized for ordering too many tests as one could also be criticized for omitting a potentially useful test. All of the incentives in medical training lean toward ordering more tests, and how the additional information improves patient care receives little consideration. This philosophy is ingrained in the culture and reinforced by patient demands and the public's perception that more care means better care.

At the time of the study, healthcare expenditures were on the order of 8 percent of the U.S. gross domestic product (GDP), and everyone expected that if healthcare expenditures reached 10 percent of GDP, things were going to change. Yet today, 30 years later, healthcare expenditures are at about 17 percent of GDP, the Medicare Trustees Report predicts that Medicare will be insolvent by 2012, and people are still speculating about when things are going to change. At least there is now some cause for optimism that some meaningful changes will take place that will lead to healthcare resources being spent more wisely. This paper examines what factors might drive such changes. The focus is on four of the main drivers of healthcare costs: demographics, limited quality measures, the third-party payment system, and technology growth.

In terms of demographics, as we live longer we become victims of our success. The population includes more older people, who, on average, make more intense use of healthcare resources than do younger people. At the same time, quality measures are limited, and it is quite challenging to measure and reward good-quality care. The result is a massive healthcare system in which some of the care is of good quality and some of bad quality. Additionally, the third-party payment system insulates some of the main drivers of healthcare costs (patients and physicians) from the actual cost of care. When one enters a store to make a purchase, the cost is clearly marked, and one can judge the value of the item relative to one's budget. In health care, by contrast, the cost to the consumer is generally unknown, and out-of-pocket costs are not related to the actual cost of care and often not related to the patient's own consumption of care. Of course, health care is a different kind of commodity from such purchases as appliances. However, a system in which copayments are the same for a very expensive and a very inexpensive test encourages increased consumption of health care without consideration of value. Generally, patients who receive a great deal of health care pay no more than those who receive only a little. A similar situation exists at the physician level. When our hospital's house staff is asked about the prices of the tests they order in the context of a discussion about why they are ordering a test and how the patient is going to benefit from its results, physicians rarely know what the tests cost. In an academic medical center, the costs of testing and new technology are invisible because doctors are removed from the payment system and insulated from the cost of health care. Similarly, house officers are often shocked to learn of the difference in cost between the latest fourth-generation antibiotic and older generics.

Of all the factors that drive up healthcare costs, however, the growth of technology can be singled out as most significant. Technology, of course, has many benefits. Numerous examples exist of advances in technology that have led to great improvements in health care. However, before a new technology is embraced, a technology assessment should be performed to determine whether it will yield actual patient benefits that outweigh any possible risks. This point is best illustrated by randomized controlled trials. The current healthcare system does not emphasize the need for evidence of benefit before widespread diffusion of new technology.

Today we are seeing a rapid proliferation of technologies for both diagnosis and treatment. A major example is imaging, whose rates have increased dramatically in the past few decades. For example, cardiac imaging used by cardiologists has increased by 24 percent per year over the past decade. Looking just at Medicare data from 1999 to 2003, cardiac imaging increased 45 percent. Computed tomography (CT) scans represent the largest part of the cardiac imaging increase; CT scans of various body parts, excluding the head, have increased by 85 percent (MedPAC, 2007). In 2005, the estimated cost for all imaging was $100 billion (Farnsworth, 2005).

It is fair to say that the benefit to patients of this increase in imaging remains unclear. There have been no tremendous declines in mortality or improvements in health outcomes that are clearly related to the increase in imaging. So what is driving the increased use of imaging? Certainly, the technology has gotten better. Pictures are much clearer, for instance. And the technology has also become easier to use. Furthermore, imaging-related entrepreneurial activity, such as freestanding CT centers, has grown, and once one has made a capital investment in a very expensive CT scanner, the incentive to use it is great. Defensive medicine, such as ordering a specific test because of concern about being sued, is always mentioned as a driver of healthcare costs in relation to technology advances. Patient demand for the use of new technologies has also increased. Patients read about these advances on the Internet, hear about them in the media, are bombarded with related direct-to-consumer advertising, and request use of the technologies from their doctors.

Pictures are very powerful, and people are driven by images they see in the media. A recent collection of media clips, for example, showed a cover story in *Time* magazine about a CT angiogram, with the headline "How to stop a heart attack before it happens."[1] Yet how these tests could prevent a heart attack is unclear. Tests appear to have become confused with prevention, but the link between the two remains undetermined. Most prevention is based on lifestyle changes—such as better diet, increased physical activity, and smoking cessation—that individuals can make to reduce their risk of disease. If people eat a heart-healthy diet, exercise regularly, and do not smoke, they can reduce their chance of having a heart attack by 50 percent. They can also get a CT scan, but doing so is not going to change their chance of having a heart attack. It is possible, of course, that taking the test might make a person more likely to eat a healthy diet, exercise, and not smoke, but there are no data indicating this is the case. Still, patients appear to hear the message that getting such tests can prevent a heart attack. When people say they are doing something for prevention, they are usually talking about getting some kind of test.

Medicare data show a tremendous increase in the use of all cardiac imaging modalities. CT has seen the biggest increase, followed by magnetic resonance imaging and then positron emission tomography. Looking at these data, one can certainly understand why the Medicare Payment Advi-

---

[1] *Time Magazine*, September 5, 2005.

sory Committee is so interested in assessing the use of imaging, since it has been a huge driver of the increase in Medicare costs per beneficiary.

Take as an example cardiac CT angiography, the technology that makes it possible to visualize the coronary arteries noninvasively. The pictures are impressive, but there are currently no data on associated clinical outcomes, so there is no way to know whether the information from the images can be used to affect patient health.

There are data, however, showing that the increased use of CT scans poses a significant radiation risk. David Brenner recently wrote in the *New England Journal of Medicine* that some 62 million scans are done annually in the United States and that this number is increasing every year (Brenner and Hall, 2007). It is estimated that 2 percent of all cancers in the United States are attributable to radiation from CT scans and that some 3 million additional cancers can be expected in the next decade because of increased use of CT scans. The obvious question, then, is how the benefits from these additional CT scans can be weighed against the associated risks. In the Medicare system, a new test tends to be used first in high-risk patients and then, as it becomes more accepted, to be used more frequently, in lower-risk patients, and repeatedly. This pattern explains the dramatic increase in the use of CT scans.

Two years ago the Medicare Coverage Advisory Committee (MCAC) evaluated data related to cardiac computed tomographic angiography (CCTA). Although most Medicare decisions are local, if the Centers for Medicare & Medicaid Services (CMS) issues a national coverage decision, it trumps all local decisions. Thus a meeting of MCAC is sometime convened to review the evidence concerning a procedure or practice. The typical process is that MCAC reviews all of the data and then votes on the evidence, after which CMS makes a decision on whether to extend or expand coverage.

Duke University was commissioned to perform the evidence review for CCTA. The conclusions of the technology assessment were that the benefits of CCTA were unproven. MCAC voted that the evidence on CCTA was insufficient to establish its benefit. However, CMS elected not to issue a national coverage decision following that meeting, which meant that coverage decisions were left to local carriers. There was tremendous interest in CCTA at that time. Colleagues from the American College of Cardiology (ACC) and the American College of Radiology (ACR) collaborated on draft text that could be used for local CCTA coverage decisions, based on the ACC and ACR consensus concerning indications for use of the technology. Just a few months after the Medicare coverage meeting in which the evidence was found to be insufficient, all 50 states had included CCTA in Medicare coverage by local decisions (Redberg, 2007).

Looking at some other diagnostic and treatment technologies, we are likely to hear more about spinal fusion, implantable cardiac defibrillators, percutaneous coronary interventions (PCIs, also known as stents), and lap banding for morbid obesity. Defibrillators, which basically prevent sudden death by firing a shock to the heart, were the focus of an MCAC meeting in February 2003. After publication of the results of Multicenter Automatic Defibrillator Implantation Trial 2, Guidant and major makers of defibrillators petitioned CMS for expanded coverage, and CMS expanded implantable cardioverter defibrillator (ICD) coverage for primary prevention. Now a much larger potential pool of ICD recipients exists because primary prevention includes anyone who has had a heart attack and a certain amount of damage to the heart muscle—a much bigger group than actual survivors of heart attacks (secondary prevention). Because of this expansion, only 1 in 11 patients derives any benefit from ICD, where benefit is defined as the device having been activated and the patient having been saved from a potentially lethal rhythm. Recently a published Medicare data analysis showed no survival benefit (at 1 year) for patients with ICD compared with conventional therapy, after adjustment for age and comorbidity. Again, then, evidence is accumulating after practice patterns have been established that casts doubt on the rationale for widespread ICD use. However, ICDs are now part of the culture in electrophysiology. Even so, to some extent the data on benefits lag behind usage, particularly in subgroups such as elderly people and women (Lin et al., 2007), and ICDs are implanted in far more patients than will ever benefit from the device (Lin et al., 2008).

PCIs show similar trends. There is tremendous geographic variation in the use of PCI. We have done some work in collaboration with colleagues at Dartmouth looking at the use of PCI across the country and documenting its appropriate use. As one might expect, we found a great deal of geographic variation and data suggesting that much PCI use is actually inappropriate, or there was no documentation of ischemia prior to its use.

A key point of this paper, therefore, is that technology use often goes far beyond what the data show with respect to patient benefit. For example, it is estimated that more than one-third of all CT scans are unnecessary. Therefore, it is easy to discern a great deal of inefficiency in the system. The implication is that there is room for improvement in our culture, our practice, and our delivery of health care. A major step would be to begin more systematic data collection and to develop more prospective registries, such as the National Cardiovascular Data Registry at the ACC. Kaiser has large registries. More systematic data collection and analysis would lead to better-informed decisions. More randomized controlled trials—which will require more funding—is in order, as is the development of more observational data. It is important that these data be gathered, analyzed, and incorporated into practice guidelines and reimbursement. Changing practice patterns is much more difficult after they have been established, even with the introduction of new evidence.

In addition, all these data must be more widely available. Currently, it can be very difficult to access large databases. More transparency is needed for these kinds of data.

Finally, there must be more consistent review of the evidence for clinical benefit prior to the routine use of new technologies. A change of culture is needed in this regard so that a technology does not see widespread adoption before the evidence review is complete. This is one crucial way to concentrate healthcare spending so that it yields the greatest possible benefit in actually improving health outcomes. Once a technology has been widely adopted, curtailing its use is extremely difficult, and there are many examples of this point in our healthcare system.

The healthcare system could benefit from a systems engineering approach whereby data collection and review are incorporated into the practice of medicine; the data collection is accessible, easily performed, and inexpensive; and with rapid turnaround, the data can be examined quickly. It is essential to align incentives and reward evidence-driven care.

A LOOK AT THE FUTURE OF CLINICAL DATA SYSTEMS AND CLINICAL DECISION SUPPORT

Michael D. Chase, M.D., Kaiser Permanente Colorado

To date, health care in the United States has not fully leveraged the available clinical data to improve the health outcomes of individuals and populations. From a technology and clinical data perspective, data too often are "locked away" on paper, in various applications, and in isolated databases. Too few practices and hospitals use electronic medical records (EMRs), and usability issues remain. Existing data standards are used inconsistently, as are interoperability standards. Thus the information needs of patients, physicians and care teams, organizations, and the healthcare system as a whole are not being met. Privacy and security concerns persist. More important, the culture of health care presents barriers to the effective use of the data and information. From a process perspective, the complexity of health care has dramatically increased. More people have chronic disease, more have multiple chronic diseases, and the treatments and technologies available have increased. In response to this increased complexity, health care has not taken full advantage of engineering principles that can be used to deal with complex processes. The healthcare environment, with its structure and financing, adds considerably to the barriers.

The above issues limit the effectiveness of clinical decision support. To create a more effective learning healthcare system, the healthcare establishment will need to direct more attention to various areas, including the people and culture, the processes, the data and technology, and the healthcare environment. Integrated delivery systems are well positioned to address these areas and can serve as a model for those that deliver care outside of such systems. Much work remains, however, before a learning healthcare system can be fully realized throughout the United States.

An editorial entitled "Is Information the Answer for Hypertension Control?," written by Eric Peterson and published in the *Archives of Internal Medicine* (Peterson, 2008), commented on a paper in that issue of the journal that reported on a study of blood pressure control in a large population of patients with cardiovascular disease. The study found a blood pressure control rate of 95 percent, significantly better than what is usually seen. The editorial suggested that the system described in the paper provided a hint as to how electronic data systems may hold the key to achieving better blood pressure control in the future. It read:

> For a moment, imagine you live in a world in which an integrated EMR system was the standard in most community practices . . . the blood pressure trajectories of hypertensive patients could be easily tracked . . . feedback reports could then quickly update busy caregivers regarding which of their patients fell short of treatment goals and needed closer follow-up. And as an intervention, such data could be used to provide various incentives for meeting blood pressure control goals. . . . Taken [one] step further, online pharmacy systems, linked to decision support, could also be used to proactively remind patients and/or alert their physicians if important therapies were consistently missed. . . . Therefore, in the future, ambulatory information systems could be applied both as a diagnostic tool and as an effective therapeutic intervention. (Peterson, 2008)

The purpose of this paper is to identify some of the barriers to fully realizing such a vision of a learning healthcare system and to discuss how they might be overcome.

The barriers to synthesizing and using information to support enhanced care delivery can be viewed in terms of four broad categories: people and culture, process, data and technology, and the healthcare environment. Challenges from the people standpoint include the prevailing culture of health care with its hierarchical, often physician-centric, and slow-to-evolve team-based approach to care. The clinical leadership needed to address the larger issues in health care is often lacking and not adequately fostered and valued. The skills and training required to use technology and information systems, as well as team skills, need further development. With respect to the process of care, health care has grown in complexity, thanks in part to its complex workflows. One of the major purposes of this workshop is to highlight the underuse of tools that could be adopted from engineering, particularly as they apply to complex systems, such as tools for system design, analysis, and control. Because of the culture and structure of health care, an end-to-end, patient-centered view of the process is often lacking. Care is viewed at the departmental level or from a disciplines frame of reference, as opposed to a continuous view of the care process. As a result, problems with transitions of care between departments or venues of care are magnified.

The healthcare industry lags behind other industries in how information technology is used. Clinical information systems often are not integrated. Data are locked away in various applications, often still on paper, and in various databases. This lack of integration occurs even within organizations; it is far worse across organizations. Data standards and interoperability standards are used inconsistently. This situation is being addressed by a number of public and private organizations, including the Office of the National Coordinator for HIT, the American Health Information Community, the Healthcare Information Technology Standards Panel, and the Certification Commission for HIT. Usability issues remain, and there is continued concern about privacy and security issues. Finally, the healthcare system in the United States presents significant barriers. Most primary care is delivered by relatively small practices, and most specialty care is delivered by individual departments with, as noted above, a lack integration among the various care venues. Healthcare financing and reimbursement reinforce this fragmented care.

In considering what is required to provide clinical decision support that will enhance the care delivered to patients, one needs to take into account both an individual patient-centered view and a population view. Accomplishing this requires getting the right information to the right team member at the right time in the workflow or the decision-making process so as to trigger the right event for the care of an individual patient as well as for a population of patients. Another way of framing this point is to ask, "What sorts of information do the patient, the clinician, and the healthcare team need to meet their agreed-upon healthcare goals?"

A review of clinical decision support published in 2005 in the *British Medical Journal* concluded that "clinical decision support systems have shown great *promise* for reducing medical errors and improving patient care. However, such systems do not always result in improved clinical practice, for reasons that are not always clear" (Kawamoto et al., 2005). This observation suggests that we are dealing with a very complex system, one that is not sufficiently understood. Engineering expertise can be applied to better understand the process of care and the application of technology so as to improve the provision of effective clinical decision support.

On this same topic, a 2004 article in the *Journal of the American Medi-*

cal Informatics Association entitled "Some Unintended Consequences of Information Technology in Health Care: The Nature of Patient Care Information System-Related Errors" (Ash et al., 2004) cautioned against unintended consequences of information technology in health care. The paper pointed to potential errors in the process of entering and retrieving information, such as human–computer interface issues and cognitive overload, and it addressed the overemphasis on structured and complete information entry or retrieval. The paper also warned about errors in the communication and coordination process, including the potential for misrepresenting collective, interactive work as a linear, clear-cut, and predictable workflow; the possibility of misrepresenting communication as information transfer; decision support overload; and the loss of prior mechanisms for catching errors. The paper highlights the fact that we do not completely understand healthcare processes and do not fully recognize the disruption that occurs when technology is introduced—underscoring the need for engineering expertise in the process of designing a better learning healthcare system.

What are some general themes regarding effective clinical decision support? Clinical decision support should be carried out in the context of a planned care model—a model that is much more patient-centric, that takes into account process redesign and a team approach, and that is enhanced by information technology. This model differs significantly from the old one-doctor, one-patient, one-exam-room, paper-record model. In approaching clinical decision support, one needs to think broadly across the care team members, including the patient; across the continuum of care; and across the tools and systems available. Some decision support opportunities include

- *reference information and guidance*—clinical evidence sources and guidelines,
- *direct-to-patient clinical decision support*—availability of information,
- *relevant data presentation*—attention to the human–computer interface,
- *documentation forms and templates*—integration into the workflow,
- *order entry facilitator*—integration of decision support at order entry,
- *protocol and pathway support*—a way to facilitate the care process,
- *reactive alert and reminders*—used judiciously, and
- *use of clinical data*—clinical registries to support the planned care model.

Use of clinical data, including clinical registries in the context of team process redesign, is one particular area in which one can often see significant improvement of care at both the individual and population levels.

What might this effective use of clinical decision support look like? Imagine a patient time line that extends for a year. On that time line is a point that represents an encounter. If one enlarges that point, one can see what some of the decision support opportunities are, many of which are currently available at Kaiser Permanente. The systems underlying decision support includes the EMR, online tools that give patients access to their medical records, and clinical registries. The patient time line starts with the appointment process and may include an appointment. A patient questionnaire can be delivered, such as a health risk appraisal or a questionnaire specific to the patient's condition or disease.

A preventive alert system is available that, at check-in, alerts the patient to needed interventions, thereby activating the patient as well as the care team as the patient moves through the healthcare system. At the rooming stage, the medical assistant can be reminded to address important risk factors, such as assessing smoking status and informing the patient about smoking cessation programs. An array of tools are available to clinicians during this encounter, including reminders for prevention issues, alerts for chronic care issues, and a variety of charting tools supporting the care process and facilitating data entry. Computerized physician order entry is a particularly powerful tool to facilitate clinical decision making. There are also alerts and reminders for those instances in which, for example, a physician may prescribe a medication to which the patient is allergic, that interacts negatively with another medication, or that is contraindicated for the patient's specific condition. As this process unfolds, one can see that it would be very easy to overload one part of the system, such as the encounter in the exam room between physician and patient. That is why one needs to think across the continuum of care and across the care team members who are available to avoid creating a bottleneck in one part of the process.

At discharge, printing of patient instructions and other visit information can be available for reinforcement and later review by the patient or family members. Decision support can also be embedded in the pharmacy information system, thereby using the pharmacist as another team member in the care delivery process.

Finally, the enhanced system uses clinical registries, which apply data from the EMR as well as other clinical systems. This is one way to enable new models of care, including outreach to patients with needed interventions that can be done outside of the usual face-to-face visit. This availability of information allows all of the care team members, including patients and their families, to participate in the care being delivered.

Now let us look at a specific example of enhanced care enabled by information technology. The editorial mentioned at the beginning of this paper referred to a process of care that exists at Kaiser Permanente Colorado (KPCO)—the Collaborative Cardiac Care Service composed of Kaiser Permanente Cardiac Rehabilitation and the Clinical Pharmacy Cardiac Risk Service. It is a service whereby nurses and clinical pharmacists coordinate the provision of cardiac risk reduction activities in patients with cardiovascular disease by supporting and working collaboratively with patients, primary care physicians, and cardiologists. The focus is on activities that have been shown to improve patient outcomes. The service assists patients in managing and monitoring antiplatelet therapy, antilipid therapy, beta-blocker medication, angiotensin-converting enzyme inhibitor medication, blood pressure control, and diabetes management, if applicable. It also provides counsel and support on lifestyle changes. The service follows more than 12,000 patients with cardiovascular disease. Performance levels obtained in this population of patients include an average low-density lipoprotein cholesterol of 78 and average blood pressure of 126/72. More important is that the cardiac mortality of this population has been reduced by 73 percent. Also of interest is that the organization has seen a financial return because fewer patients with cardiovascular disease require rehospitalization or further cardiac interventions.

The development of the KPCO Cardiac Rehabilitation and Clinical Pharmacy Cardiac Risk Service addressed and overcame many of the barriers in the areas of people and culture, process, data and technology, and the healthcare environment that were reviewed earlier, resulting in superior clinical outcomes. The service has many of the characteristics that could be considered components of a model learning healthcare system. With regard to the people issue, KPCO has developed a culture of physicians, nurses, and clinical pharmacists working together and focused on the patient. That collaboration has extended to those who work in information technology. There has been effective clinical leadership on the part of clinical pharmacists, nurses, physicians, and information technologists in the establishment of these services. Clinical staff have focused roles and clear accountability and are trained in their roles, including use of the technology. In terms of process, clear, evidence-based guidelines and clinical pathways are agreed upon by all involved and modified as needed according to new research findings or internal learning. Alternative approaches to care and communication with patients have been more fully exploited with the use of phone contacts, mail, secured messaging, group visits, and direct patient Internet access to medical records, including laboratory results, medications, and patient instructions. There are clear hand-offs and communication with other team members, including primary care clinicians and cardiologists.

On the technology side, KPCO has been using EMRs for 10 years, a necessary but not sufficient measure to support this kind of process. An information infrastructure is required with the capability to aggregate data that facilitate the identification and stratification of populations of patients into the clinical registry. This registry provides the real-time information needed by the team members to properly manage both individual patients and the population. It alerts the team members when needed interventions are due or when they have not been completed, thus ensuring long-term adherence to agreed-upon goals. The registry facilitates the tracking of the performance of the service, providing necessary feedback on its processes. A clearly defined clinical model from an engineering perspective informs the technology approach. Collaboration with information technology enables system adjustments as the clinical model transitions. KPCO is an integrated healthcare delivery system that allows a system-level view. The program design was not significantly constrained by the financing and reimbursement system that currently prevails in the United States.

Is information the answer? Yes, but it is only part of the answer. One cannot think about data and technology without also taking into account people and their culture, focusing on the process of care from the patient's perspective, and addressing the healthcare environment. In sum, the challenge and opportunity for all who want to see an improved learning healthcare system is to address all of these interrelated components.

CARE COORDINATION AND LINKAGE

Amy L. Deutschendorf, M.S., R.N., APRN-BC,
Johns Hopkins Hospital and Health System, Clinical Resource
Consultants, LLC, Johns Hopkins University School of Nursing

The current healthcare environment is characterized by escalating systems and patient complexities. The proliferation of new medical information and technologies, increased regulatory oversight, an aging population, and heightened consumer awareness and expectations are all affecting the ability to provide coherent care for patients. The dismantling of traditional care delivery models as a result of cost constraints in the early 1990s has also contributed to the disorganization, fragmentation, and discontinuity of patient care. With as many as 20 healthcare providers per patient, the need for effective communication and collaboration has become more important than ever to achieve quality and safety outcomes. The National Quality Forum has identified care coordination as one of its top national priorities (National Priorities Partnership, 2008). This paper focuses on those structure and process factors that contribute to the current state of discontinuity and fragmentation in patient care. The critical factors in effective care delivery models are discussed, as well as the need for communication models and systems that can provide the accurate and timely transfer of patient information throughout the healthcare continuum.

The current healthcare system evolved from the late 1980s and early 1990s with the broad penetration of managed care in an attempt to respond to economic pressures and manage rapidly escalating healthcare costs. Financial risk was transferred from the payer to the provider, with spending being more tightly controlled and facility service to the acutely ill being limited. To contain costs, acute care facilities sought strategies to improve efficiencies in care delivery, which resulted in widespread restructuring, reengineering, and redesign efforts. These changes had a significant effect on hospital systems, clinical staff, and resources. Hospitals could no longer afford uncoordinated patient care that resulted in ad hoc patient care decisions. Although some new patient care delivery models were proposed that centered care on patients and families, most were more closely related to industrial approaches geared to achieving efficiencies affecting the bottom line. Untested models were implemented without evidence of improved clinical quality outcomes, effective care delivery systems were frequently dismantled, and unskilled workers were substituted for professional staff. There was an exodus of experienced care providers, resulting in shortages in most healthcare disciplines. Ultimately, clinical quality and safety outcomes eroded as a result of a lack of understanding of the complexities of individual human responses to similar stimuli.

In addition to such changes in care delivery systems, other factors played a major role in creating the complexity of the current healthcare environment. New information and medical technology that must be translated into safe practice is proliferating at an extraordinarily rapid rate, making it nearly impossible to determine true priorities for implementation in evidence-based practice. As noted, each patient may have up to 20 healthcare providers, all generating assessments and treatment plans that must be coordinated and communicated. Multiple levels of care must be considered when patients are being transitioned out of the acute care setting, all with different rules for admission and reimbursement. Although the average length of a patient's hospital stay has decreased by 23 percent over the past decade, the severity of illness has increased by 12 percent, necessitating improved assessment and monitoring strategies. Twenty-five percent of a hospital's census may turn over in a 24-hour period, adding to increased patient care unit activity and the need for accurate coordination of services and resources. As many as 62 percent of hospitals report operating over capacity. The increased collection and public reporting of quality and safety data, sanctioned by regulatory agencies as a means of demonstrating organizational performance, is contributing to health systems' administrative burden and threatens to distract caregivers from a focus on the bedside.

As the average length of stay decreased, it was estimated that half of American hospitals would close by the year 2000, but this projection underestimated the effect of the aging population. Today, it is not unusual for an 85-year-old with chronic health conditions to be living at home, still driving, with a spouse who also has chronic disease and has nowhere to go after a catastrophic illness. The health needs of the aging population were not fully anticipated when the Balanced Budget Act was passed in 1997, reducing Medicare payments to skilled and long-term care providers. (Some of these cuts were reinstated under the Balanced Budget Reform Act of 1999 and the Budget Improvement and Protection Act of 2000.[2]) As a result, elderly patients may consume more acute care resources and have longer lengths of stay while awaiting appropriate transition to another level of care because no public funds are available to support assisted living and long-term care.

Today the objectives of acute care are "stabilization and transition," admitting only the sickest patients and focusing on preservation of their functionality. Although these objectives are significantly different from those of just 20 years ago, patient care delivery processes have not changed dramatically, even as the increased severity of illness demands significant transformation. As noted, it is not uncommon for a quarter of a large academic hospital's patients to have a length of stay of 24 hours or less. The impact of this shortened length of stay combined with the increased severity of illness is that healthcare practitioners must accurately assess, evaluate, and treat patients during this time frame. There is a disparity between the expectations of the acute care environment and those of the regulatory agencies. The acute care setting is frequently viewed by regulatory bodies as the point of access for all current and historical patient problems, when such attention to patient needs is more appropriately the purview of the ambulatory care environment. The healthcare provider has a more limited exposure to the patient in the acute care setting than in any other setting. Yet it is expected that all biopsychosocial, economic, and developmental problems the patient has ever experienced will be addressed and documented in this setting, at the same time that the healthcare providers are employing preventive strategies and facilitating healthy behaviors in the future. More focus is required on how to improve access to ambulatory care departments, where the appropriate objectives are health promotion, illness prevention, and stabilization or improvement of function.

The complexity of patient populations has changed radically, in part because of increased life spans, greater prevalence of chronic illness, and expanding consumer expectations. Healthcare consumers are armed with

---

[2] H.R. 2015 [105th]: Balanced Budget Act of 1997; H.R. 5661 [106th]: Medicare, Medicaid, and SCHIP Benefits Improvement and Protection Act of 2000.

Internet information and resources, arriving at appointments with their physicians well prepared with questions, background information, and specific suggestions about their preferred treatment. Often, they present their findings in the form of demands, having decided in advance what the best therapy is. Healthcare providers have not fully anticipated the implications of an elderly, sicker consumer and have not implemented methods to manage unrealistic expectations. Education needs to be provided actively to patients and families so they know that although they are likely to live longer, they will do so with chronic disease. They must be counseled about their responsibilities for healthy behaviors and understand that the current armamentarium of diagnostics and treatments cannot "cure" those chronic conditions, but will at least help preserve functional status. Preparing patients and families for realistic end-of-life decisions is more important than ever, given the increased healthcare costs associated with futile care.

The demand by payers, consumers, and purchasers for demonstration of outcomes has led to a greater prevalence of regulatory standards and oversight focused on improving quality and safety outcomes. Reduced practice variation through evidence-based care and fiscal responsibility through cost-effective strategies are expected to be transparent to the consumer and payer through the provision of specific and quantifiable information. Pay for performance, an incentive-based concept that rewards healthcare organizations that can demonstrate improvement as defined by outcome indicators, may create even more stress on an institution that has limited financial resources to divert to quality initiatives. Unfortunately, the number of mandatory initiatives and reporting requirements not only may tax an organization's financial and human resources, but also may ultimately contribute to a lack of progress in reducing adverse events—or worse, create an increase in unanticipated serious outcomes. The "risk of abundant quality" may be described as a situation in which changes conceived as important and beneficial by all stakeholders are implemented but result in unexpected new hazards, including increased direct and indirect costs, new errors and adverse events, and lost opportunities elsewhere (Warburton, 2005).

An example is the increase in redundant pneumococcal vaccinations for hospital inpatients as acute care facilities attempt to comply with Joint Commission Core Measures. Although evidence regarding the safety of multiple revaccinations is inconclusive, increased adverse events have been reported (Shih et al., 2002). Additionally, processes such as pneumococcal vaccination, smoking cessation, and influenza vaccination are more appropriately applied and measured in the primary care setting.

At the same time, both public and private payers are devising new and inventive ways to avoid payment for services that have been provided. Although the goal is to give providers incentives to ensure the medical necessity of therapies and appropriate levels of care, the result has been an expectation that providers will do more with less. Under the Medicare Modernization Act of 2003, it is expected that CMS will collect billions of dollars in perceived overpayments for services that were rendered in good faith by dedicated providers. The newest strategies to deny reimbursement for therapies for complications of illness perceived to have occurred in the hospital are ill conceived, for in many cases these complications were not truly preventable (Pronovost et al., 2008). The imperative to appeal reimbursement decisions has resulted in increased administrative burden and greater healthcare costs borne by the healthcare provider.

Few data showing true safety improvement have emerged over the past 8 years since the publication of the Institute of Medicine (IOM) report *To Err Is Human* (IOM, 2000). Failure to rescue, described as "death due to complications of serious illness and disease" (Silber et al., 1992), remains a serious problem. It is plausible that the ratio of safety–risk (adverse events related to the implementation of safety or quality initiatives) to safety–improvement may actually be increased as a result of the complexity of the environment, numerous and sometimes random regulations, and the lack of proven systems and processes to address the ways in which patients receive care. There needs to be a focus on the *provision* rather than the *demonstration* of quality care, with the application of research findings to support structures and processes linked to quality and safety outcomes.

These and related issues have combined to create a crisis in the way care is provided to patients. Operationally, care delivery may be defined as the way in which providers and services are deployed to meet patient and family needs over the continuum of care. Research that links clinical outcomes with patient care models is woefully lacking, and current models of care, characterized by a "siloed" mentality, continue to reflect the mindset of an industrial age. Fundamental processes of care have not changed to accommodate the complexities of healthcare systems and patient illnesses, which include rapid changes in condition and limited exposure. Provider shortages are evident in all specialty areas and are projected to worsen over the next 10 years, with demand significantly exceeding supply because of increased consumption of healthcare resources by an aging population. Patient care in the acute setting is frequently organized around physician service lines rather than the patient. Nurses and other providers have become task oriented as a result of the emphasis on productivity and the increased regulatory demands for documented compliance with standards. Staffing patterns that have been adopted because they are economically efficient, such as 12-hour nursing shifts, have led to care that is more fragmented and has less continuity. Patient care planning is unidimensional and uncoordinated as a result of poor communication among providers, patients, and families and across levels of care. Hand-offs between providers, from shift to shift and across transitions, are insufficient and frequently result in poor patient outcomes caused by "lost" information. The medical record, which traditionally was the one repository of all patient information and which told the patient's "story," is often incoherent as organizations try to translate a paper record into an electronic format and end up with voluminous, redundant, and inefficient information technology solutions. Other technological solutions designed to improve safety outcomes, such as physician order entry, may in fact increase errors because of the lack of a systems approach to planning and implementation.

In the final analysis, the current healthcare environment reflects an overwhelming lack of coordination and continuity of care. The plan of care is often a "secret," with different providers having discreet and important pieces of the puzzle that are known only to them and from which the patient and family are excluded. As noted earlier, the National Quality Forum has adopted *care coordination* as one of its national priorities. The forum defines care coordination as activities ensuring "that the patient's needs and preferences for health services and information sharing across people, functions and sites are met over time" (NQF, 2009). New models of care delivery must be developed to reflect future objectives, as indicated in Table 3-2.

If care delivery systems are to be redefined to meet prospective healthcare demands for improved clinical and financial outcomes, there must be a dramatic change in healthcare culture from siloed to systems thinking. All patients should expect to have their care managed. Care management should reflect a systems model defined by a multidisciplinary, collaborative practice approach integrated into patient care delivery. The major elements of redefined care delivery systems must be centered on communication, collaboration, coordination, and continuity. New structures and processes must be built to support these elements.

Strategies must be implemented that support frequent, real-time, mul-

TABLE 3-2 Patient Care Delivery Transition

Old Approach	New Approach
• Focus is on the high-risk patient	• Focus is on all patients
• Episodic acute care is the priority	• Continuity of care across the care continuum is the priority
• Healthcare professionals work in isolation	• Collaboration among healthcare team members is required
• Care planning is conceptual	• Care planning is aggressive and results oriented, and prevention is important
• Provider infrastructure is fragmented, and information systems are not integrated	• Provider infrastructure is fully integrated

tidisciplinary communication with all patients, through all transitions, including the family as well as the patient. It has been reported that 70 to 80 percent of all healthcare errors are caused by human factors associated with interpersonal interactions (IOM, 2001). Even the simple approach of having all members of provider teams take part in daily multidisciplinary rounds with all patients can improve patient care planning, expedite care delivery, and reduce fragmentation. Care planning must be truly interdisciplinary, with all providers sharing information, contributing to the coordination of care, and being accountable for patient outcomes. Although it is essential that care planning be collaborative, one physician should be identified as "team captain" and be responsible for synchronizing consulting services and the provision of resources. This physician would also be responsible for providing a sensible interpretation of information to patients and families. Traditional paternalistic approaches by healthcare providers toward patients and families need to be replaced with partnerships that empower patient and family decision making.

New models of care must be based on evidence, must reflect intra- and interepisodic domains, and must include provisions for seamless transitions between episodes. Rigorous research is needed on the relationships between care delivery models and associated quality and safety outcomes for the appropriate levels of care. Quality and safety indicators should be measured in the correct environments so they do not distract care providers from the focus of the patient's problem and the objectives of the care setting. A patient who is critically ill in the hospital is unlikely to benefit from smoking cessation education, for example, yet the provider is required to at least address this standard through documentation. Provider roles must be clearly defined and carried out according to patient characteristics and the required provision of services to improve efficiencies and avoid duplication. Procedures for ensuring competency should be consistently tested and implemented, and they should reflect the dynamic changes in medical information and technology. The idea of technology as a panacea for patient safety should be tempered with careful analysis, planning, and evaluation. Nurses and other bedside providers have become so reliant on equipment and electronic data that clinical correlation may be nonexistent, resulting in increased errors and adverse events (Bates, 2005; Karsh, 2004; Rotschild et al., 2005). Although technology is a necessary component of the armamentarium of adjunctive patient safety structures, its impact may be negligible if not actually detrimental unless there is proper clinical interpretation.

Processes of care must be realigned around the patient and family. Provider teams should be centered at the unit of care to improve communication and coordination and expedite care delivery. Traditional academic models that may result in as many as 10 medical services treating patients on 1 unit should be reevaluated so that similar patients and provider services can be aggregated in single locations. Because patient conditions are rapidly changing, increasing the frequency of monitoring and surveillance is paramount to improving safety and reducing adverse events. Typical nursing processes, such as taking vital signs every 4 hours or offering assessments every 12 hours, are no longer necessary in an environment where the patient's status is continuously changing. Assessments focused on the problem for which the patient was admitted—and which must be resolved to facilitate the next transition of care—should be performed frequently and should relate to evidence-based guidelines. Coherent documentation systems must be developed that do not merely translate a paper record into an electronic format, but rather reflect the patient's story and make it possible for that story to be shared across levels of care. The implementation of disparate documentation systems that do not "talk" to each other should be discouraged, if not eliminated altogether.

To accomplish the overarching and major systemic changes in patient care delivery required to achieve true improvements in quality and safety, certain healthcare traditions must be addressed. These traditions exist in all disciplines and in each patient care environment. Whether they have to do with academic teaching rounds or nursing reports, they reflect structures that worked in an age when patients might have been admitted to the hospital for diagnostic tests, and an average length of stay might have been 7 to 10 days. Systems engineering principles should be implemented to engage departments and professionals in the creative thinking needed to address today's patient populations in all care settings. True change can occur only with appropriate preparation that engages all stakeholders and addresses the system components that may be affected. The only constant in today's healthcare system is change, and our ability to anticipate and plan, rather than react, will determine our ultimate success in the achievement of healthcare outcomes.

TRANSFORMING HOSPITALS THROUGH REFORM OF THE CARE PROCESS

Ralph W. Muller, M.A.,
University of Pennsylvania Health System

The care and service processes in American hospitals, the most complex institutions within the American healthcare system, need to undergo a transformation. Numerous reports have shown that complexity can be reduced and performance improved through careful evaluation of the systems underlying important care and administrative processes within hospitals. This paper focuses on three successful transformations within UPHS, each in an area that causes significant patient frustration:

- *patient billing*—reorganizing billing systems for greater efficiency and improving reporting systems so as to be able to provide more effective feedback to employees;
- *patient access to physicians*—reducing patient waiting times and easing the scheduling of physician appointments; and
- *in-patient progression*—reducing complexity to streamline the course of treatment during hospital stays.

These case studies highlight several themes:

- *issue definition*—defining the issue clearly to lay the groundwork for the fundamental transformation of work required to effect lasting change in complex systems that are built within entrenched cultures;
- *constant vigilance*—monitoring progress and results on a daily basis to ensure that old patterns are not repeated; and
- *structured rewards*—using incentives to reward improvement and maintain changes in a complex system.

Billing

A common patient complaint concerns hospital billing. Patients and their families often cannot understand their bills, question the fees charged, or object to long delays between the date of service and receipt of the bill. Often the tendency within the hospital is to blame the finance office, which sends the bill, but in fact the bill generated is the result of a multistep process that commences before the patient is even provided care. As shown in Figure 3-1, the typical hospital billing process is complex, and breakdowns can and do occur at many points. For example, if incorrect insurance information is collected on admission or if there is an error in medical chart abstraction defining the patient's services, the final bill will be wrong.

Through a systematic review of the billing process, UPHS found that the component functions operate in silos, with no clear connection between the people who register patients at intake and those who prepare and send out the bill after discharge. This situation led to an enormous amount of rework and frustration among employees, who had limited tools with which to ensure that the right bill went to the right person at the right time.

Several corrective actions were taken. First, it quickly became apparent that there was a body of expertise around the billing of Medicare, Blue Cross Blue Shield, and other major insurance carriers. To interface effectively with each of these carriers, UPHS reorganized its billing function by payer, rather than by medical specialty. This redesign was complemented by

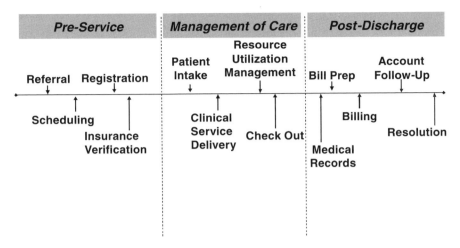

FIGURE 3-1 Revenue cycle engineering.

changes in information technology that helped organize and prioritize the work of frontline employees and their managers. In addition, productivity and quality measurements were built more explicitly into job descriptions, evaluations, and incentive systems for the staff.

Reporting systems that give feedback on performance on a daily, weekly, and monthly basis are critical. To this end, UPHS implemented a system that provides granularity of information, so that information at the level of the frontline employee completing a billing form can be evaluated by the supervisor, by the operating unit, and across the system. UPHS can summarize and drill down on particular billing information so that the information is presented at the transactional level to the frontline employee, but it can also be summarized for the chief financial officer and CEO as needed. This is a critical element added to the billing transaction system: the ability to aggregate underlying information to support different levels of review.

As a result of these changes in the UPHS billing system, annual recurring income improved by $57 million, or 2 percent of revenue—a considerable gain when hospital margins of 3 or 4 percent are difficult to secure. The process and system changes implemented also yielded productivity improvements equivalent to 20 staff.

Access to Physicians

A second transformation effort at UPHS focused on increasing patient access to physicians. With more than 1,000 physicians practicing at 150 sites, UPHS is a large regional provider of specialty physician services, and it has experienced marked increases in demand for these services. As in other large physician groups that lack standardized processes, the increasing demand was challenging UPHS's ability to serve patients. For example, a review of practice call records revealed that 22 percent of the total phone calls received (300,000 per year) were not answered by a person. Another service and efficiency issue was the high frequency of "appointment bumping," or the cancellation of a visit by a physician or patient. Analysis revealed that making appointments with long lead times, which at UPHS were often 60 days or more, resulted in a 50 percent or greater likelihood that either the physician or the patient would cancel the appointment. Rescheduling patients after a cancellation required a great deal of extra work.

To tackle such service and efficiency issues, UPHS evaluated the full continuum of its care process, including access and scheduling of appointments, availability, patient flow during and after the visit, and follow-up. The evaluation engaged all caregivers. As noted above, for appointments scheduled more than 60 days in advance, there was a 50 percent chance that either the doctor or the patient would cancel, so scheduling appointments within 6 to 10 days of a request became a key focus. The result has been increased patient satisfaction, as well as less staff time spent rescheduling appointments. UPHS also found that when a physician cancels a patient's visit, especially more than once, the chances are three to four times higher that the patient will miss the visit (Figure 3-2). UPHS educates its doctors about this statistic, and it has implemented a series of policy and process changes to reduce the frequency of cancellations.

Another focus of the effort to improve patient access to UPHS practices was an evaluation of capacity—again taking a systems approach to the processes of care. Understanding capacity use across all dimensions—examination rooms, providers (physicians, nurse practitioners), and clinical and clerical staff—helped pinpoint opportunities to increase outpatient capacity and address patient service problems. In some cases, there was a 50 percent difference between provider capacity and actual activity. For example, patient demand to see a doctor on a Tuesday or Wednesday significantly exceeded capacity, while there was excess room capacity on Friday afternoons. Incentives to encourage the use of rooms in off-peak periods have been instituted, and exam room, provider, and clerical staff capacity has been harmonized to reduce mismatches and increase effective capacity use.

In addition, patient intake processes have been redesigned so that the front office performs rapid check-in and collects all critical patient information via the EMR, including patient histories, medication management, and chief complaint lists. Patient flow within the practice has also been enhanced through the use of patient tracking systems and process changes

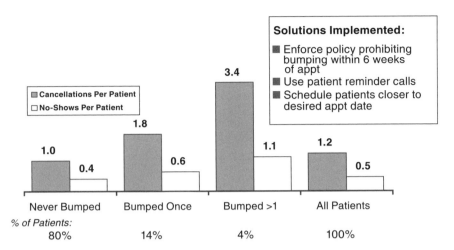

FIGURE 3-2 Impact of physician-initiated appointed rescheduling on patient-initiated cancellations and no-shows.

that encourage patients to complete all requests (e.g., prescription refills) during the visit, rather than in follow-up.

UPHS also tracks relevant metrics across various clinical departments. Sharing comparative data with physicians, most of whom strive to be among the best, has spurred internal competition to achieve and demonstrate improvement.

Inpatient Stays

As is the case with many acute care hospitals in the country, occupancy rates at UPHS are very high, with patients occupying 90 percent or more of the hospitals' beds on average. The result is bottlenecks in the emergency room and difficulty in accommodating regional referrals. Because building new beds is expensive—approximately $2 million a bed in Philadelphia—UPHS focused on optimizing the flow of patients in its hospitals. This systems change has made it possible to treat admitted patients more expeditiously, which is both better for patients and their families and consistent with demands insurers are placing on hospitals.

The complex patient flow process was broken down into its component parts, with a focus on not only the steps just prior to discharge but also the activities that occur before and during the stay. The patient flow process encompasses the initial referral, insurance verification and the logistics of obtaining a hospital bed, medical management once the patient has been admitted (e.g., the turnaround of lab and imaging results and medication management), planning for the discharge with the care team and family, and finally, turning around of the bed for the next patient.

UPHS undertook a major analysis of these processes and related bottlenecks, leveraging information technology to enhance the availability of information and streamline processes. An electronic board that tracks the status of inpatients in the hospital enables every doctor, nurse, resident, transporter, and housekeeper to access detailed information and keep track of each patient. The board displays easy-to-read icons that indicate whether a patient is in imaging, whether his or her lab results are available, whether prescriptions have been written, or whether the patient needs to be discharged. That information, once gathered by one caregiver, is now known by all, which saves time and frustration and enables caregivers to manage the process more effectively. Giving the critical information to staff members allows them to focus on being doctors, nurses, social workers, or transporters rather than wasting time tracking down information that is already available. This initiative created the equivalent of 17 new beds, avoiding $34 million in construction costs and improving the patient, family, and physician experience.

Lessons

The transformations described above offer several key lessons:

- *Use data and analysis to identify opportunities and motivate change.* It is necessary to break down complex processes to understand their component parts, to identify where breakdowns occur, and to make all members of the team aware of the issues. In the billing process, for example, the critical process steps turned out to be at the front end rather than the back end. In increasing access to physicians, the critical element was to manage the balance based on the availability of the physicians, examination rooms, nurses, and clerical staff. To advance patient care processes inside the hospital, it was critical to track the key steps in the patient journey from admission to discharge, sharing information in real time with all caregivers.
- *Redesign workflows and restructure roles, integrating information technology.* Each of these cases relied on redesigned workflows and restructured roles for the staff, with extensive use of information technology to facilitate the restructuring. For example, the restructuring of work in the patient billing process was supported by new tools that prioritize the daily work of frontline staff and aggregate decision support information for management at all levels.

The physician access initiative was integrally associated with EMR implementation, which enabled a streamlined collection of patient information. The electronic patient board that tracks patients throughout the hospital stay and provides status information to all caregivers has been a critical element in improving the management of inpatient stays.

- *Establish goals and monitor performance in real time.* In each of these efforts, critical metrics were identified and tracked on a daily basis. Any authorized staff member can access the same data at the appropriate level of granularity—per patient, per unit, or per hospital.
- *Create meaningful incentives for physicians, management, and staff.* Efforts to redesign the care processes at UPHS were integrated into the overall management plan of the organization. For example, all UPHS administrators, including the CEO, academic department chairs, and every member of senior management, have related goals that are written into their individual and team plans. Metrics related to each of the processes discussed are reflected in incentive plans for middle managers as well. Consequently, for more than 1,000 of UPHS's 13,000 employees, these processes are incentivized through compensation plans. Other recognition programs, such as quality awards, are also used to encourage doctors, nurses, and other clinical staff to move these transformation efforts forward.

The care transformation that has been achieved at UPHS is an example of how to manage the complex American healthcare system, one institution at a time, by bringing more accountability into the system.

A PERSPECTIVE ON PATIENT-CENTRIC, FEED-FORWARD "COLLABORATORIES"

Eugene C. Nelson, D.Sc., M.P.H., Elliott S. Fisher, M.D., M.P.H., and James N. Weinstein, D.O., M.S., The Dartmouth Institute for Health Policy and Clinical Practice at Dartmouth Medical School and Dartmouth–Hitchcock Medical Center

"It is important to note that clinical work doesn't have to be done at the expense of scholarly work. They should be and need to be done together."

James N. Weinstein, D.O., M.S.

This paper is intended to respond to a bold charge issued by the organizers of this workshop:

> To highlight complexities in and impediments associated with generating clinical information and knowledge, as well as to reflect on systems changes or incentives that might address the various asymmetries and barriers to use of clinical data for health learning.

The paper responds to this charge by first briefly describing the nature of the problem; then explaining the fundamental idea, providing a case study to demonstrate how the idea can work in the real world; and finally, outlining a path forward for enacting the proposed solution, taking into account some of the impediments and complexities that may arise. As suggested by the above quotation from Weinstein, a basic premise is that the intelligent design of health information systems can unite clinical practice with clinical research and contribute powerfully to a learning healthcare system, with everyone learning from his or her own practice base.

The Nature of the Problem

This section begins with a case study (fictitious name, but based on a real situation) that illustrates the nature of the problem:

> Terry Adams, author of a best-selling management book, was a 62-year-old business school professor with a history of disabling low back pain. He had experienced six prior flare-ups in the past decade. When he had an episode of back pain, he had excruciating pain that made him unable to function for days or weeks at a time. Over the years, Professor Adams had received episodic treatments by different clinicians in different practices and had concluded that nothing would work to prevent the problem. He stated: "No one knows what causes my flare-ups, treatments have not worked—except some reduced the pain in the short term. If there is such a thing as best-in-the-world care for people like me, none of the doctors or clinicians that I have seen seemed to know it! They usually respond to my questions about what works best with a phrase like, 'Well, Terry, in my experience. . . . Blah blah blah.' Where's the evidence? What actually works best for people like me? Moreover, it appears that the doctors and practitioners do not talk to each other, do not look at my past treatments, and do not know what treatments I have gotten, nor have they reviewed the results of the numerous x-rays and CT scans that I have had over the years. Every time I have a new and severe back problem, we start all over from scratch . . . history, physical, x-rays, CT scans, with no one learning anything from my earlier treatments and apparently no good research to know what treatment is likely to work best for a person with my condition. When I put on my business school hat and think about costs, I would guess that I have cost my Blue Cross plan about $55,000 on ED [emer-

gency department] visits, office visits, medications, physical therapy, and spine surgery, not to mention that my time lost from work might run about 120 days in the past 10 years, which would conservatively add another $120,000 in indirect costs associated with lost productivity.

This case represents a common situation: the presence of disconnected, partial, non-patient-centric data and information on the patient's health status and how it has evolved over time, plus limited information on prior healthcare experiences and the associated treatments and outcomes. This state of affairs is bad for patient care, bad for practice-based learning and improvement (a core competency of today's physician), and bad for clinical research and health professional education.

The case demonstrates some of the complexities and impediments associated with generating clinical information and knowledge for improvement, research, and learning. This is all too often the current state of affairs in the world of healthcare information systems. In general, (1) data do not follow the patient over time; (2) data are not turned into information to guide treatment, even though both the evidence base and information about the patient's personal preferences and values at the point of care and in the flow of care offer important guidance on treatment decisions; (3) data are not turned into information to make it possible to learn from every patient for retrospective or prospective research; (4) data systems inside organizations often are not integrated or interoperable across organizations; and (5) data entry often is not standardized, making it difficult to ascertain the diagnoses, the comorbidities, the severity, the diagnostic tests ordered, and the treatments prescribed, and to track the health outcomes and costs over time that are associated with the inputs (patient factors) and processes (treatment factors) of care. For all of these reasons, the healthcare system suffers a variety of information problems:

- inadequate information for high-quality, patient-centric clinical care;
- inadequate information with which to understand and improve the process of care;
- limited quality and cost measures to support public reporting on quality and value; and
- inadequate information for patient-based outcomes research.

If we cannot understand patients within our systems of care, how are we going to improve? Perhaps these problems can be overcome by designing data-rich, patient-centric, feed-forward information environments with real-time feedback using a novel approach that is described below. The challenge to be overcome is depicted in Figure 3-3. The feed-forward data

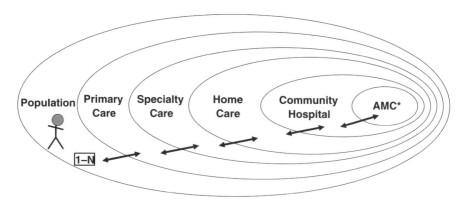

FIGURE 3-3 Feed-forward data challenge.
NOTE: AMC = academic medical center
SOURCE: Eugene C. Nelson and Trustees of Dartmouth College.

challenge is to keep the data connected to the individual patient and to the population of patients as they travel through the healthcare system. For example, during an illness patients receive services from different sites, such as primary care, specialty care, home health care, a community hospital, or an academic medical center. The objective is to turn an individual's data into useful information that can guide intelligent action and to aggregate this patient-level information to show quantifiable results within the clinical microsystem, the healthcare macrosystem, and the community.

The Fundamental Idea

The fundamental idea is to embed feed-forward information systems—with real-time feedback—into the flow of clinical care in frontline "clinical microsystems," meaning the places where patients, families, and caregivers meet—the places where care is delivered and where outcomes and costs are produced (Nelson et al., 2007a). The terms "feed forward" and "feedback" are described below:

- The term "feed forward" refers to designing an information system to collect patient data in real time as care is delivered. The data collection occurs from the first visit, and the data move with the patient as personal information. The data are always available and displayed in a useful format as the patient's healthcare experiences continue. In such a system of care, patients and providers can understand what they need to know, and patients are more likely to receive the right care at the right place at the right time, every time, based on accurate information and their own preferences.

- The term "feedback" refers to designing an information system at the level of the individual patient to accumulate these historical data in order to form subpopulations of patients, and it also refers to displaying patient and physician data for the prospective management of individual patients who are in the care system. Feedback is also necessary for the evaluation, management, and improvement of individual patient care. The information can then be rolled up to better understand populations of patients cared for by clinical programs. Furthermore, at no additional cost, the information provides a database that contributes to basic, translational, outcomes, and evaluative research and to health professional education (promoting practice-based learning and improvement as well as systems-based practice). This real-time feedback system closes the loop, with an active improvement process being part of a patient-centered, integrated clinical practice.

Figure 3-4 illustrates the feed-forward and feedback concepts in the context of a single clinical microsystem. In general, a patient enters a clinical microsystem and receives an orientation to that particular system.

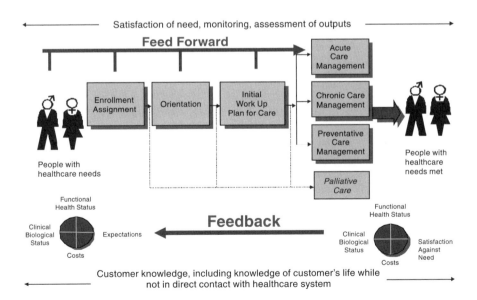

FIGURE 3-4 Feed-forward and feedback in the context of a general clinical microsystem.
SOURCE: Eugene C. Nelson and Trustees of Dartmouth College.

Then an initial health assessment is conducted, which leads to a plan of care based on that patient's health status, needs, and preferences. Many patients enter a system with appropriate indications for consideration of a diagnostic or therapeutic intervention, but appropriateness does not mean a patient prefers or wants the intervention. In "either–or" clinical situations, an approach must be used that is consistent with both best evidence and patients' preferences and values. This approach can be facilitated by feeding forward patient-based data on demographics, family history, clinical status, functional status, and expectations for desired health outcomes based on an individual patient's values and preferences, while healthcare costs are captured as important information for use in considering both the efficacy and efficiency of care. The clinician completes the assessment based on the patient's medical history, a physical examination, and diagnostic tests, all of which contribute to a patient-centric plan of care. The patient care plan will include a blend of services—preventive, acute, chronic, and palliative—based on the patient's current needs and preferences and on the success of the care plan at producing desired outcomes efficiently. These measures work best when collected longitudinally as part of normal clinical practice. They often include the patient's clinical status, functional status, and perceptions of the care received relative to the patient's needs, in addition to tracking other measures of direct and indirect costs of care for a given episode of illness. This information can then be used in a feedback mode to evaluate care for populations of patients and to improve care in specific clinical settings, and it can be incorporated in a database for research and education.

Of course, many patients with challenging and costly healthcare problems receive care from more than one clinical microsystem as the illness episode evolves. For example, a person who suffers an acute myocardial infarction (AMI) may receive care in a number of frontline microsystems, such as an ED, a coronary catheterization laboratory, a coronary care unit, and a cardiac step-down unit. This patient may receive follow-up care from a cardiac rehabilitation program, a cardiologist, and a primary care physician. Like Professor Adams in the above case study, the person may have concomitant conditions (e.g., back pain) with their own episodes. If one wishes to evaluate the success of care provided to a particular AMI patient—or for a population of patients who have comparable coronary events, such as ST[3]-elevated myocardial infarctions—one will need to follow the changes in health outcomes (clinical, functional, patient perceptions) and costs as the outcomes evolve over time (e.g., at 30 days, 3

---

[3] The ST segment is the part of an electrocardiogram immediately following the QRS complex and merging into the T wave.

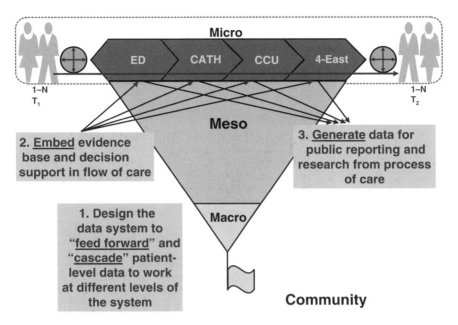

FIGURE 3-5 Data challenges: embed, feed forward, generate, and cascade.
SOURCE: Eugene C. Nelson and Trustees of Dartmouth College.

months, 6 months, 12 months after AMI) and be cognizant of concomitant illnesses and adjust for their impact.

Figure 3-5 illustrates this common illness episode situation in the context of a multilevel healthcare system serving a community. The AMI patient is moving "horizontally" through frontline clinical microsystems over time. The collection of microsystems that contribute to the care of the AMI patient can be viewed as a cardiovascular mesosystem, which is often part of a larger healthcare system (i.e., a macrosystem), such as a community hospital or academic medical center. This common situation poses several daunting challenges to the design of health information systems that contribute to patient care, research, and education while delivering the best possible results in the most efficient manner. The data challenges can be summarized by the phrase "embed, feed forward, generate, and cascade." Again referring to Figure 3-5, which portrays the healthcare system by blending "horizontally linked clinical microsystems" with "vertically organized healthcare delivery systems," we can see that there are three fundamental challenges to the design of high-utility healthcare information systems:

- Design the information system to feed forward and to cascade patient-level data to work at different levels of the healthcare system—micro, meso, macro, community, and region.
- Embed the evidence base and decision support—for patients and caregivers—in the flow of clinical care to enable the right care, consistent with patient preferences, to be delivered at the right place and at the right time, every time.
- Generate accurate data from the care process to be used for clinical program improvement, biomedical research, health professional education, and transparent public reporting on health outcomes and costs of care.

The core assumption is that in the design of high-utility EHRs it is not enough to have standardized nomenclature for the essential elements of care (tests, diagnoses, procedures, medications, and so forth). One must also have *patient-centric*, feed-forward, and feedback information systems to manage patients, improve processes, and serve as a research database for learning how to reliably produce better health outcomes, higher quality, and better value. Without this information, the EHR is not patient-centric, nor does it exemplify a learning healthcare system. The key term here is "patient-centric," which requires

- measurement of health status and outcomes that are consistent with the IOM's definition of health,
- the ability to follow patients over time as they move in and out of different parts of the healthcare system and to enable aggregation of data at different levels of the system (micro, meso, macro, community, and region), and
- use of patient reports as well as clinician reports of health status and health-related data in a consistent manner.

The term "health" is often used without an agreed-upon definition, but it is important to define exactly what the term means if one intends to design a "health" information system. The IOM has defined health in this way: "Health is a state of well-being and the capability to function in the face of changing circumstances. Health is a positive concept emphasizing social and personal resources as well as physical capabilities" (IOM, 1997). Improving health is a shared responsibility of healthcare providers, public health officials, and a variety of actors in the community who can contribute to the well-being of individuals and populations.

If one wishes to measure, study, and improve the outcomes and costs of care, it is also important to have an agreed-upon framework for defining

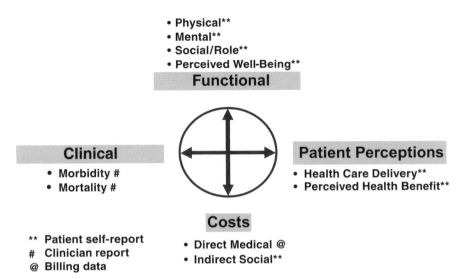

FIGURE 3-6 Value compass framework for measuring outcomes and costs of care and demonstrating the need for patient- and clinician-reported data.
SOURCE: Eugene C. Nelson and Trustees of Dartmouth College.

what is meant by outcomes and costs. One useful paradigm for defining and measuring outcomes and costs is the clinical value compass, which is shown in Figure 3-6 (Nelson et al., 1996, 2007b). The value compass approach suggests that the quality of patient care outcomes can be measured by focusing on three domains—clinical, functional, and satisfaction against need—whereas the costs of care can be captured in a fourth domain, which is measured by determining the direct costs of providing care to patients and the indirect social costs patients incur by being ill or injured and receiving care. Consequently, one way to measure the value of patient care is to assess quality in relationship to costs over time. A careful examination of the data required to measure quality in relationship to costs reveals that some areas can best be measured on the basis of clinician-reported data, some on the basis of patient-reported data, and some on the basis of billing data. These "best sources" are specified in Figure 3-6.

To summarize, the fundamental idea is that if we wish to have an information system that can generate clinical information and knowledge and that can create the conditions necessary to build a learning healthcare system, we will need to design feed-forward and feedback information systems that can

- be embedded in the flow of patient care and can enhance patient care, research, and education and capture patient- and clinician-reported data in a standardized way;
- aggregate data horizontally to capture outcomes of patients and populations over time, and aggregate data vertically to portray quality and cost outcomes at different levels of the system—micro, meso, macro, community, and region; and
- be responsive to the IOM's definition of health, which emphasizes the functional health status of the individual and reflects the social need to increase the value of care by providing better-quality results in a more efficient manner.

The next section offers a case study to demonstrate that these demanding requirements for designing this kind of information system can be met in the real world of health care.

A Case Study

To explore the fundamental idea presented above, this section presents a case study involving the Dartmouth Spine Center, the collaborative National Spine Network, and a unique randomized controlled trial sponsored by the National Institutes of Health (NIH)—along with a simultaneous observational and preference-based cohort study—that involved evaluating the effectiveness of alternative methods for treating the most common spinal problems. The case study started when James Weinstein came to Dartmouth in 1996 to lead the orthopedic surgery program. He is an orthopedic surgeon with interests in basic research on pain, outcomes research, and patient-centered, shared decision-making research (Weinstein et al., 2000).

Upon coming to Dartmouth, Weinstein had the opportunity to start an innovative interdisciplinary program for back and neck care and to design it from the ground up—such a program had not existed at Dartmouth, and even today, 12 years later, still may not exist anywhere else. Part of the plan for what would come to be called the Dartmouth Spine Center was to build a real-time, feed-forward information environment, using the clinical value compass framework, that would actively contribute to better patient care, better research, and a better learning environment. This information environment was built for primary and subspecialty care, all delivered and integrated within the same home, addressing a multidimensional set of clinical problems with an interdisciplinary, patient-centered approach and incorporating patients' values and preferences.

In planning the Spine Center, it was decided that the mission would be patient-centric: to get people back to work and back to play, one back at a time. The vision for the information system was to implement the feed-forward idea in real time, embedding standardized methods for patient- and clinician-based reporting into the flow of care. Every time a patient was seen at the center, a database would accumulate information for (1) achieving better shared decision making by both patients and clinicians; (2) accomplishing better care planning to match needs, preferences, and the evidence base to treatments selected; (3) monitoring the effect of care on individual patients using standard metrics; (4) improving the center's ability to track outcomes and to use this information for improving care; (5) contributing to the National Spine Network, a comparative database involving more than 25 clinical programs across the country; and (6) building the infrastructure to conduct leading-edge prospective and retrospective research, such as the Spine Patient Outcomes Research Trial (Weinstein et al., 2006, 2007a).

Figure 3-4 shows what a feed-forward/feedback system might look like in general, while Figure 3-7 shows how such a system was designed to work in the Spine Center. When patients come to the Spine Center, they complete a computerized survey before seeing a clinician or clinical team, and their health status and expectations are recorded. That information feeds into the assessment. The clinician, or clinical team, adds information on the severity of disease, on the patient's diagnoses, and on the tests and treatments being ordered. This information contributes to a care plan that matches health status and patient preferences with the relevant evidence base and contributes to the patient's making informed decisions in cooperation with the clinician (Weinstein et al., 2007b). Patients are then assigned to different customized tracks depending on their health needs and their willingness to adhere to (or select) a particular treatment approach consistent with their preferences and values. They are followed over time as they come back to the center and update their health status information and their perceptions of the benefits of their treatment compared with their expectations. The clinician continues to use and update the standardized, fixed-field information. Charge data are extracted from billing records and added to the information system so the patient and clinical team can see, in a quantifiable and measurable way, how the patient's health outcomes are changing over time in response to treatments and how this change is influencing the costs associated with care. This same information contributes to the National Spine Network's comparative database, used to assess the Spine Center's performance in contrast to that of its peers, and it offers a database for program improvement and for research.

In practice, patients complete their health survey either when they visit the Spine Center or on the Internet before traveling to the center. The survey is analyzed instantly, and it becomes the first page of the patient's medical record so that when the patient sees the clinician, they are literally on the same page. The patient and practitioners can view the patient's clinical and functioning status and outcomes the patient hopes to experience. This information is used to promote shared and informed decision making, which leads to a plan of care for the patient. The one-page summary includes such essential information as patient history, symptoms, the patient's perceived options for treatment and desired health benefits, and clinical and functioning status. This information is updated over time and is available for each visit, making it possible to compare visits over time. Figures 3-7 through 3-8 illustrate the process and the one-page summary report.

The Dartmouth Spine Center feed-forward information system has been running and evolving for more than a decade. With research grant support from the NIH, a similar data system was exported to 13 other medical centers in 11 states across the country to gather data for randomized controlled trials and for observational cohorts concerning back surgery; the data have resulted in numerous articles in leading clinical journals (Weinstein et al., 2007a). In addition, the feed-forward system has been adapted for several other clinical programs at Dartmouth–Hitchcock Medical Center, including breast cancer, general internal medicine, plastic surgery, bone marrow transplant, and cardiovascular care.

The Spine Center case provides a proof of principle for the patient-

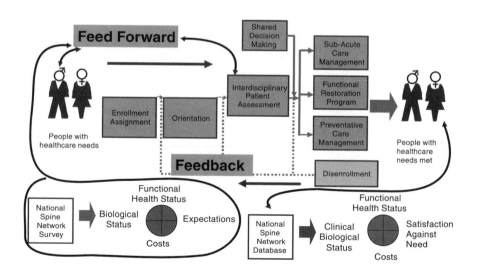

FIGURE 3-7 Spine Center process for a feed-forward and feedback information system.
SOURCE: Eugene C. Nelson and Trustees of Dartmouth College.

centric, feed-forward collaborative idea. The data system supports individualized, patient-centered care. Clinicians are now able to inform patients about their chances of success and the likelihood of complications for nonoperative vs. surgical treatment options based on research on people like them. Data are used for program evaluation and improvement as well as for comparative benchmarking. The data system contributes to the infrastructure for interdisciplinary research programs—from bench to bedside to outcomes experienced by patients. It is being used for retrospective and prospective research. Quality and cost data are published on the Dartmouth–Hitchcock website (DHMC, 2008) for transparent public reporting on important populations of patients. This initiative has helped the organization become an accountable healthcare system (Nelson et al., 2005).

One interesting footnote to the Spine Center case study is that Terry Adams, the Dartmouth business school professor mentioned earlier, had the experience of going to the Spine Center soon after it opened its doors. He did not know that the Spine Center had been designed based on his own research concerning how the world's best-in-class service organizations worked to bring quality and value to customers at the point of service, but he was moved to write a letter to the local newspaper about the wonderful care he had just received from the center. He praised the center for using innovative information technology to focus on the patient's individual and unique health state, to elicit the patient's expectations for care outcomes and explore all treatment options, to help patients make wise treatment decisions based on medical evidence and personal preferences, and to work smoothly with a full interdisciplinary team without having to go from clinic to clinic and experience frustrating waits and delays.

Discussion: A Solution, Limitations, and Conclusions

This final section of the paper proposes a solution to the challenge cited at the beginning of the paper, describes some of the limitations associated with this solution, and offers concluding remarks.

The Challenge and a Solution

If the aim is to build an information environment capable of generating clinical information and knowledge that can promote a learning healthcare system, we believe an essential part of the solution—although clearly not the full solution—is to intentionally develop what we call "patient-centric, professionally organized, feed-forward collaboratories." A few brief descriptions of the key terms in this phrase follow:

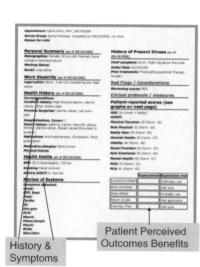
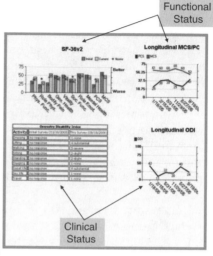

Functional Status

History & Symptoms

Patient Perceived Outcomes Benefits

Clinical Status

Appointment: 13187408; Spine Clinic; RHV; 09/19/2006
Survey: 69032; Spine Followup; completed on 09/19/2006; 19 mins
Reason for visit:

Personal Summary *(as of 09/19/2006)*
Demographics: Female; 80 yrs old; Married; Some college or technical school
Working Status:
Physical requirements of job/activity:
Social: Lives alone
Physical events since last visit: None
Psych-social events since last visit: None

Work Disability *(as of 09/19/2006)*
Legal action: None

Health History *(as of 09/19/2006)*
Current conditions:
Condition history: High blood pressure; Uterine cancer; Other chronic pain
Previous Surgeries: Uterine cancer; Not sure - pain
Hospitalizations, Cancer: 1
Family history: Asthma, Cancer, Penicillin allergy, Stroke; Uterine Cancer, Breast Cancer
Family Members w/ Breast Cancer: One sister or brother
Medications: Anti-hypertension, Cholesterol, Other prescription
Medication allergies: None known
Physical Events since last visit:

Health Habits *(as of 09/19/2006)*
BMI: 28.3 (Overweight); 155 lbs
Alcohol AUDIT: 0: non-drinker
Tobacco use: Never smoked / chew tobacco

Review of Systems
Const: Weight loss; Weakness; Fatigue, lack of energy; Fever or chills; Pain
ENT, Eyes: Dry mouth
Resp: Wheezing; Shortness of breath
Cardio: Heart palpitations (fluttering heart beat); Swelling of arms or legs

History of Present Illness *(as of 09/19/2006)*
Problem Areas: Groin, Right leg above the knee
Initial Visit: 01/18/2005
Prior treatments: Physical/Occupational Therapy, Surgery

Red Flags / Considerations
Worsening SF-36 scores: MCS

Clinical protocols / measures

Patient-reported scores (see graphs on next page)
ODI: 24 (lower = better)
AUDIT:
SF-36v2 - Physical Function: 45 (Norm: 38)
SF-36v2 - Role Physical: 32 (Norm: 40)
SF-36v2 - Bodily Pain: 55 (Norm: 45)
SF-36v2 - General Health: 46 (Norm: 47)
SF-36v2 - Vitality: 46 (Norm: 48)
SF-36v2 - Social Function: 40 (Norm: 47)
SF-36v2 - Role Emotional: 56 (Norm: 44)
SF-36v2 - Mental Health: 50 (Norm: 51)
SF-36v2 - MCS: 52 (Norm: 51)
SF-36v2 - PCS: 41 (Norm: 40)

	Expectations	Expectation met
Symptoms Relief:	Not applicable	Definitely yes
More Activities:	Not applicable	
Sleep Better:	Not applicable	Definitely yes
Return to job:	Not applicable	
Exercise / Rec:	Not applicable	Definitely yes

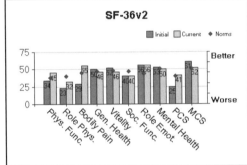

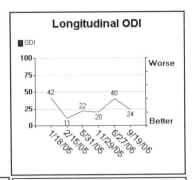

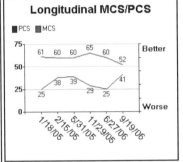

FIGURE 3-8 Patient summary report with longitudinal data: Dartmouth Spine Center.
NOTE: MCS = mental component scale, ODI = oswestry disability index, PCS = physical component scale.
SOURCE: James N. Weinstein and Trustees of Dartmouth College and Dynamic Clinical Systems, Inc.

- *Patient-centric*—The individual patient's health status, health risks, decisions based on preferences and values, perceptions of good care and good outcomes, and costs of care are at the forefront of all that is done (IOM, 2001).
- *Professionally organized*—The healthcare professionals who serve patients are expected to be responsible for the design of patient-centric delivery systems and the supporting information systems that enable them to partner with patients in delivering patient-centric care.
- *Feed forward*—Keeping patients and their data together over time requires a well-designed information system that enables key information and data to move with the patient through the healthcare

system over time to promote quality, safety, efficiency, and the best and safest match of services to patient health needs at any point in time and at any place in the system.

- *Collaboratories*—The term denotes a method for organizing virtual organizations in a complex world that combines the idea of collaboration across physically distinct settings and the idea of a scientific laboratory. The purpose is to form a community of practice that can build shared information repositories for use in advancing science and improving practice (Schneiderman, 2008).

What we are proposing, therefore, is to thoughtfully design and test innovative collaboratories that have all of the key features embedded in the Spine Center case. Some of the key characteristics of healthcare collaboratories would be

- patient-centric and focused on relevant dimensions of health outcomes for any given population of patients;
- professionally organized to fit into the flow of health care for the purpose of improving care while contributing to research and education;
- based on feed-forward methods to follow patients over time as their healthcare experience evolves and to better match patients' changing health status with an evidence-based preference-sensitive plan of care; and
- dependent on feedback methods to track health risks, health status, diagnoses, and treatments associated with health outcomes and costs and to analyze results at multiple levels of the system (patient, micro, meso, macro, community, and region).

This type of population-specific, feed-forward collaboratory could advance goals on three major fronts:

- *Health care*—Provide better care for patients by matching wants, needs, and health status with desired, effective, and efficient treatments.
- *Health research*—Provide data for observational and prospective research on the causes of disease and disability and on the effectiveness of alternative methods for treating disease and disability.
- *Health professional education*—Create better learning environments that are information rich, patient focused, outcomes driven, and engaged in advancing healthcare science as part of regular work.

The idea of patient-centric, feed-forward collaboratories is innovative, but not new. The best examples we know of today are the Dartmouth Spine Center and the National Spine Network (Weinstein et al., 2000), as well as the Karolinska Institute and the Swedish Rheumatoid Arthritis Registry. However, there are other research networks and communities of practice that have some collaboratory features, including the Cystic Fibrosis Foundation and cystic fibrosis centers in the United States; the Vermont Oxford Project and neonatal intensive care units in North America and Europe; the Autism Program at Geisinger Health System; the Northern New England Cardiovascular Group and cardiovascular programs in Maine, New Hampshire, and Vermont; and the Clinical Program Model at Intermountain Health Care (James and Lazar, 2007).

Limitations

Any effort to work with professional organizations and health systems to develop and evaluate feed-forward collaboratories will have to recognize the current reality and some of the challenges and limitations this reality imposes. A few of these are listed below:

- *Vision*—Only a few models of collaboratories in health care are available, and these are not well known.
- *Rewards*—Limited incentives and resources exist to establish collaboratories (at least in a non–Clinical Translational Science Award [CTSA] world).
- *Health Insurance Portability and Accountability Act and security*—Following patients over time and across settings requires careful attention to privacy and security issues.
- *Measurement*—Only a limited number of patient-based "gold standard" metrics exist for gathering both generic and condition-specific information.
- *Standardization*—Resistance exists among many clinicians to using standard, fixed-field data entry, and there are concerns about wasting time and doing work that is not value added.
- *Patient role*—It is a new role for the patient to act as a primary reporter of key information using standard approaches. Exercising this role will require changes in patients' expectations and an understanding that their information-providing task is essential for their own care as well as for improving care and advancing science.

These challenges suggest the need to develop demonstration programs to evaluate, validate, and refine the feed-forward collaboratory approach.

Conclusion

The time may be right for testing the patient-centric, feed-forward collaborative model. Powerful forces at work are creating a climate favorable to the development of collaboratories. These forces include communities of professional practice combining patient care and health research, the funding of research by the NIH through the new CTSA approach, the formation of regional health information organizations across the country, the emergence of new scientific paradigms that recognize complexity and the value of multiple research methods, and demands for better quality and value that are measured and transparent. An excellent example of these forces coming together can be seen in the new National Quality Forum (NQF) framework that is being considered for measuring the outcomes and efficiency of episodes of care. The NQF approach is illustrated in Figure 3-9. It calls for the collection of feed-forward, patient-centric data on populations of at-risk individuals residing in different regions of the country. Then, after the onset of an illness episode, it calls for following people over time to measure critical information, including patient factors for risk adjustment, informed decisions guided by patient preferences, treatment processes, symptoms, physical function, and emotional status. Finally,

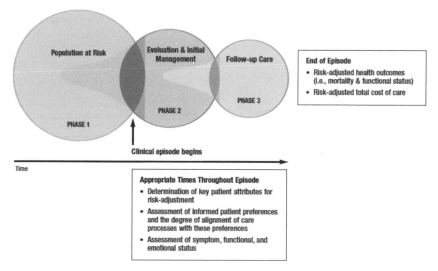

FIGURE 3-9 Generic episodes of care.
SOURCE: Reprinted with permission from the National Quality Forum (NQF, 2009).

at the end of the illness episode, it calls for completing the assessment by measuring mortality, functional status, and costs of care.

The following statement by Fisher (2008) summarizes the value of designing patient-centric, feed-forward healthcare collaboratories:

> The same underlying information system is required to improve the evidence base for both biotechnology and care delivery. We need to know:
> - Patient attributes and risks (including biologic markers).
> - Specific, targeted biologic interventions performed.
> - Attributes of the system—delivery methods—where care is provided.
> - Health outcomes and costs.
>
> We could then have a truly learning healthcare system:
>
> - *Comparative effectiveness research:* Compare biologic interventions, controlling for patient and system attributes.
> - *Comparative performance assessment:* Compare systems and care delivery methods, controlling for patient and treatment attributes.

The bold aim is to achieve better patient and population health and better healthcare outcomes by applying research and education. Accomplishing this aim will require that our health system become composed of *learning* healthcare systems. We conclude with four key points. First, the IOM definition of health stresses the functioning and well-being of the individual and requires patient-reported information to measure health status. Second, patient-centric health risks, health status, and health outcomes are an essential component of any comprehensive approach for improving health care and studying health outcomes. Third, it will be essential to design feed-forward information systems to accomplish the tripartite aim of improving healthcare outcomes, advancing biomedical research, and enhancing health professional learning. Fourth, we believe that developing and testing patient-centric, professionally organized collaboratories can help the nation achieve this bold aim.

REFERENCES

Ash, J. S., M. Berg, and E. Coiera. 2004. Some unintended consequences of information technology in health care: The nature of patient care information system-related errors. *Journal of the American Medical Information Association* 11(2):104–112.

Bates, D. W. 2005. Physicians and ambulatory electronic health records. *Health Affairs* 24(5): 1180–1189.

Brenner, D. J., and E. J. Hall. 2007. Computed tomography—an increasing source of radiation exposure. *New England Journal of Medicine* 357(22):2277–2284.

DHMC (Dartmouth Hitchcock Medical Center). 2008. *Quality reports.* http://www.dhmc.org/qualityreports (accessed June 6, 2008).

Farnsworth, C. 2005. *Testimony before the House Ways and Means Subcommittee on Health.* U.S. Congress, House of Representatives. March 17.

Fisher, E. S. 2008. Learning to deliver better health care: Rigorous study of the most effective ways to deliver care as well as what care works best can result in not only better treatment but also significant cost savings. *Issues in Science and Technology* 24(3):58–62. Spring 2008.

Gray, R. M., W. R. Newman, and A. M. Reinhardt. 1996. The effect of medical specialization on physicians' attitudes. *Journal of Health and Human Behavior* 7(2):128–132.

IOM (Institute of Medicine). 1997. *Improving health in the community: A role for performance monitoring.* Washington, DC: National Academy Press.

_____. 2000. *To err is human: Building a safer health system.* Washington, DC: National Academy Press.

_____. 2001. *Crossing the quality chasm.* Washington, DC: National Academy Press.

_____. 2007. Clinicians and the electronic health record as a learning tool. In *The learning healthcare system* (pp. 268-274). Washington, DC: The National Academies Press.

_____. 2009a. Evidence-based medicine and the changing nature of health care. In *Leadership commitments to improve value in health care: Finding common ground.* Washington, DC: The National Academies Press.

_____. 2009b. Practical frontline challenges to moving beyond the expert-based practice. In *Leadership commitments to improve value in health care: Finding common ground.* Washington, DC: The National Academies Press.

James, B., and J. Lazar. 2007. Sustaining and extending clinical improvements: A health system's use of clinical programs to build quality infrastructure. In *Practice-based learning and improvement: A clinical improvement action guide,* 2nd ed. Joint Commission Resources.

Karsh, B. T. 2004. Beyond usability: Designing effective technology implementation systems to promote patient safety. *Quality and Safety in Health Care* 13(5):388–394.

Kawamoto, K., C. A. Houlihan, E. A. Balas, and D. F. Lobach. 2005. Improving clinical practice using clinical decision support systems: A systematic review of trials to identify features critical to success. *British Medical Journal* 330(7494):765.

Lin, G. A., R. A. Dudley, and R. F. Redberg. 2007. Cardiologists' use of percutaneous coronary interventions for stable coronary artery disease. *Archives of Internal Medicine* 167(15):1604–1609.

_____. 2008. Why physicians favor use of percutaneous coronary intervention to medical therapy: A focus group study. *Journal of General Internal Medicine* 23(9):1458–1463.

MedPAC (Medicare Payment Advisory Commission). 2007. *MedPAC 2007 report to Congress.* Washington, DC: MedPAC

Miller, G. A. 1956. The magical number seven plus or minus two: Some limits on our capacity for processing information. *Psychological Review* 63(2):81–97.

National Priorities Partnership. 2008. *National priorities and goals: Aligning our efforts to transform America's healthcare.* Washington, DC: National Quality Forum.

NQF (National Quality Forum). 2009. *Measurement framework: evaluating efficiency across patient-focused episodes of care.* Washington, DC: National Quality Forum.

Nelson, E. C., P. B. Batalden, S. K. Plume, and J. J. Mohr. 1996. Improving health care, part 1: The clinical value compass. *Joint Commission Journal on Quality Improvement* 22(8):243–258.

Nelson, E. C., K. Homa, M. Mastenduno, E. S. Fisher, P. B. Batalden, E. F. Malcolm, T. C. Foster, D. S. Likosky, J. A. Guth, and P. B. Gardent. 2005. Publicly reporting comprehensive quality and cost data: A health care system's transparency initiative. *Joint Commission Journal of Quality Improvement* 31(10):573–584.

Nelson, E. C., P. B. Batalden, and M. Godfrey. 2007a. *Quality by design: A clinical microsystems approach.* San Francisco, CA: Jossey–Bass.

Nelson, E. C., P. B. Batalden, and J. Lazar. 2007b. *Practice-based learning and improvement: A clinical improvement action guide*, 2nd ed. Oakbrook Terrance: Joint Commission Resources, Inc.

Nolte, E., and C. M. McKee. 2008. Measuring the health of nations: Updating an earlier analysis. *Health Affairs (Millwood)* 27(1):58–71.

Norris, P. 2007. Skeptical patients: Performance, social capital, and culture. In D. A. Shore (ed.), *The trust crisis in healthcare: Causes, consequences, and cures* (pp. 32-46). New York: Oxford University Press.

Peterson, E. D. 2008. Is information the answer for hypertension control? *Archives of Internal Medicine* 168(3):259–260.

Pham, H. H. 2007. Care patterns in Medicare and their implications for pay for performance. *New England Journal of Medicine* 356:1130–1139.

Porter, M., and E. O. Teisberg. 2006. *Redefining health care: Creating value-based competition on results*. Boston, MA: Harvard Business School Press.

Pronovost, P. J., C. A. Goeschel, and R. M. Wachter. 2008. The wisdom and justice of not paying for "preventable complications." *JAMA* 299(18):2197–2199.

Redberg, R. F. 2007. Evidence, appropriateness, and technology assessment in cardiology: A case study of computed tomography. *Health Affairs (Millwood)* 26(1):86–95.

Rotschild, M., N. Elias, D. Berkowitz, S. Pollak, M. Shinawi, R. Beck, and L. Bentur. 2005. Autoantibodies against bactericidal/permeability-increasing protein (bpi-anca) in cystic fibrosis patients treated with azithromycin. *Clinical and Experimental Medicine* 5(2):80–85.

Schneiderman, B. 2008. Science 2.0. *Science* 319:1349–1350.

Shih, A., J. Quinley, T. K. Lee, and C. R. Messina. 2002. Assessing pneumococcal revaccination safety among New York state Medicare beneficiaries. *Public Health Reports* 117(2):164–173.

Silber, J. H., S. V. Williams, H. Krakauer, and J. S. Schwartz. 1992. Hospital and patient characteristics associated with death after surgery. A study of adverse occurrence and failure to rescue. *Medical Care* 30(7):615–629.

Warburton, R. N. 2005. Preliminary outcomes and cost–benefit analysis of a community hospital emergency department screening and referral program for patients aged 75 or more. *International Journal of Health Care Quality Assurance Incorporating Leadership in Health Services* 18(6–7):474–484.

Weinstein, J. N., P. W. Brown, B. Hanscom, T. Walsh, and E. C. Nelson. 2000. Designing an ambulatory clinical practice for outcomes improvement: From vision to reality. *Quality Management in Health Care* 8(2):1–20.

Weinstein, J. N., T. D. Tosteson, J. D. Lurie, A. N. Tosteson, B. Hanscom, J. S. Skinner, W. A. Abdu, A. S. Hilibrand, S. D. Boden, and R. A. Deyo. 2006. Surgical vs. nonoperative treatment for lumbar disk herniation: The Spine Patient Outcomes Research Trial (SPORT): A randomized trial. *JAMA* 296(20):2441–2450.

Weinstein, J. N., T. D. Tosteson, J. D. Lurie, A. N. A. Tosteson, E. Blood, B. Hanscom, H. Herkowitz, F. Cammisa, T. Albert, S. D. Boden, A. Hilibrand, H. Goldberg, S. Berven, H. An, and SPORT Investigators. 2007a. Surgical vs. nonsurgical treatment for lumbar degenerative spondylolisthesis. *New England Journal of Medicine* 356:2257–2270.

Weinstein, J. N., K. Clay, and T. S. Morgan. 2007b. Informed patient choice: Patient-centered valuing of surgical risks and benefits. *Health Affairs* 26(3):726–730.

4

Case Studies in Transformation Through Systems Engineering

INTRODUCTION

Creative approaches are necessary to meet the Roundtable's goal that "by the year 2020, 90 percent of clinical decisions will be supported by accurate, timely, and up-to-date clinical information and will reflect the best available evidence." In this section of the workshop, guidance was solicited from organizations both within and outside health care that have achieved successful elements of transformation. Presenters provided accounts of their achievements and offered insights into their organization's transformation through approaches to systems engineering. The aim was to stimulate the sense of what might be possible in health care through the lenses of three industries in particular: airlines, manufacturing, and health care.

For practitioners seeking to reform various aspects of health care, good models of the applications of principles, tools, and practices from systems engineering can be found in both business settings and healthcare systems. Four veterans of such work described their experiences to the workshop audience, discussing how complex enterprises have successfully developed systems-oriented procedures and integrated a systems orientation into practice. The session investigated how systems engineering has been successfully applied in the three industries and sought to understand which lessons might be applied to the transformation of the sociologically and technologically complex healthcare sector. Implicit in the discussions was the importance of bold leadership in driving reform, the imperative of having clarity of mission, the merits of developing strong metrics and sharing results widely, and the value of investing in people.

John J. Nance, founding member of the National Patient Safety Foundation, reported on a rich set of systems reforms that has been achieved by the aviation industry. Nance highlighted strategies that go beyond well-honed aviation practices, such as checklists and methodologies in crew resource management (CRM), which could be of benefit to healthcare systems. He described how systems engineering has been applied in sophisticated feedback systems for reporting and learning from mechanical problems, the development of robust computerized processes for many aspects of daily operations, and standardization that has been applied widely across airline operations. He also described systems that have been built around the assumption that human beings can never be perfect, and thus they are designed to be capable of absorbing anticipated levels of human failure. The discussion also touched on the importance of applying systems thinking to training, on the value of improved communication among staff at all levels, on the usefulness of minimization of variables, and on how systems interact.

To demonstrate how systems thinking can help effect deep-set, meaningful, and lasting organizational change, Earnest J. Edwards, formerly of Alcoa, Inc., focused on improvements in a specific business practice, the financial close process. Detailing how a similar change effort was applied successfully in a leading corporation, a federal government agency, and a community hospital, Edwards demonstrated how systems thinking can help organizations lower costs, improve quality, and leverage systems to yield better information for use in decision making. Moreover, he suggested, undertaking the process of change can itself help staff learn how to become solution-oriented change agents with a focus on the future—and thus become more vital partners in the enterprise, with an expanded role in strategic decisions.

Kenneth W. Kizer, chair of Medsphere Systems Corporation, began by describing the condition of the veterans healthcare system in the early 1990s. Managed by the Veterans Health Administration (VHA) in the U.S. Department of Veterans Affairs (VA), it was considered inefficient and indifferent to patient needs. Kizer described how, through a concerted reengineering effort, the VA healthcare system was transformed into a model healthcare provider. Kizer described how the VA overhauled its accountable management structure and control system, integrated and coordinated patient services across the continuum of care, improved and standardized the quality of care, improved information management, and aligned the system's finances with desired outcomes. Kizer suggested that similar interventions could help other healthcare enterprises achieve new levels of success.

In the final presentation described in this chapter, David B. Pryor, chief medical officer of Ascension Health, discussed the clinical transformation of Ascension, which is the largest not-for-profit delivery system in the United

States and the third largest system overall after the VA and the Hospital Corporation of America. Pryor described Ascension Health's "Call to Action," a program designed to reduce preventable injuries or deaths as well as to achieve certain other measurable goals. Pryor outlined a systems process for defining challenges, strategizing opportunities, focusing on goals, implementing action plans, and testing and measuring results that allowed Ascension Health to reach its goals. Pryor said that through this process Ascension Health was able to simultaneously realize outstanding clinical outcomes, achieve promising trends in financial outcomes, and develop new metrics that influence quality across its entire system.

AIRLINE SAFETY

John J. Nance, J.D., National Patient Safety
Foundation, American Medical Association

Although it would be hyperbole to say that the solution to much of what troubles American health care can be found in engineering disciplines, I truly believe that engineering and the engineering community can provide unprecedented expertise and contribute substantially, if not pivotally, to the national task of creating order out of the chaos that characterizes American health care today. This is not to demean health care. I am merely being frank about the reality that a cottage industry based on individual physician autonomy has grown to unmanageable proportions on a thoroughly inadequate organizational base. A century ago, hospitals were few and far between, and the remarkable advances in medicine and equipment achieved since that time have essentially been forced to fit the archaic mold that was established in that period. And the system clearly is not working in terms of either the reliable and safe delivery of the best care or the best value. Engineering philosophies, approaches, and discipline are not a cure-all, but where medicine has been unable to formulate a structural approach to the problem through traditional methodologies, new thinking from external disciplines may be of great benefit.

American health care needs to find a balance between two extremes. At one end of the spectrum is the clearly inadequate 19th century model of the individual doctor and the hospital as a sort of market that provides beds, nurses, and lights. At the other end is a rigid, mechanized approach to health care whereby autonomy is limited to small differences in the techniques physicians may use within the context of inflexible procedures and full employment directly by healthcare providers. Obviously, neither extreme can take advantage of both the remarkable advances in science-based medicine and the dexterity, intellect, and analytical abilities of individual physicians (as well as the human caring–based attention of nurses as the bedside eyes and ears of the physician). One extreme needs no engineering, while the other would overuse both systems engineering and the lessons from such fields as airline safety. A careful balance is needed that preserves the humanity and individual expertise of healthcare practitioners while providing an efficient and workable structure that serves the primary goal of doing the best possible job for patients and having physicians enjoy their profession.

These introductory points are important in any discussion that looks beyond medicine for answers, and this is especially true with respect to the applicable lessons from airline and aviation safety. The application of those lessons, as well as a brief look at how U.S. airlines have achieved a nearly perfect safety record, requires a basic understanding of the strategy employed and not just the tactical details of individual training programs and methods.

My professional background melds aviation and medicine and includes 18 years of experience in translating to health care the surprising human lessons we were forced to learn in the aviation industry (along with lessons from other fields such as nuclear power generation). In summary, by the late 1970s, aviation had reached the limits of its ability to improve safety significantly through merely mechanical and procedural means, and it was only by applying lessons from the human factors and performance disciplines that the airline industry was able to take the final step toward zero accidents and incidents.

In many ways this nearly unnoticed transition can be characterized as moving from a reliance on the principles of mechanical and aeronautical engineering to an acceptance of the principles and benefits of human systems engineering. The sometimes difficult transformation from a myopic focus on mechanical reliability to a focus on overall systemic reliability was guided at every step by the discipline engineering brought to bear in helping the airlines accept the realities of the potential for human failure and the resulting ability of airline safety leaders to impose better order and function. In other words, we finally had to stop believing that the only bulwark against accidents was the fine-tuning of our machines and black boxes and admit that, when even the finest airplanes could be flown into a mountain by a well-trained but confused and distracted aircrew, the failure modes of the human being would have to be addressed. The important point for the present discussion is that the same elements of transition are needed in American health care—and even more dramatically so because the procedural/mechanical side and the human systems engineering side of health care are equally undeveloped and undisciplined. To help explain why this is the case, let me focus on the experience of aviation.

For perhaps 10 years now, there has been a growing realization that aviation's experience in transitioning from a high-risk industry to a low-risk, high-reliability industry has some applicability to American health care. The problem has been oversimplification in translating that message. People in both aviation and medicine have believed that the best lessons the aviation industry can offer to health care are simply a few specific programs and methods, such as CRM courses and checklist procedures.[1] The assumption was that such tactical solutions could be transferred intact to the medical arena and yield the same dramatic improvement they achieved in aviation. In reality, while the principles of each of those tactical measures can benefit medicine if properly translated and adjusted for the realities and complexities of medical practice and application, a far richer body of lessons and benefits can be derived from aviation's experience.

Aviation, of course, is inherently no smarter about preventing disasters than is health care. But the fact that our failures were both very public and very frightening to our future customers and the fact that our death tolls reached large numbers with each major accident meant we had to address the last remaining unsolved cause of airline accidents—human mistakes— decades before health care had to face that same issue. We simply did not have the luxury of waiting for improvements to evolve. We had to figure out why dedicated, intelligent, and well-meaning air crews continued to fly mechanically perfect airliners into the ground or otherwise cause horrible accidents—so-called "pilot error" accidents.

In truth, the safety challenges the airline industry faced through the 1970s were perplexing. We had enjoyed great progress in airline safety from the dawn of commercial aviation in the late 1920s through the dawn of the jet age in the 1960s and into the 1970s. In fact, the curve of major accidents plotted against time had been declining at a remarkable rate as the machines were greatly improved, instrument flying became sophisticated, and the new jet engines introduced far greater reliability. That descending curve also represented greatly decreasing passenger fatalities, and while our metrics left something to be desired, we clearly improved by many orders of magnitude over time as mechanical failures triggering accidents became increasingly rare. Boeing, McDonnell Douglas, Convair, and later Airbus all learned how to build significant redundancy into their products, helping to pioneer the principle that no single or even dual failure of any component should ever result in the loss of control of an airplane. In fact, one of the earliest instances of human factors engineering was the decision, based on an understanding of the human propensity for failure, to have at

---

[1] CRM is a discipline that recognizes that no one leader, captain, or physician is capable of perfection. Therefore, the best defense against disaster due to human error is to utilize the professional talent and cognitive abilities of all participants through collegial communication that can be codified, taught, and required.

least two pilots in each commercial cockpit specifically to provide a human backup system. For the most part, the positive safety trends—albeit mostly mechanically based—continued into the 1980s and 1990s. With only a few exceptions—a faulty cargo-door latching mechanism (United 811, 1989, south of Honolulu); a destroyed engine and flight control system in a United DC-10 flight ending in Sioux City, Iowa, in July of the same year; the loss of the upper forward fuselage of a highly corroded Boeing 737 belonging to Aloha Airlines south of Maui in 1986; and the loss of TWA 800 due to a fuel tank explosion years later near Moriches, New York—by and large it had become a rule that when an airliner was destroyed, with or without loss of life, the primary contributing cause was human error. Indeed, records show that this was true in more than 90 percent of cases. Even the term "pilot error" (which implies a professional discretionary mistake such as making a conscious decision to violate the rules, with catastrophic results) was criticized as inadequate because being human inevitably implies being able to make errors that sometimes cause accidents.

By the 1970s, the trend curve for major airline accidents, especially in the United States, had flattened and was lying on average just a few points above zero. But it refused to descend to zero. In other words, while airline flying had become remarkably safe and reliable, especially with respect to mechanical accidents, no amount of industry effort, Federal Aviation Administration (FAA) pressure, or pilot training could completely eliminate human-caused disasters, and no accelerated application of the traditional engineering solutions appeared to improve the situation.

In the 1980s, however, a true revolution, quiet and unnoticed, began to change the equation. As a direct result, 16 years later the airline accident death rate for U.S. airlines finally hit bottom and remained at 0 for nearly 5 years—a stunning achievement. Although this 5-year 0-accident record ended with a crash in 2006 in Lexington, Kentucky, the passenger death rate in U.S. service has remained flat since then (Levin, 2009). This achievement was due to a recognition of the fact that aviation is a human system and that humans will never be able to operate without making mistakes. In other words, the path to perfect safety was through the process of building a system that fully expected and was ready to absorb human mistakes. The engineering-based disciplines that evolved in the airline business (and aviation in general) from that pivotal recognition are loosely known as human factors engineering, but they include systems engineering as well and borrow heavily from sociology, physiology, and behavioral science.

Before the industry realized in the early 1980s that it had never really addressed human failure (except to ineffectually order humans not to fail), there was a growing silence about the prospects of ever fully eliminating passenger deaths and disasters. It was quietly acknowledged that a certain number of accidents might be the cost of doing business, that accidents might be inevitable in a system that each day sent as many as 3,000 flights around the country and carried many tens of millions of passengers each year. Moreover, as the airlines came under tremendous cost pressure during the early 1980s because of deregulation and cut-rate competition, established airlines began looking desperately at ways of reducing costs. In that environment, concern grew that massive new investments in maintenance, training, and electronics would be needed to realize even an incremental improvement in safety (given that there were already so few crashes). This situation did little to generate enthusiasm for expanding safety measures or investing in new disciplines such as CRM (which was in its infancy at United at the time). The heavy price of small improvement, in other words, furthered the idea that a small number of accidents might have to be accepted as the cost of having an airline system. Of course, this was not an illogical argument at that time. In fact, one major airline executive rather infamously replied to the question of why his airline did not spend millions to establish a safety department by saying: "We don't need one. That's why we have insurance."

Before the emergence of human factors in the 1980s, the airlines had successfully applied systems engineering principles in many ways (sometimes without labeling them correctly) to develop high levels of mechanical and operational reliability. Across the industry, we had developed sophisticated feedback systems for learning rapidly about mechanical problems, systems that included the so-called Airworthiness Directives issued by the FAA (the strongest type of legal directive the FAA can issue to effect mechanical changes), as well as less urgent service bulletins transmitted to the entire commercial aviation industry within and outside the United States. In addition, there was a broad range of methods by which the airlines could communicate with each other, the FAA, and the National Transportation Safety Board, including a number of task forces and special industry groups working voluntarily with the government on problems of special concern (e.g., the revelations in the late 1980s about the susceptibility of aircraft structures to accelerated corrosion and fatigue in high-salt environments following the Aloha accident of 1986). To a certain extent, those systems have all now matured (along with individual reporting systems such as the National Aeronautics and Space Administration's Aviation Safety Reporting System), to the point that any significant problem discovered in commercial aviation can be fully discussed and communicated to every operator worldwide within hours. Aviation, in other words, worked hard to learn serious lessons about maintenance and training once the FAA pushed for airline safety by working with, instead of against, the industry.

In the same period of the 1970s through the 1990s, under Part 25 of the Federal Aviation Regulations (14 Code of Federal Regulations 25), the major airline manufacturers developed a level of redundancy in their designs such that the anticipated failure rates of most of aircraft and components had a long string of zeros to the right of the decimal point before a non-zero digit appeared. Through backup systems and preventive maintenance (pulling and replacing or overhauling components long before their first anticipated failure range), the so-called "dispatch reliability" of airliners exceeded the most optimistic expectations. In addition, airlines developed processes for the computerized tracking of maintenance, parts, and all operational elements—including crew scheduling, reservations, ship scheduling, dispatch, and coordination of all functions—optimizing the rapidly developing capabilities of computers. The airlines achieved computer-assisted standardization of nearly everything done in the maintenance hangars, in the cockpit, and even in operations. All of these elements were honed continuously because they were the most cost-effective methods of doing business. Airlines realized that in a heavily competitive environment, they simply could not afford the type of public relations catastrophe that any major accident would cause. The costs to an airline's reputation would be far beyond the direct costs of any such accident.

All of the mechanical and computerized systems were largely in place by the end of the 1970s, but, as previously noted, crashes still happened, usually because of human failure. In 1982 an Air Florida Boeing 737 crashed on takeoff in a snowstorm in Washington, DC, killing all but five of those aboard, who were rescued from the icy Potomac River. There was nothing wrong with the airplane. In 1985, an Arrow Air flight chartered to bring U.S. troops from the Middle East to Kentucky crashed in Gander, Newfoundland, killing all 256 people aboard. Although there is still controversy about that crash, it was attributed to the crew's departing with ice on the wings—again, there was nothing mechanically wrong with the airplane. A Northwest Airlines plane crashed in Romulus, Michigan, in 1987 because of the pilot's failure to extend the flaps, and all but one died. A year later, a Delta flight at Dallas–Fort Worth Airport also tried to take off with the flaps up and crashed, killing 17 people. The flight crew survived, and they were astounded at the National Transportation Safety Board's finding that all three of them had missed clear signs that the flaps had not been extended. Three highly trained, highly qualified human beings had caused a major accident, and all three had "seen"—and were willing to swear they had seen—instrument indications that the flaps were in the correct position (15-degree extension). The flaps were not in the correct position.

Given events such as these, the airline industry realized by the early 1980s that such tragedies would continue unless it adopted radically different practices and, for the first time, addressed not just advertent human failure but wholly inadvertent mistakes. To that end, the industry had to do more than adopt major changes; it had to change its philosophy and, most important, to change the entire culture of airline piloting.

Many who look at the aviation industry's excellent safety record today erroneously think it is simply the result of engineering successes based on the mechanics of the operation, on systems, and on getting people under control and completing more and more checklists. In fact, even some members of the industry are unaware of the cultural revolution that transformed our ability to prevent accidents due to human mistakes. More to the point for this workshop, the changes I refer to as a renaissance in thinking during the 1980s and 1990s have helped us create a new paradigm that can, as many have realized, be transferred to health care. In fact, I and many others have been doing exactly that with solid success for a number of years, primarily by focusing on training healthcare professionals in the discipline of how humans fail and what can be done to create a human system that can prevent those failures from hurting patients. That training is completely counter to the traditional, autonomous approach to health care, especially in relation to physicians, in holding as a fundamental tenet that although individual humans—including surgeons—are incapable of achieving perfection, interactive and collegial teams of humans can do so. Indeed, this is the primary legacy of the CRM revolution in airline cockpits, where we have saved countless lives and aircraft in the past 20 or more years by requiring more than 1 human mind to weigh in when something appears amiss and using a teamwork approach based on the common goal of flight safety to approach self-correction and safe operational decisions. Eliminated in such an atmosphere is the angry autonomous leader who disciplines a subordinate by berating, belittling, and ignoring that individual just for speaking up. Gone as well is the situation in which a subordinate has the key to save everyone but cannot pass it to the leader.

Health care today and the airline industry of yesterday are remarkably parallel in that every physician, nurse, and other healthcare professional is trained, essentially, to be perfect and never to make mistakes. Worse, the system is built the same way aviation was—on the expectation of human perfection, with few if any buffers to allow for major human mistakes. In the airline industry, thousands of work-years of engineering had been devoted (with great success) to providing backup systems for even the most arcane failure modes, but when it came to engineering for human failure, the approach taken was simply to order the human not to fail. Equally appalling in light of what we now know was the lack of emphasis on human-to-human relationships as the platform for true communication, coordination, and self-correction. Similarly in medicine, there is traditionally no expectation of human error in good doctors, nurses, and pharmacists, so there appears to be no valid reason for having backup and buffer systems to absorb mistakes.

The lesson from the airline industry, then, is that buffers against normal human error are a prime safety component in any human system. Of equal importance is the reality that the healthcare culture, as previously was the case with the airline culture, includes an expectation of hierarchical autonomy that is challenged by any subordinate speaking up to report a mistake or concern. In the airline industry, subordinates' sensitivity to the feelings of a senior created a culture-based reluctance to point out concerns, problems, or even impending disasters lest the leader become angry at the suggestion that he or she was in error. Leaders, after all, are trained never to make mistakes. But that left only one mind operating in an airplane (or an operating room), while the other qualified professionals sat in silence, even (in the airlines) if the captain was a gentle individual who wanted to hear from his or her crew. This situation kept us from improving safety levels and preventing that last tier of human mistake–driven accidents.

Perhaps the most important experience the airline industry can share with health care is its realization that no human can be perfect and that no team can function as a team without collegiality and mutual respect. We proceeded to build a system around those assumption, constructing buffers and backups for all reasonably anticipatable human failures that might otherwise lead to an incident or accident. And history shows that we have succeeded.

We learned that a safety system has three distinct tiers. Tier 1 encompasses all the training and indoctrination and agreed-upon or imposed professional methods, such as checklist compliance and "time-outs," that are designed to prevent human error. Understanding that some human error will occur despite our best efforts at standardization and training, we then must construct Tier 2, comprising those buffers and backups that will catch and cancel out the effects of human error and latent system failures. Finally, Tier 3 reflects the realization that even after accomplishing highly effective work in preventing and then screening out the effects of mistakes, we will still occasionally experience catastrophic failure unless we enter every operational sequence expecting a 50 percent chance of failure. With this expectation and through collegial teams whose members have no hesitation in communicating with each other for the good of the mission, we construct a systemic approach that ensures our leaders are ready and willing to consider even the most tenuous concern as potentially valid and "stop the line," or hold off on the operation, or abort the takeoff until the team and the leader are sure that safety is not threatened. Thus, either a junior flight engineer or a new circulating nurse would get an instant and serious audience by saying, "I'm not sure, but I think something's wrong," rather than having to overcome a group presumption of normalcy. That one change—the Tier 3 approach—can be the final key to constructing a system that protects against catastrophic patient injury or death from preventable medical *human* mistakes. But to institutionalize such procedures requires a systemic approach that is foreign to the American healthcare experience, which is why looking to the engineering community for help is so important.

Human beings fail in three basic ways—by making mistakes in perception, assumption, and communication. Perception failures include, for example, a flight crew's failure to recognize that the aircraft's wing flaps are not properly extended for takeoff. One mistaken assumption caused an accident in 1977, when two pilots assumed their Boeing 747 was cleared for takeoff when in fact it was not. Another 747 had missed a turn and was sitting sideways on the runway ahead, unseen in the fog. The decision to start the takeoff was a human mistake nurtured by a poor cockpit culture. That day it resulted in the loss of 583 lives. The third human failure is mistakes in communication, a human propensity shared by health care and aviation. Approximately 12.5 percent of the time in human verbal communication, people who otherwise understand each other fail to do so in that instance. The old phrase "I know you think you understood what you thought I said, but I am not sure you realize that what you heard wasn't what I meant" points to the universality of misunderstanding. We have learned, however, that reading back a clearance or a medical order can reduce the potential for mistakes to below half a percent.

Aviation had to learn these basic failure modes instead of fighting to deny them or ordering them to not occur. We had to learn to inculcate the expectation of such failures in everything we did. So, too, must health care. But to accept these realities operationally and culturally and integrate them into health care (with its largely autonomous tradition), we need a structured, engineered framework within which such approaches as the minimization of variables, collegial team communication, and the three tiers discussed above can be deployed as standard operating methodology. Equally important—and not just to avoid the charge of creeping cookbook medicine—is that the resulting structure must nurture physicians in using their cognitive, analog, diagnostic, and surgical skills to do what checklists, machines, and procedures alone can never accomplish. By finding the proper balance, one can create a system that enables humans—through technology and enlightened methodologies—to practice what they do best—apply judgment, skill, and reason.

We cannot incorporate an expectation of perfection in a human system without creating and nurturing disasters. We cannot fail to accommodate human attitudes, feelings, or physiological limitations without perpetuating a societally unacceptable level of patient injuries and service quality. What health care needs from the applied and unique expertise engineering can provide is a structure that legitimizes and inculcates known best practices, eliminates the need or latitude to reinvent each procedure, and provides the best possible operational buffers against inevitable human fallibility, while

at the same time providing the latitude within which healthcare professionals can practice with caring and engaged attention.

This exploration of looking to the engineering community to assist
health care probably heralds the most important advances in changing
how we have traditionally thought of the problems of patient safety, service
quality, and healthcare delivery since we first began to recognize that we
have a national problem with what George Halvorson, chief executive officer (CEO) of Kaiser Permanente, calls our nonsystem. To bring order out
of chaos, we need help that goes beyond the traditional methods applied in
the past. In aviation, both mechanical and systems engineering provided the
keys both to building reliable airplanes and to staffing them with imperfect
humans who, working together and as colleagues able to communicate
without barriers, could accomplish what a single commander could not. If
we keep that in mind and borrow liberally from other disciplines, we can
engineer a system that works, that works safely, and that can be financially
sustainable.

ALCOA'S REORIENTATION:
STREAMLINING THE FINANCIAL CLOSE PROCESS

Earnest J. Edwards, Alcoa, Inc., Martha Jefferson Health Service

World-class organizations have been breaking traditional paradigms
and achieving real value by adding to their operations the use of finance organizations that embrace and act on the following five key characteristics:

1. emphasizing high efficiency, low cost, and high quality;
2. effectively leveraging systems and providing better information for
   decision making;
3. becoming solution oriented and change agents;
4. focusing on planning the future and not reporting the past; and
5. becoming vital business partners with an expanded role in strategic
   decisions.

Although health care is different from most industries, it could benefit
by embracing these same characteristics and using finance as an example
of major change for other areas to follow. During the major change that
took place at Alcoa in the 1990s (as directed by then-CEO Paul O'Neill),
finance and other staff groups played an integral role in the transformations that were required of all business units and staff departments. Two
of the guiding principles that fostered the improvements achieved were
to make quantum-leap changes so as to close the gap in the best-in-class

where such a gap existed and to insist on "no opt out" by any function or department.

This paper reports on the streamlining of the financial closing process, which was a quality cycle-time reduction project. This project resulted in significant cost reductions and enabled other finance projects to make more rapid changes with greater benefits. This was especially true in the subsequent period of Alcoa's rapid growth strategy. The accelerated closing project also provided more timely information for business decision making, served as an example of how to improve routine processes in a major way, and was a major motivating force in the company. A similar project was undertaken and completed successfully in the U.S. Department of the Treasury, again under O'Neill's leadership, and more recently, another such project, yielding many of the same value-adding benefits and direct cost reductions, was carried out at the Martha Jefferson Hospital. This is a worthwhile leadership project that can introduce major change to any organization and serve as an example of what can be done with commitment, focus, and no major investment.

When O'Neill joined Alcoa as CEO, he was the most highly focused and dedicated-to-change person in the organization. He moved around quietly, talking with everyone and getting to know what was really happening. The first thing he introduced us all to, for about a year, was safety, quality, and quality training. That focus altered our outlook about how things should be and also changed our work behavior.

O'Neill's next move was to turn the entire Alcoa organization upside down. He created what was called the inverted pyramid. The customers were king, at the top of the pyramid. A step down were business leaders, whose job it was to make the customers happy. Functional groups, such as the one to which I belonged, were dismayed because we found ourselves near the bottom of the pyramid. But then O'Neill put the CEO at the very bottom of the pyramid. That was transforming in and of itself, as it caused all of us to change our thinking from focusing on who was at the top of the company to focusing on what function or activity was at the top in terms of importance.

O'Neill followed the introduction of the pyramid with the charge that "[w]e are going to make quantum leap changes to Alcoa's performance." He told us to identify best-in-class practices, whether in our business units or functional groups, and he said he wanted all of us to be using such practices within a couple of years. For the finance group, the challenge was clear: we needed to redirect resources while reducing costs. To that end, my group took a close look at the financial closing process, and we undertook it as a significant quality cycle-time reduction project, which is the focus of this paper. We carried out this project successfully at Alcoa, and subsequently were able to help others succeed in similar undertakings at the U.S. Department of the Treasury and at Martha Jefferson Hospital. The focus of this paper is on Alcoa.

To put this experience in perspective, when we started the project in 1991, Alcoa was a $10 billion company; by 2007, we were a $31 billion company. We had 150 locations in 20 countries when we started; that increased to 316 in 44 countries. Our net income of $0.4 billion in 1991 increased to $2.6 billion in 2007. During this growth, we were also able to achieve significant reductions in systems and processes.

At Alcoa, 70 to 80 percent of our finance people were working on transaction processes. We decided we should reduce the percentage and number of employees working on transaction processes and at the same time give more attention to decision support processes. We initially chose three projects in the controllership function for transforming the company's finance function. We wanted a common chart of accounts, including setting up a worldwide common accounting and finance language, providing consistent information, and improving communication among business units, among other strategies. We wanted an accelerated closing process, by which we meant we wanted to shorten the closing cycle to three days, significantly improve processes, and provide timely performance information to management. We also wanted to create a shared services center to better pool transaction processing for U.S. businesses, lower costs, improve service, and refocus on business analysis and support. Although people in finance would have liked to focus on shared services, O'Neill preferred accelerated closing, and as CEO he had a weighted vote, so we ended up focusing on that area first.

Our objectives for the three projects were straightforward. We wanted to improve information sharing, achieve better and more timely decision making, institute easier modeling and analysis, improve systems efficiency, ensure that we could adapt more readily to change, enable shared ledger processing, set ourselves up to be ready for growth, and ensure a certain degree of immunity to organizational change. Perhaps the core goal was readiness for growth. Immunity to organizational change was a goal because every time we changed the organization, finance had to expend a great deal of energy shuffling the books around. The accelerated closing project involved the most people and touched on most of the objectives, which made it ideal as the initial focus.

Alcoa's closing was completed at 4:30 p.m. on the eighth workday of the month. We found that a world benchmark for a comparably structured company was 3 workdays, so we wanted to strive for that. Earlier completion would increase the relevance of the information and free staff time for more value-adding work.

Frankly, our first reaction to the prospect of closing Alcoa's books in 3 days was skepticism. We thought it was impossible given the global nature of our enterprise. We had several project guidelines. We wanted to move from a closing time of 8 days to 3 days by February 1993. We set no interim targets, but said we wanted to get to the final goal as quickly as possible, with the quality of data improved. We said we would develop standard metrics that would be published worldwide throughout the company. The last guideline was new for us: publishing metrics on how well we were progressing toward the goal at each location was alien to our culture at the time, but it turned out to have great advantages.

We encountered a great deal initial resistance. People were constantly looking for ways to opt out. They kept asking us to explain the objectives and guidelines. Our response was direct. We simply said, "Here are the guidelines, and you can read them for yourselves." Then we said, "Just get it done." Our initial challenge was getting the word out, as many people were involved in the process. Beyond that, we had to overcome innate inertia and move thinking from "why it can't be done" to "how it will be done." One key was explaining the real benefits we could expect to reap if we were successful.

Ultimately, we were successful. In just 9 months, 70 percent of the operations had reached their targets. Eight months later Alcoa had matched the world standard with an in-control and capable process. One of the biggest surprises was how quickly we started to make gains in a process we had been doing every month for many years in basically the same way and taking the same amount of time. Our success demonstrates what can be done when staff are empowered and the whole organization is working on a problem.

The results were significant. We saw quality improvement at all locations. We could document productivity improvement in terms of days saved times people in the process. Communication and cooperation were much improved, while frustration with what had been a painful process was greatly reduced. In the change process, we developed advanced-quality tools that were deployed across the entire organization. We were able to get financial information out sooner and to improve performance feedback. We developed a very positive image in the financial community because of our insistence that efficiency matters. One of the most relevant lessons for health care is that we demonstrated that significant improvements can be made to administrative processes relatively quickly and inexpensively, resulting in greater satisfaction among both employees and management. Moreover, we showed the rest of the organization that an administrative process could be improved; later, the CEO used that to his advantage to keep everybody moving toward quantum change. We were then able to focus more resources on developing our new chart of accounts and creating the U.S. shared service center, which provided even more significant cost reductions and benefits to Alcoa's finance organization, as indicated in our project objectives.

More recently, we helped apply similar strategies to streamlining the financial closing process at the Department of the Treasury. This was a larger, much more complex organization in some respects, with components ranging from the Internal Revenue Service and the Customs and Border Patrol to the Bureau of Alcohol, Tobacco and Firearms, but the nature of the problem was similar. As of January 2001, the bureaus and various reporting entities were taking 20 workdays to submit monthly financial data to the Treasury's Financial Analysis and Reporting System. As we had found at Alcoa, however, world-class organizations close their monthly books in 3 days. On April 11, 2001, then-Secretary O'Neill challenged the department to achieve a 3-day close by no later than July 3, 2002. There was significant concern as to whether this was feasible in light of the size and complexity of the U.S. Treasury. However, because this was a directive from the top, with no opt-outs allowed and most of the same project guidelines as at Alcoa, the closing project was started. I am still amazed at how rapidly the number of days to close dropped in the early months of the project, given the complexity of the government. The success underscores the fact that there is a tremendous amount of know-how in an organization. People want respect. They want a challenge. Give them a stretch goal, tell them what to do, and get out of their way. Within every organization, that know-how is in place. We simply fail to call on it or fail to manage it properly with efficiency as a focus.

The benefits of the 3-day close at Treasury were significant. Data have become more timely, accurate, and meaningful. There is better communication with internal and external organizations. There is more time to perform analysis and focus on other goals. The change process brought to light and ultimately reengineered old and inefficient ways of operating. The process forced the department to work more efficiently and put the previous month "to bed" earlier. The change process identified and resolved key system fixes. Staff restructured some of their contracts so as to obtain more timely information from contractors. The process moved a monthly cost meeting one week earlier in the month, and overall it helped with budget execution and monitoring of the status of funds. The process is still in effect today, and I am told that it was a factor in the entire federal government's achieving a 45-day annual closing that President Bush had challenged them to accomplish. Ultimately, the process is all about adding value.

Finally, we applied a similar process at Martha Jefferson Hospital, a not-for-profit, 176-bed community hospital based in Charlottesville, Virginia. Fully accredited by the Joint Commission on Accreditation of Healthcare Organizations, the hospital has a caring tradition of more than 100 years, with close ties to its community. Its key services include a cancer care center, a cardiology care center, a digestive care center, a vascular center, a women's health center, an emergency department, and primary care services. The medical staff includes nearly 400 affiliated physicians representing more than 35 specialties.

The financial people at the hospital embraced an ambitious set of goals. One was a project in fiscal year (FY) 2005 to reduce the financial close process from 15 to 5 business days by FY 2007. Unlike Alcoa or the U.S. Treasury, Martha Jefferson used more detailed guidelines for other process improvements they wanted to accomplish. Specifically, they wanted to enhance the use of systems for automation by effectively utilizing a recently installed general ledger system to implement a new time and attendance system, to implement an operating budget system for automation of budget processes and management reporting, to institute firm monthly close deadlines, and to implement processes throughout the month to ensure data quality at the end of the month.

Among their challenges was the need to break from the usual "That's the way we've always done it" way of thinking. There was also an issue of converting serial steps to a parallel process where appropriate and focusing on doing what one can when one *can* vs. when one *must*. Obtaining commitment was another challenge, but it ended up being a success factor since the finance organization put it on the line.

I actually thought the hospital's project guidelines were a bit more detailed because of the added system implementation work they needed to accomplish, and they did not want to aim for a 3-day close in the initial objective. Although it took a little longer to reach the 5-day closing, they still succeeded and are extremely excited about this accomplishment. Their report on the closing progress showed the same rapid improvement in the early months as was achieved at Alcoa and the U.S. Treasury. I have recently learned that they continue to make progress and are now approaching the 3-day closing.

Key success factors at Martha Jefferson included a commitment to process improvement, deadlines, and each other, as well as to teamwork and a belief in the "possibilities." The payoffs were significant and came in the form of timeliness, transparency, and ease of access. Staff could now spend more time with information and less with data. The accuracy, reliability, and consistency of financial information were all improved. Paper-based reporting was eliminated. There was earlier and enhanced access to appropriate financial information at each level of the organization, and overall, finance personnel were better able to serve and support operating departments in financial management of the organization.

Many applications of this process could benefit health care, and similar processes could likely be applied throughout the healthcare enterprise with similar quantum-change benefits. When it comes to the problems or opportunities of health care, I think the glass is half full, not half empty.

VETERANS HEALTH AFFAIRS: TRANSFORMING THE VETERANS HEALTH ADMINISTRATION

Kenneth W. Kizer, M.D., M.P.H., U.S. Department of Veterans Affairs, Medsphere Systems Corporation, Inc., Kizer & Associates, LLC

The veterans healthcare system administered by the VA was established after World War I to provide medical and rehabilitation care for veterans having health conditions related to their military service. Today it is the nation's largest healthcare system, although it is an anomaly in American health care insofar as it is centrally administered, fully integrated, and both paid for and operated by the federal government.

As the system grew and became more bureaucratic, its performance deteriorated, and it failed to adapt to changing circumstances. By the early 1990s, VA health care was being widely criticized for providing fragmented and disjointed care of unpredictable and irregular quality that was expensive, difficult to access, and insensitive to individual needs.

Between 1995 and 1999 the VA healthcare system underwent a radical reengineering that addressed management accountability, care coordination, performance measurement, resource allocation, and information management. Numerous systemic changes were implemented, producing dramatically improved quality, service satisfaction, and efficiency. VA health care is now recognized as among the best in America, and the VA transformation is viewed as a model for healthcare reform and organizational transformation.

A Short History of the Veterans Healthcare System

The United States provides the most comprehensive benefits for military veterans of any country in the world. The special status accorded veterans dates back to colonial days (VHA, 1967; Weber and Schmeckebiar, 1934).

Veterans healthcare benefits were originally limited to infirmary care provided by the U.S. Public Health Service (USPHS) or by contract civilian hospitals. President Lincoln set the precedent for the government's providing institutional care for veterans when he established the National Asylum for Disabled Volunteer Soldiers in 1865.

The sharply increased number of veterans needing medical care after World War I prompted Congress to increase healthcare benefits for veterans, transfer 57 USPHS hospitals to the U.S. Veterans Bureau, and approve hospital care for indigent veterans without service-connected disabilities (Mather and Abel, 1986; VHA, 1967).

In 1930 President Hoover merged the Bureau of Pensions, the National Home for Disabled Volunteer Soldiers, and U.S. Veterans Bureau to establish the Veterans Administration (Mather and Abel, 1986; Weber and Schmeckebiar, 1934).[2] This new independent federal agency was charged with consolidating and coordinating the various veterans benefit programs that existed for the nation's then 4.7 million veterans. The founding of the veterans healthcare system is generally linked with the establishment of the VA (Piccard, 2005; Weber and Schmeckebiar, 1934)[3] at a time when there was essentially no public or private health insurance in the United States.

The veteran population increased suddenly and massively after June 1945. Many of the more than 12 million new veterans produced by World War II sought care from the VA. The agency was overwhelmed. Legislation was enacted in 1946 to establish a new VA Department of Medicine and Surgery to "streamline and modernize the practice of medicine for veterans"[4] (Mather and Abel, 1986; VHA, 1967).

To improve the quality and quantity of its medical staff as quickly as possible, the VA sought affiliations with university medical schools (VHA, 1946). Northwestern University and Chicago's Hines VA Hospital were the first to affiliate. This relationship was widely replicated, establishing a highly successful ongoing partnership between the VA and academic medicine.

The veterans healthcare system grew rapidly during the late 1940s and 1950s, adding more than 70 new hospitals, establishing academic affiliations and teaching programs, expanding research activities, and putting into place new venues of care (Mather and Abel, 1986; VHA, 1967). During these years the VA emphasized hospital inpatient and medical specialist care, consistent with what was then viewed as the best medical care.

As the system grew and became more complex, it became increasingly cumbersome and bureaucratic as well as increasingly underfunded and understaffed. During the 1970s and 1980s, a number of embarrassing quality-of-care incidents occurred at individual VA hospitals. Widespread media coverage of these incidents indicted the whole system. Many Vietnam veterans, already angry about what they perceived to be an unjust and unending war, as well as the public's often hostile response to them when they returned home, were alienated by the system's seemingly lackluster response

---

[2] Executive Order 5398, July 21, 1930.

[3] Although the founding of the veterans healthcare system is generally linked with formation of the VA, the system actually took form incrementally over several decades in the first half of the 20th century. Some authors cite its founding as occurring in 1946, when VA health care was restructured in the aftermath of World War II.

[4] See Public Law 79-293 (1946).

to their problems, prompting some disgruntled veterans to stage events to embarrass the VA (Klein, 1981; Longman, 2007).

Responding to the many veterans service organizations that had long sought higher status for veterans programs, President Reagan established the Cabinet-level Department of Veterans Affairs in 1989[5] (Light, 1992). The Department of Medicine and Surgery was renamed the Veterans Health Services and Research Administration, which was later renamed again to the VHA.[6]

By 1994 the VA had grown to be the country's largest healthcare provider, with an annual medical care budget of $16.3 billion, 210,000 full-time employees, 172 acute-care hospitals having 1.1 million annual admissions, 131 skilled nursing facilities housing some 72,000 elderly or severely disabled adults, 39 domiciliaries (residential care facilities) that each year cared for 26,000 persons, 350 outpatient clinics having 24 million annual patient visits, and 206 counseling facilities providing treatment for posttraumatic stress disorder (PTSD). The VHA also partnered with most states to fund state-managed skilled nursing facilities for elderly veterans, administered a contract and fee-basis care program paying for "out-of-network" services, and managed a number of nonhealthcare concerns.[7]

By this time the veterans healthcare system was highly dysfunctional. The quality of care was irregular (Associated Press, 1990; Childs, 1970; GAO, 1987, 1995; Office of the Inspector General and Department of Veterans Affairs, 1990, 1991; U.S. Congress, 1987); services were fragmented, disjointed, and insensitive to individual needs (GAO, 1994a; Light, 1992; Longman, 2007); inpatient care was overused (Booth et al., 1991; GAO, 1989; Smith et al., 1996); customer service was poor (GAO, 1994a; Longman, 2007); and care was often difficult to access, with patients sometimes traveling hundreds of miles or waiting months for routine appointments (GAO, 1993; Longman, 2007). Reflecting popular sentiment, movies

---

[5] Because of its broad public recognition, "VA" was maintained as the acronym for the new Cabinet Department, albeit now standing for "Veterans Affairs." The VA became the 14th Cabinet agency in the executive branch of the federal government per Executive Order 5398, 1989.

[6] Like the Department of Health and Human Services, which administers its programs through 11 sub-Cabinet agencies (e.g., the Food and Drug Administration, Centers for Medicare & Medicaid Services, Centers for Disease Control and Prevention), the VA administers its many health and social support programs through a number of sub-Cabinet agencies per Public Law 79-293, 1946 (e.g., the VHA, Veterans Benefits Administration, National Cemetery Administration, Board of Veterans Appeals).

[7] These nonhealthcare concerns included 32 golf courses, 29 fire departments, a national retail store system (the Veterans Canteen Service), 75 laundries, and 1,740 historic buildings, among other things. The VHA was and continues to be the largest laundry service in the world, and it oversees more historic sites than any entity except the Department of the Interior.

such as *Article 99* and *Born on the Fourth of July* portrayed VA health care as a bleak backwater of incompetence, indifference, and inefficiency.

Between 1995 and 1999, the veterans healthcare system underwent a radical reengineering that markedly improved its quality of care, service satisfaction, and efficiency. In recent years, the VA has been hailed as providing some of the best health care in the United States (Arnst, 2006; CBS Evening News, 2006; Freedberg, 2006; Gearon, 2005; Glendinning, 2007; Krugman, 2008; Rundle, 2001; Stein, 2006; Stires, 2006; Waller, 2006). The veterans healthcare system is now viewed as a model of high-quality, low-cost (i.e., high-value) health care, and a number of authors have advocated it as a model for American healthcare reform (Gaul, 2005; Haugh, 2003; NBC Nightly News, 2006; Oxford Analytica, 2007; Piccard, 2005).

Missions of the Modern Veterans Healthcare System

The VHA is a highly complex organization. Understanding its multiple missions, four of which are specified in statute, is important to understanding the changes in its strategies and tactics.

The VHA's primary mission is to provide medical care for eligible veterans in order to improve their health and functionality and reduce the burden of disability from conditions related to their military service. Initially, all honorably discharged veterans were eligible for VA health care, but as the system's cost grew, Congress limited eligibility for VA health care to those who were poor or had a service-connected condition,[8] underscoring the safety net role established for the system in 1924 (Steiner, 1971; VHA, 1967; Wilson and Kizer, 1997). This explains in large part why the VA's patient population is disproportionately older, sicker, and more socioeconomically disadvantaged than the general population or than Medicare beneficiaries (Frayne et al., 2006; Kazis et al., 1999; Rogers et al., 2004; Singh et al., 2005; Yu et al., 2003). Within the VHA's patient population, a number of groups have been identified as "special populations" because their health conditions are disproportionately prevalent among veterans or particularly related to military service. These special populations include persons with spinal cord injuries, amputations, traumatic brain injury, serious mental illness, substance abuse disorders, PTSD, or blindness; former prisoners of war; Persian Gulf War veterans; and homeless persons. The VHA has a binding obligation to serve these groups and has developed special expertise in treating them.

The VHA's second mission is to train healthcare personnel (Stevens et

---

[8] Unlike Medicare or Medicaid, which are entitlement programs that must be funded in accordance with the growth in the number of beneficiaries, veterans health care is a discretionary program that may be funded at whatever level Congress chooses.

al., 1998, 2001). Although most often associated with postgraduate medical education[9] (Longman, 2007), the VHA offers training for more than 40 types of healthcare professionals through affiliations with more than 1,100 universities and colleges. More than 100,000 trainees rotate through VHA facilities each year.

The VHA's third mission is to conduct research that will improve the care of veterans (Rutherford et al., 1999). The VHA conducts research in the basic biomedical sciences, rehabilitation, health services delivery, and quality improvement. Placing a dedicated research program within such an immense healthcare delivery system—and one with a stable patient population that has a high prevalence of chronic conditions—creates an especially fertile environment for research.

The system's fourth mission is to provide contingency support to the military healthcare system and the Department of Homeland Security. In times of national emergency, the VHA provides personnel, pharmaceuticals, supplies, and other support to the National Disaster Medical System (Kizer et al., 2000a; U.S. Congress, 2001).

The final mission of the VHA is to serve the homeless because about a third of adult homeless men in the United States are veterans. The VA is the nation's largest direct provider of services to homeless persons, providing healthcare services (and other services) to more than 65,000 homeless veterans each year (Rosenheck and Kizer, 1998).

Transforming the Veterans Healthcare System

In 1994 there was widespread consensus that the veterans healthcare system needed a major overhaul, but there was little agreement about how to effect the needed change. Under new leadership drawn from outside the system, a radical reengineering of VA health care was proposed (Kizer, 1996; Kizer and Garthwaite, 1997). The reengineering was intended to create a seamless continuum of consistent and predictable high-quality, patient-centered care that was of superior value.

The concept of value was a fundamental underpinning of the reengineering. In particular, the reengineering sought to create an organization with the following features: (1) superior quality of care that was predictable and consistent throughout the system, (2) health care that was of equal or better value than care provided by the private sector, and (3) high reliability.

---

[9] Approximately half of all American medical students and one-third of all postgraduate physician residents receive training at VA facilities each year. Two-thirds of U.S.-trained physicians have received at least some of their training at a VA medical center. About 85 percent of VA hospitals are university-affiliated teaching hospitals (i.e., 130 of 153 hospitals in 2007), and 70 percent of the VA's 14,000 staff physicians have university faculty appointments.

$$V = \int A + TQ + FS + SS \, / \, C$$

V = Value
A = Access
TQ = Technical Quality
FS = Functional Status
SS = Service Satisfaction
C = Cost (or P = Price)

FIGURE 4-1 The Veterans Health Administration value equation. Value is defined operationally as being a function of access, technical quality, patient functionality, and service satisfaction, all divided by cost or price.

It was argued that if the VHA were to continue to enjoy public support, it would have to be able to demonstrate its value to both veterans and the public. To operationalize the concept of value, a relatively objective method for determining value was needed. This method was accomplished by use of the *value equation* shown in Figure 4-1, in which value is deemed to be a function of technical quality, access to care, patient functional status, and service satisfaction, all divided by the cost or price of the care. Each of the four value domains in the numerator was linked to a menu of standardized performance measures[10] (Light, 1992).

The reengineering was based on five interrelated and mutually reinforcing strategies: (1) create an accountable management structure and management control system, (2) integrate and coordinate services across the continuum of care, (3) measure performance and create an environment supportive of improvement and high performance, (4) align the system's finances with desired outcomes, and (5) modernize information management.

Change Strategy 1: Create an Accountable Management Structure and Management Control System

The most visible steps taken to increase management accountability were (1) the establishment of a new operational structure based on the concept of integrated delivery networks, (2) the implementation of a new performance management system, and (3) decentralization of much of the operational decision making. It was envisioned that these and other

---

[10] To facilitate valid comparison with the private sector, whenever possible the performance measures are the same as those used by the private sector.

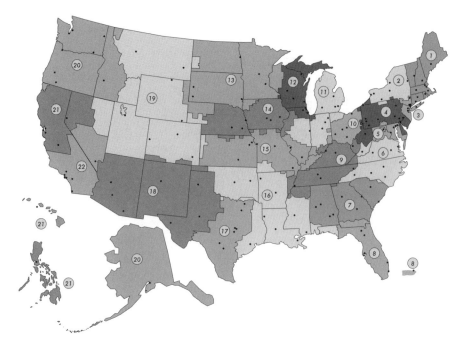

FIGURE 4-2 Map of the Veterans Health Administration's 21 Veterans Integrated Service Networks.
SOURCE: VA, 2010.

measures would provide a foundation for the emergence of a new organizational culture in which accountability would be a core value.

Establishment of Veterans Integrated Service Networks After development, vetting, and requisite congressional approval of the restructuring plan, in fall 1995 the VHA's more than 1,100 sites of care delivery were organized into 22 Veterans Integrated Service Networks (VISNs, pronounced "visions") (Kizer and Garthwaite, 1997; Kizer and Pane, 1997). The decision to have 22 VISNs was based on a judgment about how care could best be distributed, and the catchment areas of the VISNs were determined according to prevailing patient referral patterns, the ability of each VISN to provide a continuum of primary to tertiary care with VA assets, and relevant state or county jurisdictional boundaries[11] (U.S. Congress, 1987). The number of VISNs was reduced to its current 21 in 2002 (Figure 4-2).

---

[11] A typical VISN encompassed 7 to 10 VA medical centers, 25 to 30 ambulatory care clinics, 4 to 7 nursing homes, 1 to 2 domiciliaries, and 10 to 15 counseling centers. The population served by each VISN averaged 150,000 to 200,000.

The VISN became the system's basic operating unit. It provided a structural template for coordinating services, pooling resources to meet the needs of the served population, and ensuring continuity of care; reducing service duplication and administrative redundancies when appropriate; improving the consistency and predictability of services; promoting more effective and accountable management; and, overall, optimizing healthcare value (Kizer and Garthwaite, 1997).

Implementation of a new performance management system A new performance management system was instituted in 1995 (Kizer, 1996; Trevelyan, 2002). Two key elements of this new system were the measurement of performance using standardized metrics and an annual performance contract that was used to clarify management expectations, encourage managers' engagement, and hold management accountable for achieving specified results. The use of such performance contracts was novel within the federal government. In this new performance management system, the organization's missions were aligned with quantifiable strategic goals, progress toward these goals was tracked using performance measures, the performance data were made widely available, and management was held accountable for the results achieved.

Concomitant with efforts to improve the quality of care, steps were taken to increase the knowledge base concerning clinical quality improvement and to encourage innovation. These efforts included initiation of the VA National Quality Scholars Fellowship Program (Batalden et al., 2002) and the VA Faculty Fellows Program for Improved Care for Patients at the End of Life (Block, 2002; Gibson, 1998), implementation of the Quality Enhancement Research Initiative (QUERI) (Ashton et al., 2000; Bozzette et al., 2000; Demakis et al., 2000; Every et al., 2000; Feussner et al., 2000; Finney et al., 2000; Fischer et al., 2000; Hynes et al., 2004; Kizer et al., 2000b; Krein et al., 2000), and hundreds of innovations in care delivery (Beason, 2000; Charles, 2000; Kizer, 2000; VHA, 1996a).

Decentralization of operational decision making In an effort to help change the organizational culture, a substantial amount of the operational decision making that had formerly been done in headquarters was delegated to the VISNs. The goal was to decentralize decision making to the lowest, most appropriate management level. Although quality improvement targets were often determined centrally, operational strategy and tactics to achieve the goals were left up to the VISNs.

Change Strategy 2: Integrate and Coordinate Services

In 1994 the two biggest problems with the VA's delivery of care were its variable quality and its fragmentation. Fragmentation of care is a serious problem everywhere in American health care, but it was especially serious in the VA because of the system's historical bias toward providing specialist-based, inpatient care; the limited use of care management and primary care; the sociodemographics of the VA's service population; the anachronistic laws governing eligibility for care; and the high rate of "dual-eligible" patients[12] (GAO, 1994b, 1995; Tseng et al., 2004).

The VHA transformation sought to reduce care fragmentation through a number of systemic changes aimed at coordinating and integrating service delivery across the continuum of care. Particularly important were the implementation of universal primary care, revision of the laws governing eligibility for care, and creation of the VISN management structure. Unsuccessful attempts were made to gain legislative authority for VA medical centers to participate in the Medicare program to help rationalize the care of dual eligibles.

Implementation of primary care A number of primary care pilot projects had been initiated at VA medical centers in the late 1980s and early 1990s (Cope et al., 1996; Rubenstein et al., 1996a, 1996b), but only about 10 percent of VA patients were enrolled in primary care at the end of FY 1994. Universal primary care was viewed as a lynchpin for integrating and coordinating care delivery and was believed to be essential regardless of what else was done to restructure the system. Thus a primary care initiative was launched in early FY 1995 before the VISN reorganization and other reengineering plans had been finalized (Management Decision and Research Center, 1995; Yano et al., 2007).

Eligibility reform The federal laws governing eligibility for VA health care were a major cause of service delivery fragmentation. These laws often required that patients be hospitalized for procedures routinely done on an outpatient basis elsewhere. They also required that the VHA treat only a veteran's service-connected condition. Such service-related conditions were often not the veteran's greatest health care need and were sometimes being exacerbated by non-service-related conditions that the VA could not legally treat. Thus one of the keys to transforming VA health care was to change the eligibility laws so that patients could receive whatever care was needed and be treated in the most appropriate medical care setting.

---

[12] "Dual-eligible" patients are eligible for care provided by the VA and another system. Most often this is Medicare, but it also may be the Indian Health Service, Tri-Care offered by the Department of Defense, or private indemnity insurance.

Repeated attempts to change these laws over the previous decade had been unsuccessful because key congressional leaders feared the change would increase use and, consequently, costs. However, VHA leadership convincingly argued that the eligibility laws made it impossible to manage the cost of the system prudently. This argument was pivotal to gaining enactment of the Veterans Health Care Eligibility Reform Act of 1996 (Public Law 104-262, 1996). This law gave the VHA the authority needed to provide care in any medically appropriate setting, to outsource services and partner with non-VA healthcare providers, and to establish an enrollment system.

Other efforts to increase the coordination and integration of care Other steps were taken to better coordinate and integrate care. For example, between 1995 and 1999, 52 VA medical centers were merged into 25 multicampus facilities, each under single management; multi-institutional "service lines" (e.g., lines in primary care or behavioral health) were implemented in some VISNs; multidisciplinary "Strategic Healthcare Groups" were organized at VHA headquarters (Kizer, 1996); care management was implemented as a system-wide strategic initiative (Employee Education System, 1999); better continuity of care through more convenient access was pursued through the establishment of hundreds of new community-based outpatient clinics (CBOCs); and a National Formulary of prescription drugs, nonprescription products, and medical supplies was established to promote evidence-based drug prescribing and improved pharmaceutical management (IOM, 2000a; Kizer et al., 1997; Sales et al., 2005; Young, 2007).

Change Strategy 3: Measure Performance

Performance measurement and the public reporting of performance were considered critical to improving the quality of care, standardizing superior quality, and demonstrating improved performance. As part of the performance management system, clinical performance was routinely measured and tracked. Two specific instruments were developed to carry out the performance assessments: the Prevention Index and the Chronic Disease Care Index[13] (Kizer, 1999). Both were instituted in late FY 1995 to track

---

[13] The Prevention Index consists of nine clinical interventions that measure how well VHA practitioners follow nationally recognized primary prevention and early detection recommendations for eight conditions with major social consequences: influenza and pneumococcal diseases, tobacco consumption, alcohol abuse, and cancer of the breast, cervix, colon, and prostate. The Chronic Disease Care Index consists of 14 clinical interventions that assess how well practitioners follow nationally recognized guidelines for 5 high-volume diagnoses: ischemic heart disease, hypertension, chronic obstructive pulmonary disorder, diabetes mellitus, and obesity.

adherence to established clinical best practices for common preventable or chronic conditions. A Palliative Care Index was instituted in 1997 to track adherence to best practices for end-of-life care (Penrod et al., 2007; Quill, 2002).

Another important clinical quality improvement effort was the National Surgical Quality Improvement Program (NSQIP), begun in 1991 in response to a 1986 congressional mandate that the VA compare its risk-adjusted surgical results with those of the private sector (Best et al., 2002; Daley et al., 1997; Khuri, 2006; Khuri et al., 1995, 1998). The intent and methods of the NSQIP, which were already in place, essentially mirrored the reengineering strategies, and NSQIP was embraced as part of the transformation effort.

Other quality improvement initiatives were launched to address specific clinical conditions or operational issues, including pain management (Cleeland et al., 2003; Schuster, 1999), end-of-life care (Block, 2002; Gibson, 1998; Penrod et al., 2007; Quill, 2002), cancer (Wilson and Kizer, 1998), HIV/AIDS (Bozzette et al., 2000; Korthuis et al., 2004), pressure ulcers (Berlowitz and Halpern, 1997; Berlowitz et al., 1999, 2001), acute myocardial infarction (Landrum et al., 2004; Petersen et al., 2000, 2001, 2003; Popescu et al., 2007; Fihn et al., 2009), and hepatitis C (Holohan et al., 1999; Mitchell et al., 1999; Roselle et al., 2002; Wright et al., 2000). The use of evidence-based clinical guidelines was strongly encouraged (Kizer, 1998; Management Decision and Research Center, 1998; VHA, 1996b). The VHA partnered with the Institute for Healthcare Improvement on "breakthrough collaboratives" for reducing waiting times, improving operating room performance, and improving access to primary care, among other things (Carver, 2002; Kizer, 1998; Management Decision and Research Center, 1998; Mills and Weeks, 2004; Mills et al., 2003; Roselle et al., 2002). Clinical Programs of Excellence were established,[14] and a knowledge management tool modeled after the U.S. Army's Lessons Learned Center, known as the VA Lessons Learned Project, was created along with an intranet-based Virtual Learning Center (VLC) to promote rapid-cycle learning from actual successes and errors that had occurred in the system (Wahby et al., 2000). By the end of 2000, the VLC had 730 learning cases. In this same vein, a high-performance employee development model was also instituted (American Health Consultants Inc., 2002; VHA, 1996c).

The VHA took a leadership role in the emerging national patient safety movement and worked closely with other national organizations on patient safety issues (Davis, 1998; Leape et al., 1998; Luciano, 2000; NYT, 1999; Shapiro, 1999; Stalhandske et al., 2002). It launched its pioneering

---

[14] Under Secretary of Health's Information Letter, Designating Clinical Programs of Excellence, February 10, 1997.

patient safety initiative in 1997. This five-pronged initiative was intended to build an organizational infrastructure to support patient safety (e.g., establishing the VA National Center for Patient Safety in 1998), to create an organizational culture of safety, to implement safe practices, to produce new knowledge about patient safety through research, and to partner with other organizations to promote more rapid problem solving for patient safety issues.

Change Strategy 4: Align System Finances with Desired Outcomes

Another systemic problem with veterans health care in 1995 was that the Resource Planning and Management Resource Allocation Methodology used to distribute congressionally appropriated funds to the medical centers was neither predictable nor easily understandable, and it perpetuated inefficiencies. Thus another central reengineering strategy was to align funding with operational efficiency and clinical quality improvement.

Creation of the Veterans Equitable Resource Allocation methodology To allocate funds in a predictable, fair, and easy-to-understand manner, a new global, fee-based resource allocation system known as VERA—the Veterans Equitable Resource Allocation methodology—was developed (The Lewin Group and PricewaterhouseCoopers, 1998; VHA, 1997a, 1997b, 1998; Wasserman et al., 2001, 2003). This methodology took into account the veteran population shifts that had occurred in the 1970s and 1980s (e.g., migration from the Rust Belt to the Sun Belt), as well as the high degree of morbidity prevalent in the veteran population.[15]

Expansion of the funding base Historically, funding for the veterans healthcare system came only from the annual congressional appropriation. As part of the transformation, a greater effort was made to collect and retain private insurance reimbursement.

---

[15] VERA was designed to allocate funds to the VISN level, not to individual medical centers or clinics. Under VERA, VA patients are divided into 2 categories based on the types of services required in the preceding 3 years (i.e., Basic Care and Complex Care). Each category is assigned a national per-patient price based on the average of expenditures for the services provided. These prices are then adjusted according to several variables specific to each VISN (e.g., cost of labor and research activity). Approximately 95 percent of VA patients fall into the Basic Care category, which provides a scope of benefits comparable to Medicare Advantage and accounts for about 65 percent of total VA medical care expenditures. The 5 percent of patients falling into Complex Care, which includes services generally not covered by Medicare, account for the remaining expenditures. Although the Basic Care benefit package is comparable to Medicare Advantage, its annual rate is about half the Medicare Advantage rate.

Change Strategy 5: Modernize Information Management

The success of any healthcare delivery system today depends on its ability to manage information originating from many different sources successfully. From the outset of the program, one of its critical goals was to improve the VHA's information management capability through the implementation of a system-wide electronic health record (EHR). The VHA was well positioned to take this step.

Implementation of CPRS/VistA The VHA began to develop a computerized patient record to support clinical care in about 1980 and by the early 1990s was well ahead of the private sector in the use of information technology (IT) (Groen, 2005). In 1996 the VHA launched a major initiative to upgrade its IT infrastructure to create a communications platform robust enough to support the VISNs and to ensure a minimum level of system-wide connectivity and responsiveness. Once the IT infrastructure had been upgraded, the VHA was able to move forward quickly with nationwide implementation of the Computerized Patient Record System (CPRS) in 1997. When CPRS was combined with a new graphical user interface, the VHA's new EHR became known as the Veterans Health Information Systems and Technology Architecture, or VistA (Brown et al., 2003; Conn, 2004; Morgan, 2005; Parrino, 2003; Versel, 2003). Implementation of CPRS/VistA began at selected medical centers in February 1997 and was rolled out to all facilities in six phases. The last of the 172 medical centers went "live" with CPRS/VistA in December 1999.

CPRS includes, among many other functions, an enterprise-wide, computer-based patient record; clinical decision support with clinical reminders, a real-time order checking and clinical alert system, a notification system, and disease management features; computerized provider order entry; a clinical data repository; privacy protections; and a means to facilitate clinical workflow by providing real-time data across the entire enterprise (Brown et al., 2003; Hynes et al., 2004; Morgan, 2005).

Other information management initiatives In addition to CPRS/VistA, other IT enhancements included development and implementation of a bar-code medication administration system (Johnson et al., 2002), use of a semi-smart registration and access card, and implementation of a uniform, validated cost accounting and decision support system.

Funding for the transformation No specific funding was provided for the VHA's reengineering. However, the system's global budget allowed funds to be redirected within the budget to support new initiatives (e.g., establishing CBOCs) as savings were realized from reducing excess capacity (e.g., closing acute-care beds), negotiating more favorable pricing (e.g., the National Formulary), or providing care in lower-cost settings (e.g., moving more care to the outpatient setting).

Between FY 1995 and FY 1999, inclusive, the VA's medical care budget increased by $1 billion (rising from $16.3 to $17.3 billion), for a total 5-year aggregate increase of 6 percent. Medical care inflation was averaging 5 to 7 percent per annum during these years. By contrast, in the 5 FYs preceding the transformation (i.e., FY 1990 to FY 1994), the medical care budget increased 41 percent, and in the 5 years after the transformation (i.e., FY 2000 to FY04), it increased 58 percent.[16]

The VA Healthcare System Transformed

Over a relatively short time, nearly every major management system in the VHA was fundamentally changed and its operational performance improved. Box 4-1 lists some of the changes.

Improved Clinical Performance and Quality of Care

Documentation of the improved clinical performance of the "new VA" comes from varied sources. Jha and colleagues (2003) showed that from 1995 to 2000, the VHA markedly improved its performance on a standardized panel of quality-of-care performance measures. They further showed that the VA's performance was superior to fee-for-service Medicare on all 11 performance measures used by both systems from 1997 to 1999 and on 12 of 13 measures in 2000.

Jha and colleagues (2007) further showed that the VA's compliance with recommendations for influenza and pneumococcus vaccinations rose from 27 and 28 percent, respectively, in 1995, to 70 and 85 percent in 2003. Variation in vaccination rates (e.g., due to geography, clinical indication, site of treatment) disappeared. These changes were associated with a 50 percent drop in VA hospital admissions for community-acquired pneumonia compared with a 15 percent increase for Medicare patients, among whom vaccination rates had increased only minimally.

Kerr and colleagues (2004) compared diabetes management in the VA with that in commercially managed care organizations according to seven process, three outcome, and four care-satisfaction measures. VA patients scored better on all process measures and also on cholesterol and blood glucose control. Hypertension control and patients' satisfaction with their care were comparable in both populations. Similar findings were reported by Singh and Kalavar (2004). Ward and colleagues (2004) observed that the

---

[16] During the latter 5 years, the number of patients served by the system doubled.

BOX 4-1
Veterans Health Administration: Changes That Occurred
During Fiscal Years 1995 to 1999

- Implemented the new Veterans Integrated Service Network operating structure and its 22 new integrated service networks.
- Designed and implemented a National Formulary.
- Implemented universal primary care.
- Completed the largest ever deployment of an electronic health record in less than 3 years.
- Developed and deployed a universal "semi-smart" access and identification card.
- Closed 28,986 acute-care hospital beds.
- Decreased bed-days of care per 1,000 patients by 68 percent.
- Admitted 350,000 fewer patients to hospitals in fiscal year (FY) 1999 compared with FY 1995, even though >700,000 more patients received hands-on care in FY 1999 than in FY 1995 (a 24 percent increase in patients treated).
- Reduced staffing by 25,867 full-time equivalents (a 12 percent decrease).
- Established 302 new community-based outpatient clinics.
- Merged 52 medical centers into 25 multicampus facilities.
- Eliminated 2,793 forms (72 percent) and automated the remainder.
- Designed and implemented a new global fee-based resource allocation system.
- Increased the proportion of surgeries performed on an ambulatory basis from 35 percent to more than 80 percent, significantly decreased 30-day surgical morbidity and mortality, and increased the total number of surgeries performed by 10 percent.
- Decreased per patient expenditures by 25.1 percent (in constant dollars).
- Dramatically improved quality of care; performance on standardized quality of care indicators higher than that of Medicare on all but one measure.
- Developed and implemented customer service standards; markedly improved service satisfaction, with veterans healthcare service rating higher than that of the private sector every veteran since 1999, according to the annual American Customer Satisfaction Index.
- Launched the largest ever translational research initiative (i.e., the Quality Enhancement Research Initiative).
- Realigned the system's $1 billion research program to better address veterans' needs.
- Realigned postgraduate physician residency and other educational programs; increased the proportion of the Veterans Health Administration 9,000 residency positions dedicated to primary care from 34 percent in 1994 to 49 percent in 2000.
- Established the Bachelor of Science in Nursing as the required entry-level degree for the system's 60,000-nurse workforce, and committed $50 million to help currently employed nurses achieve this level of education.

VA's improved adherence to diabetes care guidelines was associated with frequent feedback to frontline caregivers, more effective communication between physicians and nurses, and other organizational characteristics. Proper management of diabetes is especially important for the VA because 25 percent of its patients are diabetic, and this population has an exceptionally high rate of comorbidity, as well as being heavy users of services (Ashton et al., 2003a).

Using RAND's quality assessment instrument of 348 indicators covering 26 conditions, Asch and colleagues compared VA patient care in 12 VISNs with care in 12 matched communities for the years 1997 through 2000. The VA's overall quality, chronic disease management, and preventive care were found to be significantly better, while its acute care was essentially the same as that provided in the matched communities (Asch et al., 2004a). Although the differences were greatest for conditions for which the VHA had established performance measures and actively monitored performance, better quality of care was not confined to the areas targeted for quality improvement (Asch et al., 2004b).

The nationally representative 2000 and 2004 surveys of the Behavior Risk Factor Surveillance System indicated that persons receiving care at VA medical centers were substantially more likely than insured adults treated at private healthcare facilities to receive recommended ambulatory care services for cancer prevention, cardiovascular risk reduction, diabetes management, and infectious disease prevention (Ross et al., 2008).

Selim and colleagues (2006) compared risk-adjusted mortality in persons cared for by the VA with that of those cared for by the Medicare Advantage Program for the period 1999 to 2004. They found that the average male and female patients cared for by the VA had, respectively, a 40 percent and 24 percent lower risk of death over 2 years than the average male and female patients in the Medicare Advantage Program. The researchers were unable to determine what differences in care structures and processes contributed to the lower mortality in the VA patients.

The NSQIP's linkage to improved surgical outcomes attracted the attention of the private sector in 1999. Since the feasibility of implementing NSQIP in the private sector was first demonstrated (Fink et al., 2002), this quality improvement program has been found to be fully applicable to private-sector surgical programs and is being used increasingly by private healthcare providers (Khuri et al., 2008).

Implementation of the National Formulary largely resolved the problem of varying availability of drugs (which previously had been a major source of patient complaints and physician frustration) and appears to have been effective in improving evidence-based drug prescribing, while at the same time making it possible to obtain sizable price reductions from manufacturers (Selim et al., 2006). Likewise, by using the Barcode Medication

Administration, automated prescription filling, and other measures implemented to improve medication management (Gebhart, 1999; Huskamp et al., 2003), the VHA has achieved unparalleled accuracy rates in medication administration. For instance, in 2005 the VHA filled 231 million prescriptions with an accuracy rate of 99.993 percent (Nicholson, 2006).

Higher Service Satisfaction

Service satisfaction among VA healthcare users improved dramatically from 1995 to 1999. Two of the factors most closely associated with increased service satisfaction were the CBOCs and the heightened focus on primary care (Armstrong et al., 2006; Chapko and Van Deusen Lukas, 2001; Rosenheck, 2000; Schall et al., 2004). Four years after the launch of the primary care initiative, essentially all patients in the VA healthcare system had been assigned to a primary care team, and more than 80 percent of them could name their primary caregiver.[17]

In 1999, 80 percent of VA healthcare users believed care had improved from 2 years earlier, and overall satisfaction with the VA's service received a rating of 79 on the American Customer Satisfaction Index (ACSI), compared with 70 for private-sector hospitals (National Quality Research Center, 1999). And from 1999 to 2003, the number of veterans using VA health care rose from 3.4 million to more than 7 million, suggesting that veterans had recognized the improvement and were "voting with their feet" (Fong, 2003). The VHA's service satisfaction ratings on the ACSI have been higher than those of the private sector every year since 1999 (Freedberg, 2006; National Quality Research Center, 2007a, 2007b), and VA healthcare users are reported to be 2 to 8 times more satisfied with their outpatient care than non-VA users (Harada et al., 2002).

Greater Operational Efficiency

Between 1995 and 2000, the VHA substantially improved access and efficiency (Box 4-1) (GAO, 1998, 1999). Steps were taken to decrease inpatient lengths of stay, close excess acute-care beds, increase ambulatory capacity, shift care to an ambulatory setting when medically appropriate, and make better use of nonphysician, independent licensed practitioners in primary care and other clinically appropriate settings.[18]

The General Accounting Office (now the Government Accountability Office) reported that from 1996 to 1998, the VHA reduced annual operat-

---

[17] VHA internal service satisfaction survey data, 1998.
[18] Under Secretary for Health's Information Letter: Utilization of Nurse Practitioners and Clinical Nurse Specialists. July 7, 1997.

ing costs by more than $1 billion. As a result, it realized a nonappropriated revenue surplus of $496 million (GAO, 1999).

Ashton and colleagues (2003b) reported on decreased hospital use for nine cohorts of the VHA's most vulnerable patients. This landmark study found that hospital bed day rates and urgent clinic visits for the 9 cohorts fell by 50 and 35 percent, respectively, from 1995 through 1998. A moderate increase in medical clinic visits did occur, but there was an overall substantial reduction in the amount of care provided. In all 9 cohorts, the 1-year survival rates stayed the same or significantly improved (i.e., for congestive heart failure, angina, and major depression).

In treating persons with substance abuse disorders, one of the VA's special populations, the VA substantially increased outpatient care and decreased its historical reliance on inpatient care (Chen et al., 2001; Humphreys and Horst, 2002; Office of the Inspector General, 1997). The change was described as "nothing short of dramatic" (Humphreys et al., 1999).

Recent years have also seen an improvement in access to and the quality of VA mental health care (Bhatia and Fernandes, 2008). The VHA's spending for inpatient mental health decreased by 21 percent from 1995 to 2001, while spending for specialized outpatient care rose 63 percent (Chen et al., 2003). Although this shift from inpatient to outpatient mental health care was accompanied by substantial increases in outpatient medication costs, it resulted in a 22 percent reduction in the overall average per-user cost of mental health care and a 35 percent increase in the number of persons receiving care (Chen et al., 2003). The CBOCs accounted for at least some of the increased access to mental health services (Wooten, 2002). Service-line implementation of mental health services was associated with significant improvement in the continuity of care and readmission rates (Greenberg et al., 2003). In this same vein, Long and colleagues (2005) observed that the VHA has increasingly been serving veterans who have trouble accessing private health care (e.g., for mental health services).

For veterans with PTSD, Rosenheck and Fontana (2001) found significantly decreased inpatient care but no deterioration in treatment effectiveness caused by the shortened inpatient stays, although there were mixed effects in residential treatment programs.

VERA markedly simplified the VHA's budgetary process and provided financial incentives for coordinating care in the most appropriate setting. Between FY 1994 and FY 1999, the VHA's systemwide average annual expenditure per patient decreased from $5,479 to $4,105, a 25.1 percent decrease in constant dollars.[19]

---

[19] In this calculation, Basic and Complex Care patients post-VERA were combined to allow comparison with expenditures pre-VERA.

Thibodeau and colleagues (2007) documented a significant decreased cost per patient and an improved quality of services in the VHA from 1992 to 1998. They attributed this mainly to reductions in excess capacity and a more intense use of remaining capacity. Yaisawarng and Burgess (2006) found that the average VA hospital in FY 2000 operated at 94 percent efficiency, compared with 90 percent in private hospitals.

Implementation of VistA has been linked with improved quality of care, increased productivity, and enhanced operational capability (Brown, 2007; Pizziferri et al., 2005). Although it was feared that use of the EHR would require more time from physicians during a clinical session, this was found not to be the case (Pizziferri et al., 2005). To the contrary, clinicians using VistA have increased their productivity by nearly 6 percent per year since 1999. However, what has been truly transformative[20] is the synergism among the EHR, performance measurement, increased accountability, aligned financial incentives, a quality improvement environment, and a delivery system focused on population health (Anderson, 2005; Greenfield and Kaplan, 2004; Jackson et al., 2005; Kupersmith et al., 2007; Young et al., 1997).

Education and Research Missions

Substantial changes were made in the VHA's education and research programs, although space does not allow them to be discussed here. Suffice it to say that the research program was realigned to better address veterans' needs (Rutherford et al., 1999), as illustrated by QUERI, and the education programs were realigned to comport better with the VHA's new focus on ambulatory care and chronic disease management (Stevens et al., 1998, 2001). An example of this change is that the proportion of primary care positions among the 9,000 residency positions funded by the VHA increased from 34 percent in 1994 to 49 percent in 2000.

Lessons Learned

Much can be learned from the VHA's reengineering, and it has been the subject of a number of dissertations, case studies, and reviews (Armstrong et al., 2001; DeLuca, 2000; Edmondson et al., 2006; Kee and Newcomer, 2007; Kizer, 2001; Knopman et al., 2003; Mitkowski and Feinstein, 2007; Oliver, 2007; Perlin, 2006; Perlin et al., 2004; Skydell, 1998; Young, 2000a,

---

[20] The VA's ability to provide uninterrupted care for veterans evacuated from New Orleans after Hurricane Katrina in 2006—in stark contrast to other regional healthcare providers, whose paper records were destroyed by the floodwaters—was a graphic illustration of the value of the EHR for continuity of operations.

BOX 4-2
Veterans Health Administration Transformation:
Observations and Lessons Learned

- Rapid and dramatic change is possible in health care, even in large, politically sensitive, financially stressed, publicly administered healthcare systems.
- Improved healthcare quality, better service, and reduced cost can all be achieved at the same time.
- Articulation of a clear vision of the new future and how things will be different is essential for any effort at major change.
- The vision must be combined with a pragmatic strategic plan that includes concrete goals, defined responsibilities, and performance measures to assess progress toward achieving the goals.
- Measuring and publicly reporting performance data using standardized performance measures is a powerful lever for change.
- Performance data must be fed back to those who can make improvements.
- To improve performance or quality, leaders must show that improvement is an organizational priority and make sure that everyone in the organization knows it.
- Decentralization of authority must be coupled with a full understanding of mission-critical activities, clear delineation of responsibility and accountability, and monitoring of performance to help prevent things from "falling through the cracks."
- Automated information management is a critical tool for healthcare transformation and quality improvement; the electronic health record is an essential tool today.
- An integrated system of health care can be achieved with either vertical or virtual integration, or both. The information management system, contracts, and similar arrangements are the glue that holds a virtually integrated system together.
- Focusing on changing organizational performance and processes is more productive than focusing on poorly performing individuals.
- If healthcare change is to be successful, frontline clinicians must continuously be part of the planning and implementation from the beginning.
- Much of what is needed to accomplish and sustain change needs to be in place before the change effort is initiated.
- When major changes are being undertaken, there is no such thing as too much communication about the proposed changes.
- Training and education to prepare personnel to function in a new way are critical components of the change process.
- Regardless of how good or extensive the planning is, every problem that may require midcourse correction cannot be foreseen. Therefore, in planning for change, the perfect must not be allowed to become the enemy of the good.
- Healthcare organizations are complex adaptive systems governed by the rules of complexity theory. Healthcare change agents must understand chaos and complexity theory.
- Alignment of finances with desired outcomes is essential in any change effort.
- Leaders must maintain an unwavering focus on the ultimate goal despite being distracted by situational circumstances.

2000b). Selected lessons learned about healthcare reform and organizational transformation are listed in Box 4-2.

THE CLINICAL TRANSFORMATION OF ASCENSION HEALTH

David B. Pryor, M.D., Ann Hendrich, M.S., R.N., Sanford F. Tolchin, M.D., Robert J. Henkel, M.P.H., James K. Beckmann, Jr., M.B.A., and Anthony R. Tersigni, Ed.D.
Ascension Health

Ascension Health is the largest nonprofit healthcare system in the United States, the largest Catholic healthcare system, and the third largest system overall (after the VA and Hospital Corporation of America). Ascension Health operates in 20 states and the District of Columbia. It encompasses more than 200 places where care is provided, including 67 acute-care hospitals. Working in these hospitals are 30,000 affiliated physicians and 106,000 associates, including more than 20,000 nurses. The hospitals see 660,000 discharges a year.

Ascension Health's "Call to Action," established in October 2002, promised "Health Care That Works, Health Care That Is Safe, and Health Care That Leaves No One Behind." The goal for the Health Care That Is Safe initiative, as established in 2003, was: "The care we deliver will be safe and effective. We commit to having excellent clinical care with no preventable injuries or deaths by July 2008." The primary metric was mortality. It was estimated that 15 percent of all deaths not occurring in patients admitted for end-of-life care were preventable (900 lives annually across the Ascension Health system). In addition to mortality, seven other Priorities for Action were identified: adverse drug events, the Joint Commission on Accreditation of Healthcare Organizations' national patient safety goals, nosocomial infections, perioperative complications, pressure ulcers, falls and fall injuries, and birth trauma. Progress in the system has been remarkable, with results far exceeding the initial goals. This paper describes results through December 2007 and the approaches used across the system to achieve those results. Additional details, including the membership of the "clinical excellence team" that oversaw the creation and development of the strategy, have been presented elsewhere (Berriel-Cass et al., 2006; Butler et al., 2007; Ewing et al., 2007; Gibbons et al., 2006; Hendrich et al., 2007; Lancaster et al., 2007; Mazza et al., 2007; Pryor et al., 2006; Rose et al., 2006; Tolchin et al., 2007).

By setting a goal of *no* preventable injuries or deaths, Ascension Health committed itself to achieving a transformational goal. Transformational change, by definition, occurs at a more rapid pace than that seen in the typical incremental change process. Ascension Health identified five challenges that needed to be addressed to make rapid and sustainable change possible: (1) culture, (2) the business case, (3) infrastructure, (4) standardization, and (5) how we worked together across the organization. Specific strategies for meeting each of the challenges were implemented but are not presented here (Berriel-Cass et al., 2006; Butler et al., 2007; Ewing et al., 2007; Gibbons et al., 2006; Hendrich et al., 2007; Lancaster et al., 2007; Mazza et al., 2007; Pryor et al., 2006; Rose et al., 2006; Tolchin et al., 2007).

The focus of the work around the eight Priorities for Action was essential to the success of the efforts. At the time the work was begun, more than 240 different quality indicators were considered for use in at least 1 of our hospitals (provided by different payers, employers, and accreditation or other quality groups), and the number would be substantially larger now. Even today, however, studies demonstrating clearly improved outcomes as a result of improving a specific indicator are largely lacking. Ascension Health used a different approach to identify the key areas of focus. The 8 Priorities for Action were identified by a rapid-design planning team of 38 individuals from across the system (plus our strategic partners from the Institute for Healthcare Improvement) who were asked to address the question of what work needed to be done to eliminate all preventable injuries and deaths.

The team's work was independently validated by having 2 of our larger hospitals (and, shortly afterward, a number of our other hospitals) review the charts of their last 50 deaths and answer 3 questions: (1) Was the death in a patient not admitted for end-of-life care? (2) Was the death preventable or "potentially preventable (not necessarily an error)"? (3) If the death was potentially preventable and did not occur in a patient admitted for end-of-life care, did the admission have at least one of our Priorities for Action in addition to mortality? The initial reviews suggested that 15 percent of the deaths occurring in patients not admitted for end-of-life care were potentially preventable (translating to 900 lives saved across our system). Moreover, when we extrapolated the results of the New York and Colorado/Utah autopsy studies (Brennan et al., 1991; Thomas et al., 2000), which are described in the Institute of Medicine report *To Err Is Human* (IOM, 2000b), we estimated that between 8 and 22 percent of the deaths in patients not admitted for end-of-life care might have been related to errors. This indicated that avoiding all unnecessary deaths in patients not admitted for end-of-life care—which, by our calculation, would result in a 15 percent reduction in the death rate—was a reasonable, albeit ambitious, goal. We were encouraged to find that all of the unnecessary deaths in our review were associated with at least one of our Priority for Action events (in addition to mortality), suggesting that the strategy of focusing on the eight Priorities for Action was sound. Further validation of the focus on the eight Priorities for

Action subsequently occurred in 2004 when the Institute for Healthcare Improvement's 100,000 Lives campaign chose to focus on similar events (Institute for Healthcare Improvement, 2006).

Initially we selected the percentage decline in the mortality rate among patients not admitted for end-of-life care as our primary outcome metric. This metric was measured by having all hospitals examine the charts of all deaths (or at least a random sample of 50) during the last quarter of the baseline year and each subsequent year and identify the proportion of patients not admitted for end-of-life care. This proportion was then multiplied by the total number of deaths for the year and divided by the number of discharges to create a "rate of death" among patients not admitted for end-of-life care. In our assessments, there were approximately 660,000 discharges, including 15,000 deaths. Of those deaths, 37 to 40 percent were among patients not admitted for end-of-life care. Reducing by 15 percent the 6,000 deaths among patients not admitted for end-of-life care (40 percent of 15,000 deaths total) would mean that 900 deaths would be prevented annually (15 percent of 6,000). This became the primary goal to be achieved by July 2008.

We seriously underestimated our potential. What we found was that mortality rates among patients not admitted for end-of-life care after our first year of focus on the Priorities for Action had declined by 21 percent. With the initial success, we also decided to explore other approaches for measuring progress that did not require manual chart reviews. We looked at a number of approaches for correcting mortality rates to take into account the severity of illness, and we selected the Care Science model (Pauly et al., 1996) (now part of Premier). Changes in the mortality rates measured using the two approaches had a correlation coefficient greater than 0.85, and we believed this was close enough. The new outcome measure became the observed minus the expected mortality rate per 100 discharges (the difference, rather than the ratio, was selected to maintain a constant relationship between the number of deaths avoided and the percentage decline in the mortality rates each year).

Using this model, we estimate that more than 3,000 deaths have been prevented in the 4 years since the baseline year (through March 2008). The yearly incremental progress for each year (measured from April of one year to March of the subsequent year) is shown in Figure 4-3. Because the y axis is the observed minus the expected mortality rate, improvements are represented by falling numbers. For the final year, April 2007 through March 2008, the estimated number of deaths avoided vs. the baseline year (April 2003 through March 2004) was 3,275, reflecting a slight increase in the number of admissions in the final year.

Figure 4-4 offers another way of looking at this information. Here, the declines in observed mortality (not adjusted for severity of illness, ex-

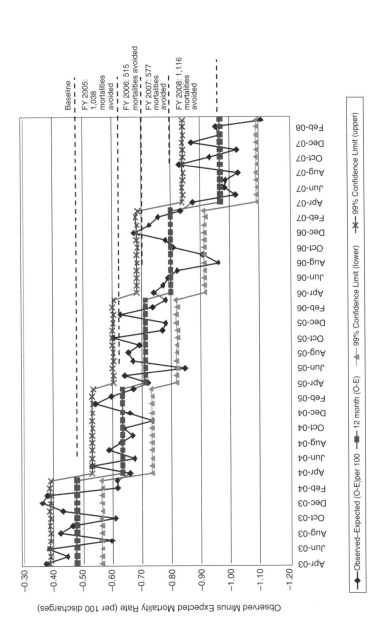

FIGURE 4-3 Observed mortality minus expected mortality from April 2003 through March 2008. Shown are the yearly average and the subsequent incrementally avoided mortalities estimated for each year from the baseline year.

NOTE: FY = fiscal year.

SOURCE: Reprinted with permission from Ascension Health. © 2008 Ascension Health. This work, including its content, may not be used, reproduced, duplicated, displayed, or distributed absent express written permission from Ascension Health.

cept that known hospice patients are excluded) for each of our FYs (July through June) are plotted against one y axis, and the increasing case mix index over time is plotted against the other y axis. Although the majority of deaths have occurred in patients expected to die during their hospitalization, the declines have been significant enough to show an improvement in the observed mortality rates despite the increasing severity of illness among patients admitted (measured by the case mix index).

One important factor contributing to our success has been how the work has been shared across Ascension Health. For each of our Priorities for Action, one to three of our hospitals have served as the alpha or lead site(s), testing and trying different improvement approaches. In all of our hospitals, for each Priority for Action, affinity groups (composed of key individuals at each hospital for each Priority for Action) have formed with steering committees to identify key strategies, standardize key outcome measures, and foster learning communities that have met both in person and virtually.

One example of how this has worked is our approach to perinatal safety (i.e., eliminating birth trauma). Forty-three sites at Ascension Health deliver about 75,000 babies a year. The alpha sites working with the steer-

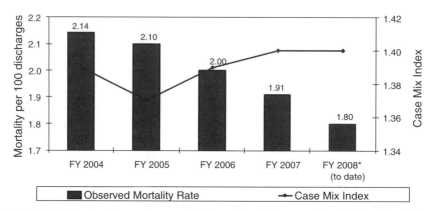

FIGURE 4-4 Yearly observed mortality (unadjusted for severity of illness) and the case mix index for fiscal years (July through June) 2004 through 2007 and fiscal year 2008 through December. Unadjusted mortality declined by more than 1,500 lives with adjusted mortality decreasing by over 2,800 lives.
NOTE: FY = fiscal year.
SOURCE: Reprinted with permission from Ascension Health. © 2008 Ascension Health. This work, including its content, may not be used, reproduced, duplicated, displayed, or distributed absent express written permission from Ascension Health.

ing committee identified five important elements that needed to be adopted. They called the program HANDS (for Handling All Neonatal Deliveries Safely). The five elements were (1) an elective induction bundle, (2) an augmentation bundle, (3) common physician and nurse training programs for communication and interpretation of fetal monitoring strips, (4) SBAR (Situation, Background, Assessment, and Recommendation) communication standards for communication among clinical team caregivers, and (5) crisis simulation training using mannequins to help teams become used to working efficiently together in high-risk, critical situations.

The steering committee planned an in-person kick-off meeting (which subsequently became an annual meeting) that included five individuals from each Ascension Health hospital where babies are delivered. Attendees typically included a lead obstetrician, a lead nurse, a lead administrator, and two other key care team members. These individuals were asked to commit to all five elements of the program and take them back to each of their hospitals. It was a moving moment when the 220 attendees demonstrated their commitment to the program by signing a self-drawn tracing of their hands (referring to the program title, HANDS, of course) on a big sheet of paper hung on the wall.

The results have been exceptional. Standardized reporting for all the Priority for Action measures from all sites began midway in the work in January 2006. Figure 4-5 shows the monthly rate of birth injuries since that time. The 2 years of experience shown include 144,688 live births. In January 2006 the birth trauma rate was close to 3 per 1,000 live births. Since then rates across Ascension Health have steadily fallen to the current rate of less than 0.5 per 1,000 live births. Figure 4-6 is a graph that is transparently shared across Ascension Health, giving the experience of each hospital shown. The y axis shows the rate for an entire year (in this case, calendar year 2007) for each hospital positioned along the x axis. For reference, the national rate of 2.6 birth traumas per 1,000 live births is also shown. Although the same definitions are used, the Ascension Health numbers represent self-reported clinical results for 2007, while the rate from the Agency for Healthcare Research and Quality is based on claims data for 2004 (and current national results may be lower). Using the national reference rate of 2.6, current Ascension Health performance for 2007 (0.69 per 1,000 live births) is 74 percent lower than the national reference rate.

Figure 4-7 shows the neonatal mortality rates per 1,000 live births for the individual hospitals. Across all of Ascension Health, the rate for 2007 was 0.95, or 79 percent lower than the national rate reported in 2004.

Pressure ulcers are a frequent and often serious or even disabling occurrence in hospitals (particularly Braden stage 3 and 4 ulcers). A pressure ulcer initiative led by Ascension Health nursing was the subject of the first Priority for Action national affinity group meeting. About 240 individuals

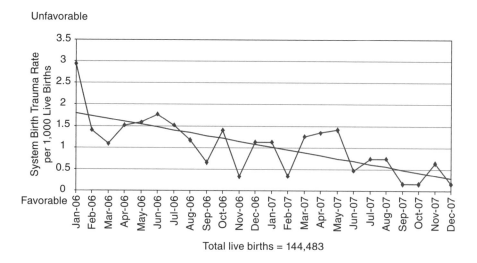

FIGURE 4-5 Ascension Health System birth trauma rates from January 2006 through December 2007.
SOURCE: Reprinted with permission from Ascension Health. © 2008 Ascension Health. This work, including its content, may not be used, reproduced, duplicated, displayed, or distributed absent express written permission from Ascension Health.

from across our 67 acute-care hospitals attended. In the 2-day meeting, participants agreed on standardized approaches for measurements and developed a single care plan for use across the system called SKIN—for Surfaces, Keep turning, Incontinence, and Nutrition management. Surfaces referred to the fact that many patients spend too much time on mattresses or frames that are not skin-injury sparing, either because they are outdated or because they are designed for units not expecting to accommodate prolonged stays (e.g., the emergency room, perioperative recovery units). The proposed elimination of preventable pressure ulcers across Ascension Health represented a significant commitment by the organization, as it would entail such actions as the replacement of all inappropriate mattresses and frames (a $60 million capital investment) to ensure that every patient would always be on an appropriate surface.

The results of the initiative are shown in Figures 4-8 and 4-9. Figure 4-8 shows the monthly decline across the system for calendar years 2006 and 2007. Figure 4-9 shows the results for each hospital for the entire calendar year of 2007. It is difficult to offer a comparison with national benchmarks, as no comparable data exist. However, available evidence suggests

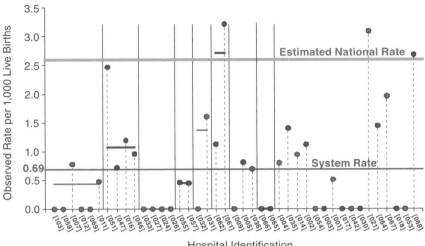

Hospital Identification

FIGURE 4-6 Individual hospital birth trauma rates for calendar year 2007.
NOTE: The graph represents data that are self-reported and self-validated in accordance with the definitions and guidelines adopted by the Ascension Health Perinatal Safety Affinity Group.[a]

[a] Birth trauma is unintentional harm to a newborn that occurs during birth and requires medical intervention. Ascension Health uses the Agency for Healthcare Research and Quality (AHRQ) birth trauma patient safety indicator definition and clinical case review. Estimated national rate: the Healthcare Cost and Utilization Project (HCUP) rate for 2004 was 2.6 birth traumas per 1,000 live births, (AHRQ, 2004). (The national data collection methodology may not be identical to Ascension Health methodology.) System rate is 0.6882 birth traumas per 1,000 live births (based on the AHRQ birth trauma patient safety indicator definition and clinical case review).
SOURCE: Reprinted with permission from Ascension Health. © 2008 Ascension Health. This work, including its content, may not be used, reproduced, duplicated, displayed, or distributed absent express written permission from Ascension Health.

that pressure ulcers occur in 7 to 8 percent of discharges from American hospitals. When this figure is converted to rates per 1,000 patient days, estimates of occurrence would be on the order of 18 to 22 facility-acquired pressure ulcers. Measured against this rate, the current performance across Ascension Health is 95 percent lower.

Figures 4-10 to 4-13 show the rates of hospital-acquired infections across Ascension Health: Figures 4-10 and 4-11 provide similar results for ventilator-associated pneumonia; and Figures 4-12 and 4-13 show results

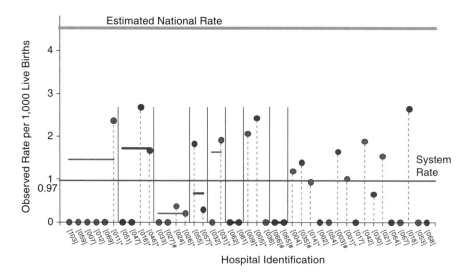

FIGURE 4-7 Individual hospital neonatal mortality rates for calendar year 2007. NOTE: This graph represents data that are self-reported and self-validated in accordance with the definitions and guidelines adopted by the Ascension Health Perinatal Safety Affinity Group.[a]

[a]Neonatal mortality is a death during the first 28 days after birth and prior to discharge of a live-born inborn infant ≥ 24 weeks of gestational age born without lethal malformation or abnormality. The estimated national rate is 4.52 neonatal mortalities per 1,000 live births based on 2004 data (CDC, 2007). The system rate is 0.9528 neonatal mortalities per 1,000 live births.
SOURCE: Reprinted with permission from Ascension Health. © 2008 Ascension Health. This work, including its content, may not be used, reproduced, duplicated, displayed or distributed absent express written permission from Ascension Health.

for central line–associated bloodstream infections in the intensive care unit. Compared with national rates, Ascension Health's performance is 56 and 32 percent lower for pneumonia and bloodstream infections, respectively. Despite the improvements shown in these figures, however, we believe further progress still needs to be made.

Figure 4-14 shows performance across the system for falls resulting in serious injury. Given that appropriate care management strategies (e.g., early ambulation) require patients to walk even when they may be weakened, it is impossible to prevent falls completely. It is possible, however, to reduce significantly not only the number of falls that occur but also the number of serious injuries that result. By screening patients for their fall risk and adopting strategies that identify such patients (e.g., "Ruby Slippers,"

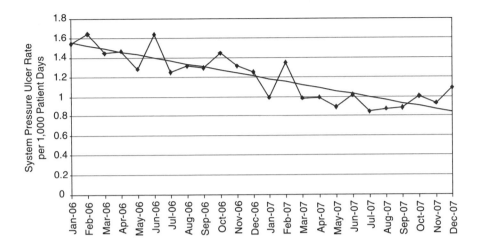

FIGURE 4-8 Ascension Health System pressure ulcer incidence rates system-wide from January 2006 through December 2007.
SOURCE: Reprinted with permission from Ascension Health. © 2008 Ascension Health. This work, including its content, may not be used, reproduced, duplicated, displayed, or distributed absent express written permission from Ascension Health.

which provides all high-risk patients with colored, ribbed socks), associates working on a floor can quickly identify and aid patients who require assistance and who may be trying to ambulate on their own. Strategies such as these have resulted in a significant improvement across the system. The system rate for falls with serious injury is 0.097 per 1,000 patient days. National benchmarks are again difficult to find, but an estimate is 6 percent of the median falls index, or 0.21 per 1,000 patient days. Ascension Health's rate is 54 percent lower.

Figure 4-15 provides a summary of performance across all of the measures for calendar year 2007 vs. the national benchmarks cited. Although comparisons with national benchmarks in many cases require significant extrapolation, the results clearly demonstrate that it is possible to make remarkable progress in improving patient safety in a large, geographically dispersed health system.

Strategies for addressing each of the challenges cited earlier have been important contributors to our success. One question that frequently arises is the effect on financial operations (the business case for quality). The leadership across Ascension Health has been committed to improving quality and safety, but it has also believed that such work will contribute positively

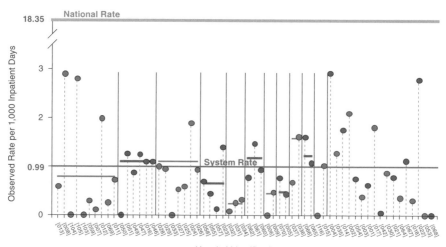

FIGURE 4-9 Individual hospital pressure ulcer incidence for calendar year 2007. NOTE: This graph represents data that are self-reported and self-validated in accordance with the definitions and guidelines adopted by the Ascension Health Pressure Ulcers Affinity Group.[a]

[a] A facility-acquired pressure ulcer is an observable pressure-related alteration of intact skin that was not identified and documented within the first 24 hours after admission. The estimated national incidence rate is 7 percent of discharges or ~18.35 facility-acquired pressure ulcers per 1,000 inpatient days (Whittington and Briones, 2004). (The national data collection methodology used by Whittington and Briones may not be identical to Ascension Health methodology.) The system rate is 0.9831 facility-acquired pressure ulcers per 1,000 inpatient days (metric excludes obstetrics, behavioral health, and exempt rehabilitation units).

SOURCE: Reprinted with permission from Ascension Health. © 2008 Ascension Health. This work, including its content, may not be used, reproduced, duplicated, displayed, or distributed absent express written permission from Ascension Health.

to operational performance by reducing costs associated with avoidable injuries. Figure 4-16 offers one example of how this works. Malpractice costs—shown in terms of total cost and cost per equivalent discharge—have declined significantly since FY 2004. In FY 2007, costs were 56 percent lower than they were in FY 2004. Although many risk management strategies contributed to this performance, the reduction in avoidable injuries and other negative events has been a very important contributor.

Ascension Health is nearing completion of a coordinated, committed 5-year effort to eliminate all preventable injuries and deaths occurring in

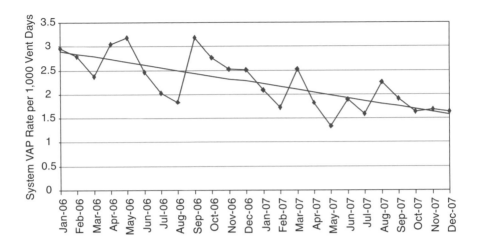

FIGURE 4-10 Ascension Health System ventilator-associated pneumonia (VAP) rates system-wide from January 2006 through December 2007.
SOURCE: Reprinted with permission from Ascension Health. © 2008 Ascension Health. This work, including its content, may not be used, reproduced, duplicated, displayed, or distributed absent express written permission from Ascension Health.

our hospitals. Through focused and sustained efforts involving thousands of committed associates and physicians across our hospitals, we have made remarkable progress. Although our results have exceeded our initial expectations, we remain humbled by the amount of work remaining. Clearly, greater reductions are possible, as evidenced by some of the variability still present in our system and by the average performance of Ascension Health on other indicators and measures. We believe we have been focusing on the most important factors, such as accountable goals; transparency across our system in reporting results; addressing the five challenge areas, including the business case for quality; and the deep organizational commitment across our boards of directors, senior management, and clinicians with mutual accountability. Many individuals have requested that we share our results for their motivational value and as a demonstration of the rapid improvements that are possible across a large system. Although the results speak for themselves, it is important to recognize that we chose self-reporting methodologies that have not been independently validated and that some national benchmark comparisons are problematic, requiring significant extrapolation.

Internally across our system, we have borrowed Churchill's quote after El Alamein to refer to our work: "This is not the end. This is not even the

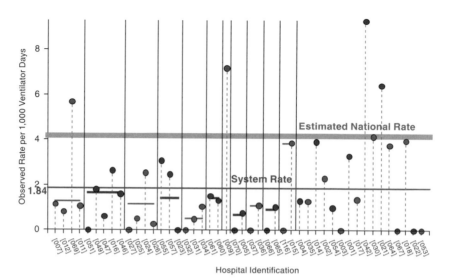

FIGURE 4-11 Individual hospital ventilator-associated pneumonia rates for calendar year 2007.
NOTE: This graph represents data that are self-reported and self-validated in accordance with the definitions and guidelines adopted by the Ascension Health Nosocomial Infections Affinity Group.[a]
[a] Ventilator-associated pneumonia (VAP) is a pneumonia infection that a patient acquires while on a mechanical ventilator. The PFA metric includes ICU patients only. The estimated national rate in 2006 was 4.12 VAPs in the ICU per 1,000 ventilator days (excluding burn and pediatric ICUs); 4.17 VAPs in the ICU per 1,000 ventilator days (including burn and pediatric ICUs (Edwards et al., 2007). The system rate is 1.812 VAPs in the ICU per 1,000 ventilator days.
SOURCE: Reprinted with permission from Ascension Health. © 2008 Ascension Health. This work, including its content, may not be used, reproduced, duplicated, displayed, or distributed absent express written permission from Ascension Health.

beginning of the end, but it may be the end of the beginning." Viewed in the context of this workshop, many of our approaches have focused on standardizing specific processes in high-risk areas, using systems engineering methods where possible. We have recently begun work that focuses not simply on sustaining our current performance, but also on extending the improvement by adopting strategies that have been developed, particularly in other industries, around a high-reliability culture. In these approaches, our focus shifts to a coordinated analysis of every event and near-miss that occurs, while we continue to promote and refine the teamwork and individual behaviors necessary to ensure that the inevitable individual errors that occur in human processes do not result in harm to a patient.

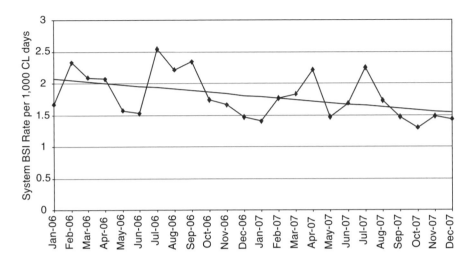

FIGURE 4-12 Ascension Health System intensive care unit central-line bloodstream infection rates system-wide from January 2006 through December 2007.

NOTE: BSI = bloodstream infection; CL = central line.

SOURCE: Reprinted with permission from Ascension Health. © 2008 Ascension Health. This work, including its content, may not be used, reproduced, duplicated, displayed, or distributed absent express written permission from Ascension Health.

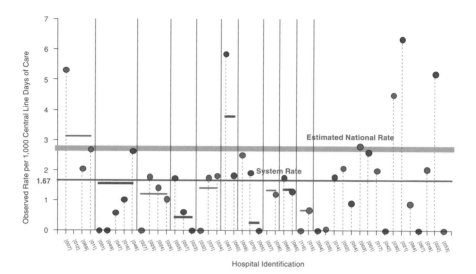

FIGURE 4-13 Individual hospital ICU central-line bloodstream infection rates for calendar year 2007.

NOTE: This graph represents data that are self-reported and self-validated in accordance with the definitions and guidelines adopted by the Ascension Health Nosocomial Infections Affinity Group.[a]

[a] Bloodstream infection (BSI) is a hospital-acquired infection as a result of an arterial or venous line IV. The PFA metric includes ICU patients only. The estimated national rate for 2006 data was 2.57 BSIs in the ICU per 1,000 central-line days (excluding burn and pediatric ICUs); 2.80 BSIs in the ICU per 1,000 central-line days (including burn and pediatric ICUs) (Edwards et al., 2007). The system rate is 1.764 BSIs in the ICU per 1,000 central-line days.

SOURCE: Reprinted with permission from Ascension Health. © 2008 Ascension Health. This work, including its content, may not be used, reproduced, duplicated, displayed, or distributed absent express written permission from Ascension Health.

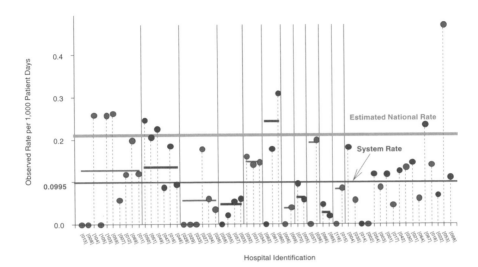

FIGURE 4-14 Ascension Health System falls with serious injury rate system-wide for calendar year 2007.

NOTE: This graph represents data that are self-reported and self-validated in accordance with the definitions and guidelines adopted by the Ascension Health Falls and Fall Injuries Affinity Group.[a]

[a] Fall with serious injury is an unplanned descent to the floor or against an object (assisted or unassisted) that requires medical intervention. Ascension Health uses the National Database of Nursing Quality Indicators Falls and Falls with Serious Injury definitions, which exclude certain units. The estimated national rate is (median of "All Falls" indexes) (0.06) = 0.21 falls with serious injury per 1,000 patient days. Six percent is the estimated percent of "All Falls" resulting in serious injury. (The national data methodology may not be identical to Ascension Health methodology (Hitcho et al., 2004; Page, 2005). The system rate is 0.0972 falls with serious injury per 1,000 patient days (metric excludes pediatric, obstetrics, and behavioral health units).

SOURCE: Reprinted with permission from Ascension Health. © 2008 Ascension Health. This work, including its content, may not be used, reproduced, duplicated, displayed, or distributed absent express written permission from Ascension Health.

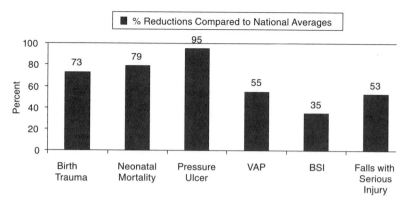

FIGURE 4-15 Summary reductions in overall calendar year 2007 compared with extrapolated benchmarks.

NOTE: BSI = bloodstream infection; VAP = ventilator-associated pneumonia.

SOURCE: Reprinted with permission from Ascension Health. © 2008 Ascension Health. This work, including its content, may not be used, reproduced, duplicated, displayed, or distributed absent express written permission from Ascension Health.

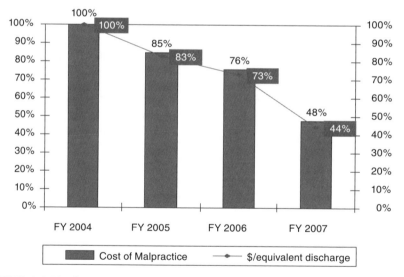

FIGURE 4-16 Risk management program reductions in the overall cost of malpractice and the cost per equivalent discharge from fiscal year (FY) 2004 through FY 2007. Operational performance and clinical performance are related.

NOTE: Percentage costs are compared with FY 04.

SOURCE: Reprinted with permission from Ascension Health. © 2008 Ascension Health. This work, including its content, may not be used, reproduced, duplicated, displayed, or distributed absent express written permission from Ascension Health.

REFERENCES

AHRQ (Agency for Healthcare Research and Quality). 2004. *HCUP nationwide inpatient sample (NIS)*. Rockville, MD: AHRQ. www.hcup-us.ahrq.gov/nisoverview.jsp (accessed September 7, 2007).

American Health Consultants, Inc. 2002. New performance model helps transform veterans health agency: Delivery of health care and management structure change radically. *Healthcare Benchmarks and Quality Improvement* 9(12):61–64.

Anderson, M. 2005. Lessons learned from the Veterans Health Administration. *Healthcare Papers* 5(4):30–37.

Armstrong, E. G., J. W. Barron, and A. Bender. 2001. *Creating a culture of patient safety: Three large-scale organizational examples*. Cambridge, MA: Risk Management Foundation of the Harvard Medical Institutions.

Armstrong, B., O. Levesque, J. B. Perlin, C. Rick, G. Schectman, and P. M. Zalucki. 2006. Reinventing Veterans Health Administration: Focus on primary care. *Healthcare Quarterly* 9:80–85.

Arnst, C. 2006. The best medical care in the U.S. *Business Week* July 17:50–56.

Asch, S. M., E. A. McGlynn, M. M. Hogan, R. A. Hayward, P. Shekelle, L. V. Rubenstein, J. Keesey, J. Adams, and E. A. Kerr. 2004a. Comparison of quality of care for patients in the Veterans Health Administration and patients in a national sample. *Annals of Internal Medicine* 141(12):938–945.

Asch, S. M., E. A. McGlynn, M. M. Hogan, R. A. Hayward, P. Shekelle, L. V. Rubenstein, J. Keesey, J. Adams, and E. A. Kerr. 2004b. Is better quality in VHA confined to areas of performance measurement? Paper presented at Health Services Research & Development National Meeting, Washington, DC.

Ashton, C. M., B. Bozkurt, W. B. Colucci, C. I. Kiefe, D. L. Mann, B. M. Massie, M. T. Slawsky, W. M. Tierney, J. A. West, D. J. Whellan, and N. P. Wray. 2000. Veterans Affairs quality enhancement research initiative in chronic heart failure. *Medical Care* 38(6 Suppl. 1):I26–I37.

Ashton, C. M., J. Septimus, N. J. Petersen, J. Souchek, T. J. Menke, T. C. Collins, and N. P. Wray. 2003a. Healthcare use by veterans treated for diabetes mellitus in the Veterans Affairs medical care system. *American Journal of Managed Care* 9(2):145–150.

Ashton, C. M., J. Souchek, N. J. Petersen, T. J. Menke, T. C. Collins, K. W. Kizer, S. M. Wright, and N. P. Wray. 2003b. Hospital use and survival among Veterans Affairs beneficiaries. *New England Journal of Medicine* 349(17):1637–1646.

Associated Press. 1990. Rating group finds veterans' hospitals lagging in quality. *The New York Times*, June 4.

Batalden, P. B., D. P. Stevens, and K. W. Kizer. 2002. Knowledge for improvement: Who will lead the learning? *Quality Management in Health Care* 10:3–9.

Beason, C. F. 2000. Creating an innovative organization. *Nursing Clinics of North America* 35(2):443–451.

Berlowitz, D. R., and J. Halpern. 1997. Evaluating and improving pressure ulcer care: The VA experience with administrative data. *Joint Commission Journal of Quality Improvement* 23(8):424–433.

Berlowitz, D. R., J. J. Anderson, G. H. Brandeis, L. A. Lehner, H. K. Brand, A. S. Ash, and M. A. Moskowitz. 1999. Pressure ulcer development in the VA: Characteristics of nursing homes providing best care. *American Journal of Medical Quality* 14(1):39–44.

Berlowitz, D. R., G. J. Young, G. H. Brandeis, B. Kader, and J. J. Anderson. 2001. Health care reorganization and quality of care: Unintended effects on pressure ulcer prevention. *Medical Care* 39(2):138–146.

Berriel-Cass, D., F. W. Adkins, P. Jones, and M. G. Fakih. 2006. Eliminating nosocomial infections at Ascension Health. *Joint Commission Journal of Quality and Patient Safety* 32(11):612–620.

Best, W. R., S. F. Khuri, M. Phelan, K. Hur, W. G. Henderson, J. G. Demakis, and J. Daley. 2002. Identifying patient preoperative risk factors and postoperative adverse events in administrative databases: Results from the Department of Veterans Affairs National Surgical Quality Improvement Program. *Journal of the American College of Surgeons* 194(3):257–266.

Bhatia, S. C., and P. P. Fernandes. 2008. Quality outcomes management: Veterans Affairs case study. *Psychiatric Clinics of North America* 31(1):57–72.

Block, S. D. 2002. Medical education in end-of-life care: The status of reform. *Journal of Palliative Medicine* 5:243–250.

Booth, B. M., R. L. Ludke, D. S. Wakefield, D. C. Kern, L. F. Burmeister, E. M. Fisher, and T. W. Ford. 1991. Nonacute days of care within Department of Veterans Affairs medical centers. *Medical Care* 29(8 Suppl.).

Bozzette, S. A., B. Phillips, S. Asch, A. L. Gifford, L. Lenert, T. Menke, E. Ortiz, D. Owens, and L. Deyton. 2000. Quality enhancement research initiative for human immunodeficiency virus/acquired immunodeficiency syndrome: Framework and plan. HIV-QUERI Executive Committee. *Medical Care* 38(6 Suppl. 1):I60–I69.

Brennan, T. A., L. L. Leape, N. M. Laird, L. Hebert, A. R. Localio, A. G. Lawthers, J. P. Newhouse, P. C. Weiler, and H. H. Hiatt. 1991. Incidence of adverse events and negligence in hospitalized patients. Results of the Harvard Medical Practice Study I. *New England Journal of Medicine* 324(6):370–376.

Brown, D. 2007. VA takes the lead in paperless care: Computerized medical records promise lower costs and better treatment. *The Washington Post*, April 10. http://www.washingtonpost.com/wp-dyn/content/article/2007/04/06/AR2007040601911.html (accessed September 20, 2010).

Brown, S. H., M. J. Lincoln, P. J. Groen, and R. M. Kolodner. 2003. VistA—U.S. Department of Veterans Affairs national-scale HIS. *International Journal of Medical Informatics* 69(2–3):135–156.

Butler, K., P. Mollo, J. L. Gale, and D. A. Rapp. 2007. Eliminating adverse drug events at Ascension Health. *Joint Commission Journal of Quality and Patient Safety* 33(9):527–536.

Carver, P. 2002. *The Veterans Health Administration and the Institute for Healthcare Improvement's advanced clinic access initiative 2001–2002.* Boston, MA: Institute for Healthcare Improvement.

CBS Evening News. 2006 (December 8). *VA: High-quality health care at low cost.* http://www.cbsnews.com/stories/2006/12/08/eveningnews/main2243606.shtml (accessed September 20, 2010).

CDC (Centers for Disease Control and Prevention). 2007. *National vital statistics reports, vol. 55, no. 19.* Washington, DC: U.S. Government Printing Office.

Chapko, M. K., and C. Van Deusen Lukas. 2001. VA community-based outpatient clinics improve access to care and increase patient satisfaction. *Forum* June:4–5.

Charles, R. 2000. The challenge of disseminating innovations to direct care providers in health care organizations. *Nursing Clinics of North America* 35(2):461–470.

Chen, S., T. H. Wagner, and P. G. Barnett. 2001. The effect of reforms on spending for veterans' substance abuse treatment, 1993–1999. *Health Affairs (Millwood)* 20(4):169–175.

Chen, S., M. W. Smith, T. H. Wagner, and P. G. Barnett. 2003. Spending for specialized mental health treatment in the VA: 1995–2001. *Health Affairs (Millwood)* 22(6):256–263.

Childs, C. 1970 (May 22). From Vietnam to a VA hospital: Assignment to neglect. *Life* 68(19):24–33.

Cleeland, C. S., C. C. Reyes-Gibby, M. Schall, K. Nolan, J. Paice, J. M. Rosenberg, J. H. Tollett, and R. D. Kerns. 2003. Rapid improvement in pain management: The Veterans Health Administration and the Institute for Healthcare Improvement collaborative. *Clinical Journal of Pain* 19(5):298–305.

Conn, J. 2004. A veteran IT system. *Modern Healthcare* 34(47):30–31.

Cope, D. W., S. Sherman, and A. S. Robbins. 1996. Restructuring VA ambulatory care and medical education: The Pace model of primary care. *Academic Medicine* 71(7):761–771.

Daley, J., S. F. Khuri, W. Henderson, K. Hur, J. O. Gibbs, G. Barbour, J. Demakis, G. Irvin, III, J. F. Stremple, F. Grover, G. McDonald, E. Passaro, Jr., P. J. Fabri, J. Spencer, K. Hammermeister, J. B. Aust, and C. Oprian. 1997. Risk adjustment of the postoperative morbidity rate for the comparative assessment of the quality of surgical care: Results of the national Veterans Affairs surgical risk study. *Journal of the American College of Surgeons* 185(4):328–340.

Davis, R. 1998. Veterans facilities air medical errors and take action. *USA Today*, October 18, 4D.

DeLuca, M. A. 2000. *Trans-Atlantic experiences in health reform: the United Kingdom's National Health Service and the United States Veterans Health Administration.* Washington, DC: The PricewaterhouseCoopers Endowment for The Business of Government.

Demakis, J. G., L. McQueen, K. W. Kizer, and J. R. Feussner. 2000. Quality Enhancement Research Initiative (QUERI): A collaboration between research and clinical practice. *Medical Care* 38(6 Suppl. 1):I17–I25.

Edmondson, A. C., B. R. Golden, and G. J. Young. 2006. *Turnaround at the Veterans Health Administration.* Boston, MA: Harvard Business School Publishing.

Edwards, J. R., K. D. Peterson, M. L. Andrus, J. S. Tolson, J. S. Goulding, M. A. Dudeck, et al. (2007). National healthcare safety network (NHSN) report, data summary for 2006, issued June 2007. *American Journal of Infection Control* 35(5):290–301.

Employee Education System. 1999. *Care management in VA—Coordinating care across all settings.* Washington, DC: Department of Veterans Affairs.

Every, N. R., S. D. Fihn, A. E. Sales, A. Keane, and J. R. Ritchie. 2000. Quality enhancement research initiative in ischemic heart disease: A quality initiative from the Department of Veterans Affairs. QUERI IHD Executive Committee. *Medical Care* 38(6 Suppl. 1): I49–I59.

Ewing, H., G. Bruder, P. Baroco, M. Hill, and L. P. Sparkman. 2007. Eliminating perioperative adverse events at Ascension Health. *Joint Commission Journal of Quality and Patient Safety* 33(5):256–266.

Feussner, J. R., K. W. Kizer, and J. G. Demakis. 2000. The quality enhancement research initiative (QUERI): From evidence to action. *Medical Care* 38(6 Suppl. 1):I1–I6.

Fihn, S. D., M. Vaughan-Sarrazin, E. Lowy, I. Popescu, C. Maynard, G. E. Rosenthal, A. E. Sales, J. Rumsfeld, S. Piñeros, M. B. McDonell, C. D. Helfrich, R. Rusch, R. Jesse, P. Almenoff, B. Fleming, and M. Kussman. 2009. Declining mortality following acute myocardial infarction in the Department of Veterans Affairs Health Care System. *BMC Cardiovascular Disorders* 9:44.

Fink, A. S., D. A. Campbell, Jr., R. M. Mentzer, Jr., W. G. Henderson, J. Daley, J. Bannister, K. Hur, and S. F. Khuri. 2002. The National Surgical Quality Improvement Program in non-Veterans Administration hospitals: Initial demonstration of feasibility. *Annals of Surgery* 236(3):344–353; discussion, 353–354.

Finney, J. W., M. L. Willenbring, and R. H. Moos. 2000. Improving the quality of VA care for patients with substance-use disorders: The quality enhancement research initiative (QUERI) substance abuse module. *Medical Care* 38(6 Suppl. 1):I105–I113.

Fischer, E. P., S. R. Marder, G. R. Smith, R. R. Owen, L. Rubenstein, S. C. Hedrick, and G. M. Curran. 2000. Quality enhancement research initiative in mental health. *Medical Care* 38(6 Suppl. 1):I70–I81.

Fong, T. 2003. An army of patients. *Modern Healthcare* (March 19) 33(20):48–50, 62.

Frayne, S. M., V. A. Parker, C. L. Christiansen, S. Loveland, M. R. Seaver, L. E. Kazis, and K. M. Skinner. 2006. Health status among 28,000 women veterans. The VA Women's Health Program Evaluation Project. *Journal of General Internal Medicine* 21(Suppl. 3): S40–S46.

Freedberg, S. J. 2006. Veterans' care praised, finally. *National Journal* 38(6):65–66.

GAO (General Accounting Office). 1987. *VA health care: VA's patient injury control program not effective*. Washington, DC: General Accounting Office.

———. 1989. *Better patient management practices could reduce length of stay in VA hospitals*. Washington, DC: General Accounting Office.

———. 1993. *VA health care: Restructuring ambulatory care system would improve services to veterans*. Washington, DC: General Accounting Office.

———. 1994a. *Veterans health care: Veterans' perceptions of VA services and VA's role in health care reform*. Washington, DC: General Accounting Office.

———. 1994b. *Veterans health care: Use of VA services by Medicare-eligible veterans*. Washington, DC: General Accounting Office.

———. 1995. *VA health care, physician peer review identifies quality of care problems but actions to address them are limited*. Washington, DC: General Accounting Office.

———. 1998. *VA health care status of efforts to improve efficiency and access*. Washington, DC: General Accounting Office.

———. 1999. *Veterans affairs: Progress and challenges in transforming health care*. Washington, DC: General Accounting Office.

Gaul, G. M. 2005. Revamped veterans' health care now a model. *The Washington Post*, August 22. www.washingtonpost.com/wp-dyn/content/article/2005/08/21/AR2005082101073.html (accessed May 30, 2010).

Gearon, C. J. 2005. Military might: Today's VA hospitals are models of top-notch care. *U.S. News and World Report*, July 18:100–106. http://health.usnews.com/usnews/health/articles/050718/18va.htm (accessed May 30, 2010).

Gebhart, F. 1999. VA facility slashes drug errors via barcoding. *Drug Topics* 143:44.

Gibbons, W., H. T. Shanks, P. Kleinhelter, and P. Jones. 2006. Eliminating facility-acquired pressure ulcers at Ascension Health. *Joint Commission Journal of Quality and Patient Safety* 32(9):488–496.

Gibson, R. 1998. The Robert Wood Johnson Foundation grant-making strategies to improve care at the end of life. *Journal of Palliative Medicine* 1(4):415–417.

Glendinning, D. 2007. VA health care quality: The road to recovery. *American Medical News* 50(46). www.ama-assn.org/amednews/2007/12/10/gvsa1210.htm (accessed May 30, 2010).

Greenberg, G. A., R. A. Rosenheck, and M. P. Charns. 2003. From profession-based leadership to service line management in the Veterans Health Administration: Impact on mental health care. *Medical Care* 41(9):1013–1023.

Greenfield, S., and S. H. Kaplan. 2004. Creating a culture of quality: The remarkable transformation of the Department of Veterans Affairs health care system. *Annals of Internal Medicine* 141(4):316–318.

Groen, P. J. 2005. *A history of health information technology (IT) in the VA: 1955–2005*. Washington, DC: P.J. Groen.

Harada, N. D., V. M. Villa, and R. Andersen. 2002. Satisfaction with VA and non-VA outpatient care among veterans. *American Journal of Medical Quality* 17(4):155–164.

Haugh, R. 2003. Reinventing the VA: Civilian providers find valuable lessons in the once-maligned health care system. *Hospitals & Health Networks* (77):50–52, 55.

Hendrich, A., A. R. Tersigni, S. Jeffcoat, C. J. Barnett, L. P. Brideau, and D. Pryor. 2007. The Ascension Health journey to zero: Lessons learned and leadership. *Joint Commission Journal of Quality and Patient Safety* 33(12):739–749.

Hitcho, E. B., M. J. Krauss, S. Birge, D. W. Claiborne, I. Fischer, S. Johnson, P. A. Nast, E. Costantinou, and V. J. Fraser. 2004. Characteristics and circumstances of falls in a hospital setting. *Journal of General Internal Medicine* 19:732–739.

Holohan, T. V., T. Mitchell, and K. W. Kizer. 1999. At war with hepatitis C, part 2: Evaluation, screening and diagnosis in the VHA. *Federal Practitioner* 16:12–15.

Humphreys, K., and D. Horst. 2002. Datapoints: Moving from inpatient to residential substance abuse treatment in the VA. *Psychiatric Services* 53(8):927.

Humphreys, K., P. D. Huebsch, R. H. Moos, and R. T. Suchinsky. 1999. Alcohol and drug abuse: The transformation of the Veterans Affairs substance abuse treatment system. *Psychiatric Services* 50(11):1399–1401.

Huskamp, H. A., A. M. Epstein, and D. Blumenthal. 2003. The impact of a national prescription drug formulary on prices, market share, and spending: Lessons for Medicare? *Health Affairs (Millwood)* 22(3):149–158.

Hynes, D. M., R. A. Perrin, S. Rappaport, J. M. Stevens, and J. G. Demakis. 2004. Informatics resources to support health care quality improvement in the Veterans Health Administration. *Journal of the American Medical Informatics Association* 11(5):344–350.

Institute for Healthcare Improvement. 2006. *100k lives campaign.* http://www.ihi.org/IHI/Programs/Campaign/100kCampaignOverviewArchive.htm (accessed June 21, 2010).

IOM (Institute of Medicine). 2000a. *Description and analysis of the VA National Formulary.* Washington, DC: National Academy Press.

———. 2000b. *To err is human: Building a safer health system.* Washington, DC: National Academy Press.

Jackson, G. L., E. M. Yano, D. Edelman, S. L. Krein, M. A. Ibrahim, T. S. Carey, S. Y. Lee, K. E. Hartmann, T. K. Dudley, and M. Weinberger. 2005. Veterans Affairs primary care organizational characteristics associated with better diabetes control. *American Journal of Managed Care* 11(4):225–237.

Jha, A. K., J. B. Perlin, K. W. Kizer, and R. A. Dudley. 2003. Effect of the transformation of the Veterans Affairs health care system on the quality of care. *New England Journal of Medicine* 34:2218–2227.

Jha, A. K., S. M. Wright, and J. B. Perlin. 2007. Performance measures, vaccinations, and pneumonia rates among high-risk patients in Veterans Administration health care. *American Journal of Public Health* 97(12):2167–2172.

Johnson, C. L., R. A. Carlson, C. L. Tucker, and C. Willette. 2002. Using BCMA software to improve patient safety in Veterans Administration medical centers. *Journal of Healthcare Information Management* 16(1):46–51.

Kazis, L. E., X. S. Ren, A. Lee, K. Skinner, W. Rogers, J. Clark, and D. R. Miller. 1999. Health status in VA patients: Results from the Veterans Health Study. *American Journal of Medical Quality* 14(1):28–38.

Kee, J. E., and K. E. Newcomer. 2007. *Leading change, managing risk: The leadership role in private sector transformation.* Washington, DC: George Washington University School of Public Policy and Public Administration.

Kerr, E. A., R. B. Gerzoff, S. L. Krein, J. V. Selby, J. D. Piette, J. D. Curb, W. H. Herman, D. G. Marrero, K. M. Narayan, M. M. Safford, T. Thompson, and C. M. Mangione. 2004. Diabetes care quality in the Veterans Affairs health care system and commercial managed care: The Triad Study. *Annals of Internal Medicine* 141(4):272–281.

Khuri, S. F. 2006. Safety, quality, and the National Surgical Quality Improvement Program. *American Surgeon* 72(11):994–998; discussion 1021–1030, 1133–1148.

Khuri, S. F., J. Daley, W. Henderson, K. Hur, J. O. Gibbs, G. Barbour, J. Demakis, G. Irvin, J. F. Stremple, F. Grover, G. McDonald, E. Passaro, P. J. Fabri, J. Spencer, K. Hammermeister, and J. B. Aust. 1997. Risk adjustment of the postoperative mortality rate for the comparative assessment of the quality of surgical care: Results of the National Veterans Affairs Surgical Risk Study. *Journal of the American College of Surgery* 185(4):315–327.

Khuri, S. F., J. Daley, W. Henderson, K. Hur, J. Demakis, J. B. Aust, V. Chong, P. J. Fabri, J. O. Gibbs, F. Grover, K. Hammermeister, G. Irvin, III, G. McDonald, E. Passaro, Jr., L. Phillips, F. Scamman, J. Spencer, and J. F. Stremple. 1998. The Department of Veterans Affairs' NSQIP: The first national, validated, outcome-based, risk-adjusted, and peer-controlled program for the measurement and enhancement of the quality of surgical care. National VA Surgical Quality Improvement Program. *Annals of Surgery* 228(4):491–507.

Khuri, S. F., W. G. Henderson, J. Daley, O. Jonasson, R. S. Jones, D. A. Campbell, Jr., A. S. Fink, R. M. Mentzer, Jr., L. Neumayer, K. Hammermeister, C. Mosca, and N. Healey. 2008. Successful implementation of the Department of Veterans Affairs' National Surgical Quality Improvement Program in the private sector: The Patient Safety in Surgery study. *Annals of Surgery* 248(2):329–336.

Kizer, K. W. 1996. *Prescription for change: The strategic principles and objectives for transforming the Veterans Health Administration.* Washington, DC: Veterans Health Administration.

———. 1998. Clinical practice guidelines. *Federal Practitioner* 15:52–58.

———. 1999. The "New VA": A national laboratory for health care quality management. *American Journal of Medical Quality* 14(1):3–20.

———. 2000. Promoting innovative nursing practice during radical health system change. *Nursing Clinics of North America* 35(2):429–441.

———. 2001. Reengineering the veterans healthcare system. In P. Ramsaroop, M. J. Ball, D. Beaulieu, and J. V. Douglas (eds.), *Advancing federal sector healthcare* (pp. 79–96). New York: Springer-Verlag.

Kizer, K. W., and T. L. Garthwaite. 1997. Vision for change: An integrated service network. In *Computerizing large integrated health networks: The VA success* (pp. 3–13). New York: Springer-Verlag.

Kizer, K. W., and G. A. Pane. 1997. The "New VA": Delivering health care value through integrated service networks. *Annals of Emergency Medicine* 30(6):804–807.

Kizer, K. W., J. E. Ogden, and J. E. Ray. 1997. Establishing a PBM: Pharmacy benefits management in the Veterans Health Care System. *Drug Benefit Trends* August:24–27, 47.

Kizer, K. W., T. S. Cushing, and R. Y. Nishimi. 2000a. The Department of Veterans Affairs' role in federal emergency management. *Annals of Emergency Medicine* 36(3):255–261.

Kizer, K. W., J. G. Demakis, and J. R. Feussner. 2000b. Reinventing VA health care: Systematizing quality improvement and quality innovation. *Medical Care* 38(6 Suppl. 1): I7–I16.

Klein, R. 1981. *Wounded men, broken promises.* New York: McMillan.

Knopman, D., S. Resetar, P. Norling, R. Rettig, and I. Brahmakulam. 2003. *Innovation and change management in public and private organizations: Case studies and options for EPA.* Washington, DC: RAND Corporation.

Korthuis, P. T., H. D. Anaya, and S. A. Bozzette. 2004. Quality of HIV care within Veterans Affairs health system: A comparison using outcomes from the HIV cost and services utilization study. *Journal of Clinical Outcomes Management* 11:766–774.

Krein, S. L., R. A. Hayward, L. Pogach, and B. J. Boots-Miller. 2000. Department of Veterans Affairs' Quality Enhancement Research Initiative for diabetes mellitus. *Medical Care* 38(6 Suppl. 1):I38–I48.

Krugman, P. 2008. Health care confidential. *The New York Times*, January 27. http://select. nytimes.com/2006/01/27/opinion/27krugman.html?_r=1 (accessed February 23, 2010).

Kupersmith, J., J. Francis, E. Kerr, S. Krein, L. Pogach, R. M. Kolodner, and J. B. Perlin. 2007. Advancing evidence-based care for diabetes: Lessons from the Veterans Health Administration. *Health Affairs (Millwood)* 26(2):w156–w168.

Lancaster, A. D., A. Ayers, B. Belbot, V. Goldner, L. Kress, D. Stanton, P. Jones, and L. Sparkman. 2007. Preventing falls and eliminating injury at Ascension Health. *Joint Commission Journal of Quality and Patient Safety* 33(7):367–375.

Landrum, M. B., E. Guadagnoli, R. Zummo, D. Chin, and B. J. McNeil. 2004. Care following acute myocardial infarction in the Veterans Administration medical centers: A comparison with Medicare. *Health Services Research* 39(6 Pt. 1):1773–1792.

Leape, L. L., D. D. Woods, M. J. Hatlie, K. W. Kizer, S. A. Schroeder, and G. D. Lundberg. 1998. Promoting patient safety by preventing medical error. *JAMA* 280(16):1444–1447.

Levin, A. 2009. Airlines go two years with no fatalities. *USA Today*. January 11. www.usatoday. com/travel/flights/2009-01-11-airlinesafety_N.htm (accessed February 23, 2010).

The Lewin Group and PricewaterhouseCoopers. 1998. Veterans equitable resource allocation assessment. *Final Report Task Order 24*. Washington, DC.

Light, P. C. 1992. *Forging legislation*. New York: W. W. Norton & Co.

Long, J. A., D. Polsky, and J. P. Metlay. 2005. Changes in veterans' use of outpatient care from 1992 to 2000. *American Journal of Public Health* 95(12):2246–2251.

Longman, P. 2007. *Best care anywhere. Why VA health care is better than yours*. Sausalito, CA: PoliPointPress.

Luciano, L. 2000. A government health system leads the way. *Accelerating Change Today* February:9–11.

Management Decision and Research Center. 1995. *Primary care in VA primer*. Washington, DC: Veterans Health Administration.

———. 1998. *Clinical practice guidelines primer*. Washington, DC: Veterans Health Administration.

Mather, J. H., and R. W. Abel. 1986. Medical care of veterans—a brief history. *Journal of the American Geriatrics Society* 34(10):757–760.

Mazza, F., J. Kitchens, S. Kerr, A. Markovich, M. Best, and L. P. Sparkman. 2007. Eliminating birth trauma at Ascension Health. *Joint Commission Journal of Quality and Patient Safety* 33(1):15–24.

Mills, P. D., and W. B. Weeks. 2004. Characteristics of successful quality improvement teams: Lessons from five collaborative projects in the VHA. *Joint Commission Journal of Quality and Patient Safety* 30(3):152–162.

Mills, P. D., W. B. Weeks, and B. C. Surott-Kimberly. 2003. A multihospital safety improvement effort and the dissemination of new knowledge. *Joint Commission Journal on Quality and Patient Safety* 29(3):124–133.

Mitchell, T., T. V. Holohan, L. W. Wright, and K. W. Kizer. 1999. At war with hepatitis C: Part 1: The VA's strategic initiative. *Federal Practitioner* 16(11):12–15.

Mitkowski, A., and J. Feinstein. 2007. *Veterans Health Administration: Dr. Kizer considers radical surgery on an ailing system*. New Haven, CT: Yale University School of Management.

Morgan, M. W. 2005. The VA advantage: The gold standard in clinical informatics. *Healthcare Papers* 5(4):26–29.

National Quality Research Center, Federal Consulting Group. 1999. *Veterans Health Administration—Inpatients, Veterans Affairs customer satisfaction study: Final report 1999.* Ann Arbor, MI.

National Quality Research Center, Federal Consulting Group, CFI Group. 2007a. *Veterans Health Administration—Inpatients, Veterans Affairs customer satisfaction study: Final report 2007.* Ann Arbor, MI.

———. 2007b. *Veterans Health Administration—Outpatients, Veterans Affairs customer satisfaction study: Final report 2007.* Ann Arbor, MI.

NBC Nightly News. 2006 (March 15). *A healthcare system seen as model for reform.*

NYT (New York Times). 1999. Progress on medical records (editorial). *The New York Times.* December 29. www.nytimes.com/1999/12/28/opinion/progress-on-medical-errors.html?pagewanted=1 (accessed February 23, 2010).

Nicholson, R. J. 2006. VA blazes path to preventing drug errors. *USA Today*, July 31. www.usatoday.com/news/opinion/editorials/2006-07-31-letters-va_x.htm (accessed February 23, 2010).

Office of the Inspector General. 1997. *The impact of downsizing inpatient substance abuse rehabilitation programs on homeless veterans and other frequent users.* Washington, DC: Department of Veterans Affairs.

Office of the Inspector General and Department of Veterans Affairs. 1990. *Audit of Veterans Health Services and Research Administration surgical complication reporting procedures.* Washington, DC: VA Office of the Inspector General.

———. 1991. *Audit of VA's control system for credentialing and privileging physicians.* Washington, DC: VA Office of the Inspector General.

Oliver, A. 2007. The Veterans Health Administration: An American success story? *The Milbank Quarterly* 85(1):5–35.

Oxford Analytica. 2007. *VA could be model for health system.* http://www.forbes.com/2007/04/19/veterans-health-care-biz-cx_0420oxford.html (accessed April 20, 2007).

Page, L. 2005. *Getting a handle on patient falls.* www.matmanmag.com (accessed January 25, 2005).

Parrino, T. 2003. Information technology and primary care at the VA: Making a good thing better. *Forum* October:1–2.

Pauly, M. V., D. J. Brailer, G. Kroch, O. Even-Shoshan, J. C. Hershey, and S. V. Williams. 1996. Measuring hospital outcomes from a buyer's perspective. *American Journal of Medical Quality* 11(3):112–122.

Penrod, J. D., T. Cortez, and C. A. Luhrs. 2007. Use of a report card to implement a network-based palliative care program. *Journal of Palliative Medicine* 10(4):858–860.

Perlin, J. B. 2006. Transformation of the U.S. Veterans Health Administration. *Health Economics, Policy and Law* 1(2):99–105.

Perlin, J. B., R. M. Kolodner, and R. H. Roswell. 2004. The Veterans Health Administration: Quality, value, accountability, and information as transforming strategies for patient-centered care. *American Journal of Managed Care* 10(11 Pt. 2):828–836.

Petersen, L. A., S. L. Normand, J. Daley, and B. J. McNeil. 2000. Outcome of myocardial infarction in Veterans Health Administration patients as compared with Medicare patients. *New England Journal of Medicine* 343(26):1934–1941.

Petersen, L. A., S. L. Normand, L. L. Leape, and B. J. McNeil. 2001. Comparison of use of medications after acute myocardial infarction in the Veterans Health Administration and Medicare. *Circulation* 104(24):2898–2904.

Petersen, L. A., S. L. Normand, L. L. Leape, and B. J. McNeil. 2003. Regionalization and the underuse of angiography in the Veterans Affairs health care system as compared with a fee-for-service system. *New England Journal of Medicine* 348(22):2209–2217.

Piccard, A. 2005. U.S. veterans' health care healed itself: So can our Medicare system. *The Globe and Mail*, March 3.

Pizziferri, L., A. F. Kittler, L. A. Volk, M. M. Honour, S. Gupta, S. Wang, T. Wang, M. Lippincott, Q. Li, and D. W. Bates. 2005. Primary care physician time utilization before and after implementation of an electronic health record: A time-motion study. *Journal of Biomedical Informatics* 38(3):176–188.

Popescu, I., M. S. Vaughan-Sarrazin, and G. E. Rosenthal. 2007. *Declines in VHA mortality in association with organizational efforts to improve care of patients with acute coronary syndrome*. Paper presented at Health Service Research and Development National Meeting, Washington, DC.

Pryor, D. B., S. F. Tolchin, A. Hendrich, C. S. Thomas, and A. R. Tersigni. 2006. The clinical transformation of Ascension Health: Eliminating all preventable injuries and deaths. *Joint Commission Journal of Quality and Patient Safety* 32(6):299–308.

Quill, T. E. 2002. In-hospital end-of-life services: Is the cup 2/3 empty or 1/3 full? *Medical Care* 40(1):4–6.

Rogers, W. H., L. E. Kazis, D. R. Miller, K. M. Skinner, J. A. Clark, A. Spiro, III, and R. G. Fincke. 2004. Comparing the health status of VA and non-VA ambulatory patients: The veterans' health and medical outcomes studies. *Journal of Ambulatory Care Management* 27(3):249–262.

Rose, J. S., C. S. Thomas, A. Tersigni, J. B. Sexton, and D. Pryor. 2006. A leadership framework for culture change in health care. *Joint Commission Journal of Quality and Patient Safety* 32(8):433–442.

Roselle, G. A., L. H. Danko, S. M. Kralovic, L. A. Simbartl, and K. W. Kizer. 2002. National Hepatitis C Surveillance Day in the Veterans Health Administration of the Department of Veterans Affairs. *Military Medicine* 167(9):756–759.

Rosenheck, R. 2000. Primary care satellite clinics and improved access to general and mental health services. *Health Services Research* 35(4):777–790.

Rosenheck, R., and A. Fontana. 2001. Impact of efforts to reduce inpatient costs on clinical effectiveness: Treatment of posttraumatic stress disorder in the Department of Veterans Affairs. *Medical Care* 39(2):168–180.

Rosenheck, R., and K. W. Kizer. 1998. Hospitalizations and the homeless. *New England Journal of Medicine* 339(16):1166; author reply, 1167.

Ross, J. S., S. Keyhani, P. S. Keenan, S. M. Bernheim, J. D. Penrod, K. S. Boockvar, A. D. Federman, H. M. Krumholz, and A. L. Siu. 2008. Use of recommended ambulatory care services: Is the Veterans Affairs quality gap narrowing? *Archives of Internal Medicine* 168(9):950–958.

Rubenstein, L. V., J. Lammers, E. M. Yano, M. Tabbarah, and A. S. Robbins. 1996a. Evaluation of the VA's pilot program in institutional reorganization toward primary and ambulatory care: Part II, A study of organizational stresses and dynamics. *Academic Medicine* 71(7):784–792.

Rubenstein, L. V., E. M. Yano, A. Fink, A. B. Lanto, B. Simon, M. Graham, and A. S. Robbins. 1996b. Evaluation of the VA's pilot program in institutional reorganization toward primary and ambulatory care: Part I, Changes in process and outcomes of care. *Academic Medicine* 71(7):772–783.

Rundle, R. L. 2001. Oft-derided veterans health agency puts data online, saving time, lives. *Wall Street Journal*, December 10.

Rutherford, G. W., T. R. Gerrity, K. W. Kizer, and J. R. Feussner. 1999. Research in the Veterans Health Administration: The report of the Research Realignment Advisory Committee. *Academic Medicine* 74(7):773–781.

Sales, M. M., F. E. Cunningham, P. A. Glassman, M. A. Valentino, and C. B. Good. 2005. Pharmacy benefits management in the Veterans Health Administration: 1995 to 2003. *American Journal of Managed Care* 11(2):104–112.

Schall, M. W., T. Duffy, A. Krishnamurthy, O. Levesque, P. Mehta, M. Murray, R. Parlier, R. Petzel, and J. Sanderson. 2004. Improving patient access to the Veterans Health Administration's primary care and specialty clinics. *Joint Commission Journal on Quality and Patient Safety* 30(8):415–423.

Schuster, J. L. 1999. Addressing patients' pain. Veterans Health Administration's addition of fifth vital sign may have far-reaching effects. *The Washington Post*, February 2:8.

Selim, A. J., L. E. Kazis, W. Rogers, S. Qian, J. A. Rothendler, A. Lee, X. S. Ren, S. C. Haffer, R. Mardon, D. Miller, A. Spiro, III, B. J. Selim, and B. G. Fincke. 2006. Risk-adjusted mortality as an indicator of outcomes: Comparison of the Medicare advantage program with the Veterans' Health Administration. *Medical Care* 44(4):359–365.

Shapiro, J. P. 1999. Doctoring a sickly system: Deadly medical mistakes are rampant. *U.S. News & World Report* 127(23):60–61.

Singh, H., and J. Kalavar. 2004. Quality of care for hypertension and diabetes in federal-versus commercial-managed care organizations. *American Journal of Medical Quality* 19(1):19–24.

Singh, J. A., S. J. Borowsky, S. Nugent, M. Murdoch, Y. Zhao, D. B. Nelson, R. Petzel, and K. L. Nichol. 2005. Health-related quality of life, functional impairment, and healthcare utilization by veterans: Veterans' quality of life study. *Journal of the American Geriatric Society* 53(1):108–113.

Skydell, B. 1998. *Restructuring the VA health care system: Safety net, training, and other considerations*. Washington, DC: National Health Policy Forum.

Smith, C. B., R. L. Goldman, D. C. Martin, J. Williamson, C. Weir, C. Beauchamp, and M. Ashcraft. 1996. Overutilization of acute-care beds in Veterans Affairs hospitals. *Medical Care* 34(1):85–96.

Stalhandske, E., J. P. Bagian, and J. Gosbee. 2002. Department of Veterans Affairs patient safety program. *American Journal of Infection Control* 30:296–302.

Stein, R. 2006. VA care is rated superior to that in private hospitals. *The Washington Post*, January 20. www.washingtonpost.com/wp-dyn/content/artcle/2006/01/19/AR2006011902936.html (accessed February 23, 2010).

Steiner, G. 1971. *The state of welfare*. Washington, DC: The Brookings Institution.

Stevens, D. P., K. W. Kizer, T. W. Elwood, and G. L. Warden. 1998. VA aligns health professions education with healthcare priorities. *Journal of Allied Health* 27(3):123–127.

Stevens, D. P., G. J. Holland, and K. W. Kizer. 2001. Results of a nationwide Veterans Affairs initiative to align graduate medical education and patient care. *JAMA* 286(9):1061–1066.

Stires, D. 2006 (May 15). How the VA healed itself. *Fortune* 153(9):130–136. http://money.cnn.com/magazines/fortune/fortune_archive/2006/05/15/8376846/ (accessed February 23, 2010).

Thibodeau, N., J. H. Evans, N. J. Nagarajanh, and J. Whittle. 2007. Value creation in public enterprises: An empirical analysis of coordinated organizational changes in the Veterans Health Administration. *The Accounting Review* 82:483–520.

Thomas, E. J., D. M. Studdert, H. R. Burstin, E. J. Orav, T. Zeena, E. J. Williams, K. M. Howard, P. C. Weiler, and T. A. Brennan. 2000. Incidence and types of adverse events and negligent care in Utah and Colorado. *Medical Care* 38(3):261–271.

Tolchin, S., R. Brush, P. Lange, P. Bates, and J. J. Garbo. 2007. Eliminating preventable death at Ascension Health. *Joint Commission Journal of Quality and Patient Safety* 33(3):145–154.

Trevelyan, E. W. 2002. *The performance management system of the Veterans Health Administration*. Cambridge, MA: Harvard School of Public Health.

Tseng, C. L., J. D. Greenberg, D. Helmer, M. Rajan, A. Tiwari, D. Miller, S. Crystal, G. Hawley, and L. Pogach. 2004. Dual-system utilization affects regional variation in prevention quality indicators: The case of amputations among veterans with diabetes. *American Journal of Managed Care* 10(11 Pt. 2):886–892.

U.S. Congress, House of Representatives, Committee on Government Operations. 1987. *Patients at risk: A study of deficiencies in the Veterans Administration quality assurance program.* Washington, DC: U.S. Government Printing Office.

U.S. Congress, House of Representatives, Committee on Veterans Affairs. 2001. *Need to consider VA's role in strengthening federal preparedness.* October 15. Washington, DC: Government Accountability Office.

Versel, N. 2003. Wired and ready. *Modern Physician* August 1.

VHA (Veterans Health Administration). 1946 (January 30). *Policy memorandum no. 2.* Washington, DC: Department of Veterans Affairs.

———. 1967. *Medical care of veterans.* Washington, DC: Department of Veterans Affairs.

———. 1996a. *VA innovations in ambulatory care.* Washington, DC: Department of Veterans Affairs.

———. 1996b (August 29). *Directive 96-053. Roles and definitions for clinical practice guidelines and clinical pathways.* Washington DC: Department of Veterans Affairs.

———. 1996c. *VHA employee development report: High performance development model.* Washington, DC: Department of Veterans Affairs.

———. 1997a. *Veterans equitable resource allocation system: Initial briefing booklet.* Washington, DC: Department of Veterans Affairs.

———. 1997b. *Veterans equitable resource allocation: Equity of funding and access to care across networks.* Washington, DC: Department of Veterans Affairs.

———. 1998. *Veterans equitable resource allocation system.* Washington, DC: Department of Veterans Affairs.

Wahby, V. S., T. L. Garthwaite, and N. A. Thompson. 2000. The VA lessons learned project. *Focus on Patient Safety* 3:1–2.

Waller, D. 2006 (September 4). How VA hospitals became the best. *Time* 168(10):36–37.

Ward, M. M., J. W. Yankey, T. E. Vaughn, B. J. Boots-Miller, S. D. Flach, K. F. Welke, J. F. Pendergast, J. Perlin, and B. N. Doebbeling. 2004. Physician process and patient outcome measures for diabetes care: Relationships to organizational characteristics. *Medical Care* 42(9):840–850.

Wasserman, J., J. Ringel, K. Ricci, J. Malkin, M. Schoenbaum, B. Wynn, J. Zwanziger, S. Newberry, M. Suttorp, and A. Rastegar. 2001. *An analysis of the Veterans Equitable Resource Allocation (VERA) system.* Santa Monica, CA: RAND Corporation.

———. 2003. *An analysis of potential adjustments to the Veterans Equitable Resource Allocation (VERA) system.* Santa Monica, CA: RAND Corporation.

Weber, G. A., and L. F. Schmeckebiar. 1934. *The Veterans' Administration—Its history, activities and organization.* Washington, DC: The Brookings Institution.

Whittington, K. T., and R. Briones. 2004. National prevalence and incidence study: 6-year sequential acute care data. *Advances in Skin and Wound Care* 17:490–494.

Wilson, N. J., and K. W. Kizer. 1997. The VA health care system: An unrecognized national safety net. *Health Affairs (Millwood)* 16(4):200–204.

———. 1998. Oncology management by the "New" Veterans Health Administration. *Cancer* 82(10 Suppl.):2003–2009.

Wooten, A. F. 2002. Access to mental health services at Veterans Affairs community-based outpatient clinics. *Military Medicine* 167(5):424–426.

Wright, T., L. Jeffers, T. Mitchell, T. V. Holohan, and K. W. Kizer. 2000. At war with hepatitis C, part 3: Managing chronic infection. *Federal Practitioners* (17):24–29.

Yaisawarng, S., and J. F. Burgess, Jr. 2006. Performance-based budgeting in the public sector: An illustration from the VA health care system. *Health Economics* 15(3):295–310.

Yano, E. M., B. F. Simon, A. B. Lanto, and L. V. Rubenstein. 2007. The evolution of changes in primary care delivery underlying the Veterans Health Administration's quality transformation. *American Journal of Public Health* 97(12):2151–2159.

Young, D. 2007. VA's 10-year journey to one formulary concludes. *American Journal of Health-System Pharmacy* 64(6):578, 580.

Young, G. J. 2000a. Managing organizational transformations: Lessons from the Veterans Health Administration. *California Management Review* 43:66–82.

———. 2000b. *Transforming government: The revitalization of the Veterans Health Administration.* Arlington, VA: The PricewaterhouseCoopers Endowment for The Business of Government.

Young, G. J., M. P. Charns, J. Daley, M. G. Forbes, W. Henderson, and S. F. Khuri. 1997. Best practices for managing surgical services: The role of coordination. *Health Care Management Review* 22(4):72–81.

Yu, W., A. Ravelo, T. H. Wagner, C. S. Phibbs, A. Bhandari, S. Chen, and P. G. Barnett. 2003. Prevalence and costs of chronic conditions in the VA health care system. *Medical Care Research and Review* 60(3 Suppl.):146S–167S.

5

Fostering Systems Change to Drive Continuous Learning in Health Care

INTRODUCTION

The vision of the Institute of Medicine's (IOM's) Roundtable on Evidence-Based Medicine (now the Roundtable on Value & Science-Driven Health Care) is "the development of a learning healthcare system that is designed to generate and apply the best evidence for the collaborative health care choices of each patient and provider; to drive the process of discovery as a natural outgrowth of patient care; and to ensure innovation, quality, safety, and value in health care" (Charter pp. xi–xii). How to realize the vision of continuous learning was the focus of the fourth session of the workshop.

The publication *The Learning Healthcare System: Workshop Summary* (IOM, 2007), based on an earlier Roundtable workshop, identified several common characteristics of a system with continuous learning, including a culture that emphasizes transparency and learning through continuous feedback loops, care as a seamless team process, best practices that are embedded in system design, information systems that reliably deliver evidence and capture results, and results that are bundled to improve the level of practice and the state of the science. With those characteristics in mind, the contributors in this chapter looked closely at how specific aspects of feedback and performance can be improved in the healthcare organizational culture, in the development of accessible knowledge, in the management of information and technology, and in the organization of information systems.

Steven J. Spear, senior lecturer at Massachusetts Institute of Technology and a Senior Fellow at the Institute for Healthcare Improvement, observed that in many sectors of the service and manufacturing economies a few high-performance organizations seem to be the leaders, and their competitors essentially compete for second place. These pioneers deliver value with less effort and cost, even though they have similar—or identical—tools, customers, suppliers, labor, and regulations. Spear said that these organizational leaders continue to push the envelope through differences in systems management and that the lessons from their success might offer perspectives on value, efficiency, quality, and other areas that are important to producing a learning, team-oriented, patient-centric culture within health care. Based on his close observations of Toyota, Southwest Airlines, Alcoa, and other industry leaders, Spear reported that, in contrast to organizations that address systems anomalies with workarounds, industry leaders carefully analyze adverse events and use them as sentinels for investigation into causes. Spear hypothesized that by adopting similar techniques, healthcare systems may be able to deliver better care to more people at less cost and with less effort—on the order of twice as good for twice as many people at half the cost.

Examining the value of knowledge management, access, and use, Donald E. Detmer, president and chief executive officer (CEO) of the American Medical Informatics Association (AMIA) and professor of medical education at the University of Virginia, argued that improved management of information applied to clinical decision support (CDS) will require structured policies and complementary agendas for informatics education and research. Detmer discussed the CDS Roadmap for National Action developed by the AMIA, which is based on the principles of (1) best knowledge available when needed, (2) high adoption and effective use, and (3) continuous improvement of CDS methods and knowledge. Detmer also discussed the Morningside Initiative, which seeks to share information broadly for CDS. Detmer highlighted the AMIA–Association of Academic Health Centers' (AAHC's) current collaboration to develop enhanced informatics curriculums for health professional and continuing education students. He also discussed current developments in CDS policy and infrastructure and identified areas for further investigation and efforts. Looking to the future, he emphasized the importance of determining the appropriate mechanism for integrating personal health records with electronic health records (EHRs).

Stephen J. Swensen, director of quality for the Mayo Clinic and professor of radiology at the Mayo Clinic College of Medicine, said the healthcare industry must address specific elements of technology management in order to drive systems change. He described work in technology management at the Mayo Clinic to develop networks that embody optimal reliability, permit nimble and effective diffusion of best practices, have built-in safety nets, and support optimal organizational learning and communication. Swensen emphasized that technology management should leverage human capital and should embody a decision-making process whereby decisions are made with an organizational perspective by cross-functional, physician-led teams. Swensen's discussion encompassed five facets of technology management—policy, appropriateness, reliability, diffusion, and social capital. In ensuring appropriate care, for example, Swensen observed that health systems face the complex task of first making sure that the right policies are in place to encourage medical centers, physicians, and other providers to use technology and deliver the appropriate care in the best setting, and then they must ensure that patients are connected in the most efficient way with the technology assets most appropriate to their needs.

Discussing the link between the organization and management of information systems and the quality and safety of patient care, David C. Classen, a physician at Computer Sciences Corporation, described current approaches to the evaluation of clinical information systems. He detailed a new simulation tool that has been developed and used by healthcare organizations to evaluate the effectiveness of clinical information systems implementations in improving the safety of care for patients. Classen demonstrated how such tools have been used by organizations to learn about the capabilities of their implemented clinical information systems and to assess system shortfalls, and he showed how organizations have used these tools to improve clinical information systems.

CHASING THE RABBIT: WHAT HEALTHCARE ORGANIZATIONS CAN LEARN FROM THE WORLD'S GREATEST ORGANIZATIONS

Steven J. Spear, D.B.A., M.S., M.S., , Massachusetts Institute of Technology, Institute for Healthcare Improvement

In manufacturing, heavy industry, high tech, services, aviation, the military, and elsewhere, a small number of organizations always race to the front of the pack in their sector, leaving everyone else competing for runner-up. Although these organizations use similar science and technology to meet the needs of a similar customer base, are dependent on the same group of suppliers, hire from the same labor pools, and are subject to the same regulations as their competitors, they deliver far more value with much less effort and at lower cost. They gain and sustain leadership by managing the complex systems of work on which they depend in markedly different ways. Healthcare organizations can learn—and have learned—from these exemplars, with outstanding results in efficacy, efficiency, safety, and quality of care.

The proposition considered here is that it is possible to deliver much better care then we currently do, to many more people than we currently do, and at much less cost and with less effort than is currently the case. The envisioned improvements are not incremental; instead, I am speaking of a product that is twice as good for twice as many people at half the cost. The proposition is not based on hypothesis or conjecture, but is supported by good clinical evidence. This paper begins by examining what needs to be done and in particular, the lessons healthcare organizations can learn from other complex, high-performing organizations in other industries so as to achieve the goal of better care for more people at less cost.

Twenty years ago I was an employee of Congress at one of the congressional agencies. At the time, the competitiveness of U.S. manufacturing with that of Japan was a major concern, focused on the idea that the Japanese were gaining an advantage from what was essentially unfair competition. People sensed that financing arrangements, competition, and domestic and international markets were being manipulated. There were accusations of dumping of various types of goods, steel not the least of these. The notion was that the appropriate response to declining competitiveness on the part of American companies was for Congress, regulators, and the executive branch to act similarly to how they perceived the Japanese to be acting.

A few years later, there was a fundamental shift in what people saw as the causes of competitive differences. Replacing the focus on large macronational elements was recognition that the differences between the countries were rooted in the differences between companies—that what was being done in companies such as Sony, Toshiba, and Hitachi was fundamentally different from what was happening in their U.S. counterparts and that what was taking place at Toyota and Honda was fundamentally different from what was going on at General Motors (GM), Chrysler, and Ford.

This realization was good news because it meant that the solution to the problem did not depend on consensus among the Majority Leader of the Senate, the President, and the Speaker of the House on the source of the problem or the solution. This good news, however, meant that U.S. companies bore a great responsibility, and that managers of individual companies and of business units within those companies had enormous influence on the outcome of their organizations' efforts.

To link this discussion to health care, let us start with a statement of the problem: too few people have access, the costs are too high, and so on. Much of the discussion among politicians focuses on whether more resources should be committed to the system. But if we pursue the parallels with the manufacturing sector, that may not be the answer. I am not going to argue against spending altogether. Certain changes are needed in terms of how information is reported and how coverage is provided for those who are least able to care for themselves. There are also separate issues of transfer of wealth and caring for the least well in our society.

Continuing the focus on the delivery of care, the experience from manufacturing suggests that presidents of hospitals, presidents of systems, managers of hospitals, and deliverers of care—from small practices to very large organizations such as the Office of Veterans Affairs—can have an enormous influence on outcomes. That is good news because it means that improving the quality of health care will not depend on a confluence of interest and perspective among three people, but can arise from the efforts of thousands or tens of thousands of people who work together to move the system in the right direction.

Returning to the perception of the competition between the United States and Japan, originally the perception was that the key competition was between Tokyo and the Diet (Japan's legislative body) and Washington and Congress. In a sense, the idea was that somehow the Japanese had unleveled the playing field, that they were not playing by the same rules or were playing by the same rules but cheating. But this perception changed, and people started to recognize that the playing field was in fact quite level.

Consider that to compete today, industries must compete in every region around the world. When they do so, they compete head to head with all of their competitors, so they cannot lock up markets, regions, or customers. For example, many towns have the equivalent of Boston's "Auto Mile," where one can walk into a Buick dealer, and if that dealer does not have what one wants, one can visit the Chrysler dealer next door and, if necessary, move on to the Ford dealer, the Toyota dealer, and so forth—all literally within walking distance. Given this phenomenon, major auto companies cannot lock up customers. How, then, can they gain a competitive advantage?

If a monopolistic relationship with one's customers is impossible, a company might try to lock up its suppliers. That cannot be done with automobiles, however, and, generally speaking, all automobile manufacturers are subject to the same regulations and innate market preferences. Customers are paying the same price for a gallon of gasoline whether they put that gas into a Ford or a Toyota or a Chrysler. The playing field is extraordinarily level. And when the playing field is level, this parity of rules can be expected to lead to a parity of outcomes. When everything is the same in terms of customers, suppliers, labor pools, and so forth, people can be expected to gain and lose leadership, gain and lose profits, in a very fluid, dynamic situation.

In the automobile industry, Ford, Chrysler, GM, Volkswagen, and their competitors do indeed fluctuate between very hot and very cold years. They are engaged in intense competition, but they are all competing for second place. In first place is Toyota, which has experienced extraordinary profitability and growth in market share and revenue. By other measures, such as market capitalization vs. profitability, there is an enormous disproportion between Toyota and U.S. companies. Not only has Toyota grown, but if one looks at the ratios, the market expects it to continue to grow at a sustained rate over many years.

One might think Toyota is an anomaly and decide to look at another playing field—say, commercial aviation. To make an apples-to-apples comparison, players in this field fly the same planes out of the same airports, hire from the same labor pool, pay the same price for jet fuel, and are subject to the same regulations. By and large, the playing field is level with parity of contest and parity of outcomes. Accordingly, in this competitive environment, Delta, Northwest, Continental, United, and American regularly have good and bad years, and they regularly gain and lose share. It turns out, though, that this is a competition for second place because there is Southwest, with some 35 years of profitable growth, year after year. Even when things go bad at Southwest, they go bad on a much smaller scale than at other companies. For example, when Southwest and American failed similar Federal Aviation Administration inspections, Southwest paid a fine and kept flying, while American essentially shut down for a week.

In terms of parity of playing field and parity of outcome, one can see such anomalous patterns in industry after industry—automobile manufacturing, the aluminum and steel industries, commercial aviation, government services, and on and on. One begins to realize that there are not just anomalies, but a population of anomalous outcomes. When one examines what the leaders—Toyota, Southwest, Alcoa, the Navy's nuclear reactor program—have in common, one finds that they have solved a problem that plagues every industry—complexity.

For any product or service, the number of elements necessary to make it function is far greater than it was 5, 10, or 20 years ago. The number of interdependencies and interconnections among those elements is far greater than ever before. The basic problem with a complex system is that, at some point, once there are enough elements and connections and interdependences, it is nearly impossible to understand the structure of the system and to understand or predict its behavior perfectly. This is where the divide begins between the companies or organizations that are in first place and those that are stuck competing for second place.

Two fundamental differences in behavior have direct application to health care, which, of course, is a complex system of work to deliver care to patients. The first is that those who are competing tend to organize themselves functionally around specialty silos, whereas those who are highly successful tend to place tremendous emphasis on building functional technical skill because they need it to compete, but this skill is in service of the process by which they deliver value to customers or patients or users. The difference is between a functional view and a functional view plus service of process and system.

The second difference is that those who are less successful put a lot of effort into the design of systems. I am not going to try to diminish that effort. But once a complex system is running and operating, its behavior is going to be somewhat unpredictable because of the problem, noted earlier, of the inevitable limits on understanding the system and the way its parts interrelate. Those who focus on designing systems tolerate things going contrary to expectations, as is inevitable with a complex system, and they dismiss this as the inevitable noise of what they do.

In contrast, when highly successful companies design and start operating systems, they do not dismiss such chatter as noise. They do not live in a world of signal and noise, where the signal is what they wanted to get and the noise is something contrary to that. Instead, they live in a world of signal and signal. The expected signals are things that happen that confirm what they believed about the system's structure and behavior; the chatter or noise points them to the things they did not understand.

A key difference between the highly successful organizations and the others is that the others tolerate, encourage, and depend on an environment where fighting fires, working around problems, coping, and otherwise making do is how work is accomplished. The problem with that approach for the people who work in those organizations is it means that every day they know they are going to go to work and fail to some degree.

Another basic problem with complex systems is that sometimes these little failures come together in idiosyncratic fashion. Not only are there the normal daily annoyances of doing work in a flawed system, but sometimes these things combine catastrophically. In contrast, those who are very good at dealing with complexity will design a system, but when they operate it, they place tremendous emphasis on identifying things that go contrary to expectations. Those signals tell them where they have to invest in building more knowledge. When they see that something has gone wrong, they are quick to deal with the problem because they know that the time to address problems is when they are still hot. Think, for example, of doctors rushing to a patient who is crashing or detectives getting to a crime scene while the evidence is still fresh. It is in dealing with problems while they are still hot that new knowledge can be generated about how the system behaves. When that knowledge is gained locally by an individual, great effort can be made to ensure that this knowledge is shared with everyone else involved.

As an example, the nuclear navy has modeled very well the behavior of constant dynamic discovery, of creating a high-velocity organization. The navy thinks about it in terms of an operator sitting down to run a nuclear reactor on board a submarine. The person may be just 22 years old, perhaps just graduated from Annapolis with a year's training in the Nuclear Reactor Program. This person is not running the reactor as if he or she has had just a year's experience, but as if he or she has had the 5,700 reactor-years of experience the navy has accumulated over the past 50 years of running reactors on board warships.

I started looking at the anomalies in manufacturing first at Toyota and then at Alcoa. I also got involved in the Pittsburgh Regional Health Initiative. Our first effort in Pittsburgh was to look at medication administration. This is a process problem because it involves doctors making diagnoses and writing prescriptions, prescriptions going to the pharmacy, orders being filled and delivered, nurses providing medication, and so on. It turned out there was a problem with how orders were being transmitted and delivered.

People in the pharmacy and in nursing came up with a solution to the problem that would save a tremendous amount of nursing time and reduce and nearly eliminate any chance of error that would result in giving the wrong medication to a patient—a particularly serious problem in a transplant case. They tried this solution in a low-cost way, then tested it again through a variety of pilots and realized it was a great idea. They wanted to institutionalize it and make their learning valuable to the organization, so they tried to find the person who owned the bridge between nursing and pharmacy. They knew this was not someone in nursing or in pharmacy or in their particular domain, so they started looking elsewhere in the organization. It was not the charge nurse or the person who played a similar role in the pharmacy, and it turned out it was not even the president of the hospital who owned the bridge between the two because the hospital was part of a larger system. Eventually they found that the first person who had formal authority over the bridge between this pharmacy and this nursing unit in a much larger system was the CEO of the hospital. Everything else was managed through functional silos and disciplines—orthopedics, obstetrics, and so on; nursing separate from medicine, medicine from surgery. Consider how difficult it is to institutionalize all the micro-changes necessary so an organization has on a daily basis a homeostatic self-correcting, self-improving dynamic. In that case it was impossible.

To return to my original proposition, it is possible to deliver much better care to many more people with much less cost and effort than is currently the case. We need not wait for the President, the Majority Leader, and the Speaker of the House to come to some kind of agreement. What we do need is for people who are responsible for systems and organizations to understand that although managing functions is necessary, it is not sufficient. They need to manage processes—not just pharmacy and nursing, but also medication administration, and not in a static fashion whereby one designs a process and hopes it will run well, but in a dynamic fashion so that chatter is not treated as inevitable noise, but as an indication of where one needs to improve.

KNOWLEDGE MANAGEMENT FOR CLINICAL CARE

Donald E. Detmer, M.D., M.A.,
University of Virginia, Charlottesville

Knowledge management for CDS requires a policy framework as well as an education and research agenda. In its CDS Roadmap for National Action, the American Medical Informatics Association (AMIA) recommended a structure with the following three pillars: (1) best knowledge available when needed, (2) high adoption and effective use, and (3) continuous improvement of CDS methods and knowledge. The roadmap led to the Morningside Initiative, which aims to develop a Knowledge Management Repository for CDS through a public–private partnership. The goal is to create a shared repository of executable knowledge for CDS that will be broadly available. The hope is that these and related initiatives funded recently by the Agency for Healthcare Research and Quality (AHRQ) will eventually result in a sustainable infrastructure.

Educational initiatives and relevant informatics research are needed. The AMIA, in collaboration with the AAHC Affiliate Roundtable, will collaborate to create a two-stage, integrated, multimodular informatics curriculum for all students studying to become health professionals. The initial course will be appropriate for students entering professional education, and the second is to be pursued just before students begin professional practice. These initiatives, combined with AMIA's 10 × 10 program for those in practice, will help address basic professional educational needs, especially in applied clinical informatics. Finally, there are major informatics research issues that need attention. One critical research and development area, for instance, concerns patients' use of their own EHRs for chronic illness management in collaboration with their clinicians via secure Web portals.

The AMIA is clearly interested in trying to foster change for purposes of improving both health and healthcare delivery. In particular, we are challenged to integrate the carbon dimensions with the silicone dimensions—that is, to bring informatics to bear on the problem. Today, we lack the right policy infrastructure to accomplish this integration. This paper looks briefly at some relevant IOM work and a project that the AMIA carried out for the Office of the National Coordinator on Clinical Decision Support, and then offers some ideas about what a national roadmap for knowledge management should look like.

The 1991 IOM study *Computer-Based Patient Record: An Essential Technology for Health Care* (reissued in 1997) (IOM, 1997) identified EHRs as an essential technology for health care. It is fascinating that this remains the case 17 years later, yet one would not think so based on the usage of EHRs in the United States today. While the 1991 report emphasized the importance of EHRs for quality improvement and for clinical decision support, these dimensions of EHRs were not really obvious at the time in terms of widely held national policy perspectives.

Whereas the 1991 report addressed essential skills needed in the workforce, the IOM's 2001 *Crossing the Quality Chasm* report firmly tied policy to how EHRs and EHR systems and communications technologies should be used to move from a costly, inefficient, and highly variable system to a system that is equitable, safe, patient centered, efficient, effective, and timely (IOM, 2001).

Another crucial IOM effort that has not received as much attention as it deserves is the Health Professions Education Summit. That meeting and the ensuing report, entitled *Health Professions Education: A Bridge to Quality 2003*, addressed many relevant dimensions of health care, including the need for aligned reimbursement incentives and regulatory requirements, robust information infrastructure, widespread use of evidence-based medicine, and a workforce skilled in evidence-based medicine, information technology (IT), and process improvement (IOM, 2003).

From the perspective of a policy background, a national roadmap for knowledge management with decision support is clearly lacking. In fact, although many developed economies around the world have put in place a good basic information infrastructure, decision support remains immature. Even Denmark has a long way to go.

The AMIA developed the CDS Roadmap for National Action between 2005 and 2007 with the support of many groups and individuals (AMIA, 2006). Some findings have just recently been approved by the American Health Information Community (AHIC) as a guide for U.S. policy in this domain. Essentially, the roadmap was intended to create a blueprint for coordinated nationwide action to ensure that usable and effective CDS will be widely used by clinicians and patients. The challenge was seen as developing decision support that is equally usable by patients and their clinicians to improve health care. Three pillars were envisioned as the foundation of the model:

> A system must continually develop the best knowledge available and make that knowledge available at the point and time it is needed. Knowledge must be both current, "right" to the best standards of the day (ideally both generally and locally), and accessible. There needs to be high adoption and effective use—performance is key to this. Methods must be improved continuously in addition to the knowledge base.

With these three pillars in mind, a coherent structure will enable progress. The following objectives are crucial: develop practical, standard formats for representing CDS knowledge and interventions; establish standard approaches for collecting, organizing, and distributing CDS; address policy, legal, and financial barriers, and create additional support and enablers; compile and disseminate best practices for usability and implementation; develop methods for collecting, learning from, and sharing national experience with CDS; and use EHR data systematically to advance knowledge.

The roadmap recommends a series of activities to improve the development, implementation, and use of CDS. It identifies work products. Objectives include organizing and facilitating the creation of a convening coordinating body and establishing a CDS technical assistance center. (Whether this should be one center or a cluster is not clear, but the goal is to establish consensus groups to answer key questions that arise on roadmap development.) We wish to assemble a best-practice synthesis, conduct training and education, and develop prototypes. Many pilot demonstrations are recommended, including supporting and facilitating related nationwide initiatives, developing practical standard formats to share knowledge and interventions, and collecting and disseminating best practices for usability and implementation.[1]

Looking at current policy and national structure, one can see that the roadmap has had an impact. AHRQ is supporting some activities through its national resource center and Centers for Education and Research on Therapeutics grants, including knowledge management CDS grants. There have been presentations to the National Committee on Vital and Health Statistics, and the Morningside Initiative begun by the Telemedicine and Advanced Technology Research Center (TATRC) is now gaining some institutional linkage to the AMIA.

The Department of Health and Human Services (HHS) AHIC meeting on April 22, 2008, approved recommendations of the ad hoc CDS workgroup; AHIC considers the AMIA's CDS Roadmap for National Action to be a foundational document. At the meeting, three priorities were identified: (1) drive measurable progress toward priority performance goals for healthcare quality improvement, (2) explore options to establish or leverage a public–private entity to facilitate collaboration across CDS development and deployment, and (3) accelerate CDS development and adoption through federal programs and collaborations. All activities relate to seeking measurable progress through quality improvement. Another recommendation was that by October 31, 2008, HHS and relevant partners should have explored options for establishing or leveraging a public–private entity (e.g., AHIC 2.0) to convene public and private organizations and stakeholders for the purpose of promoting effective CDS development and adoption and addressing gaps in CDS capabilities through planning, facilitation, and coordination of activities across diverse constituencies.

---

[1] More CDS Roadmap Information is available at www.amia.org/inside/initiatives/cds/ (accessed September 20, 2010).

In 2008, the federal government created a collaboratory for CDS. Its goal is to coordinate internal activities across AHRQ, the HHS Personalized Healthcare Initiative, and the Office of the National Coordinator. Its role is to scan and then try to leverage what is happening across the government in these areas. At the same time, as mentioned above, the Morningside Initiative has been supported by TATRC and others. (Current Morningside collaborators include the AMIA, Arizona State University, the Henry Ford Health System, the Veterans Health Administration–Office of Information, the Department of Defense, Kaiser Permanente, Partners Healthcare System, TATRC, and Intermountain Healthcare.) The goal of creating the collaboratory was to explore possibilities for developing a national knowledge management repository for CDS so that CDS information can be available in computer-executable language and thereby shared and made broadly available.

It is too early to say whether or how the above efforts will relate to AHIC 2.0, but there are signs of progress. At the same time, regulations need to be monitored to ensure we do not backslide, intentionally or not. Regulations relating to the Food and Drug Administration guidance document on CDS bear watching, as do efforts to change the Health Insurance Portability and Accountability Act in light of developments in personal health records.

This domain presents an educational challenge. Again referring to the health professions education *Bridge to Quality 2003* report, the AMIA has sought to address the challenge that report highlighted (IOM, 2003). Through its Academic Strategic Leadership Council, the AMIA is undertaking an activity with the Affiliate Roundtable of the AAHC, plus a few representatives from other organizations, whose aim is to create a common multidisciplinary approach to entry-level education for all health professional students on knowledge management CDS, as well as a second course that would be taken prior to entering professional practice. Furthermore, AMIA's 10 × 10 program aims to train 10,000 healthcare professionals to serve as local informatics leaders and champions by 2010, particularly in the area of applied clinical informatics, on which much of knowledge management focuses. Thus far, more than 1,000 people have graduated from the program.

Clearly research is highly important as well. Informatics is an emerging discipline. The AMIA recently conducted a survey of the top research issues for informaticians, and the results showed this order of importance: interoperability, workflow, quality and patient safety, decision support, and information filtering and aggregation. The emphasis on interoperability is probably no surprise, but more interesting perhaps is the attention to workflow and process design.

Regarding decision support, its impact has been relatively limited to date. Understanding of how to develop, maintain, and integrate centralized decision support resources is insufficient. Context awareness of decision support technology needs to be improved. Ultimately, this technology needs to reach the patient through secure Web portal integration, and patients need to be encouraged to work on monitoring and managing their own health care.

With respect to research information and filtering, we need to be able to better manage electronic medical literature, summarize information from clinical literature, summarize patient medical history from large volumes of data, mine data to identify patterns, and present information in the context of individual patients.

Looking to the future, in terms of people issues, we need to focus on the organization and management of complex adaptive systems and to improve policies and procedures that will provide better access to patient data. With regard to technology, our focus should be on data repositories and scaling of research methods and standards. We need human- and machine-readable protocols and results. There are also hybrid issues to be addressed.

In the United States in the near future, I think the issue will come down to where AHIC V2 (or A2) is going. Obviously, technology continues to advance in such areas as genomics, handheld computing, and so forth, and these advances are likely to shape the way the future unfolds.

One current issue in this country is the need to ensure that our basic investment in EHRs goes beyond results reporting and record keeping to encompass the really important value-added dimension of decision support. Decision support will provide the major leverage for quality and efficiency. A key question is how the personal health record and the EHR can be integrated so they inform one another. This is why the AMIA strongly supports patients' access to their EHRs via secure Web portals, along with patients' ability to comment on the findings shown.

Mario Andretti has said, "If everything is under control, you are going too slow." With this in mind, I would recommend that everyone look regularly at Daniel Masys's *Annual Reviews of Informatics* (Masys, 2007), as well as Russ Altman's *Annual Review of Translational Bioinformatics.*[2] Finally, I would stress that leadership from the National Academies in the area of knowledge management for CDS is crucial.

---

[2] See http://rbaltman.wordpress.com/ (accessed September 20, 2010).

TECHNOLOGY MANAGEMENT

Stephen J. Swensen, M.D., M.M.M., F.A.C.R., and
James Dilling, Mayo Clinic

Technology management is an important issue for the healthcare business sector. Approximately 50 percent of cost growth in health care over the past 40 years has been the result of technology innovation (CBO, 2008). Technology growth takes many forms, including the development of new pharmaceuticals, devices, and services.

Technology management has many facets, five of which are addressed in this paper:

1. policy,
2. appropriateness,
3. reliability,
4. diffusion, and
5. social capital.

Policy

Public policy and health insurance programs are powerful drivers of technology management. Choices about what is incentivized and paid for play a central role in determining what is performed and prescribed. Public policy and health insurance programs are among the reasons we have such high expenditures related to technology today.

For example, American healthcare policy is driven largely by fee for service. Most of our healthcare system pays for more exams, which in turn drive technology use. We do not pay for value (outcomes, safety, or service divided by cost over time). We pay the same to an endoscopic practice that has an accuracy rate of 90 percent as we do to a practice that has an accuracy rate of 60 percent. We pay the same to two practices even if one has a complication rate twice that of the other. We pay for use, not value.

So from a societal perspective, policy and programs that encourage self-referral and overuse achieve exactly the result one would expect, even if this was not the intent. U.S. policy and programs are dominant forces in technology purchase and management. In fact, when physicians own their own imaging equipment, the tendency is to order more exams and to charge more for poorer quality (Hillman et al., 1990, 1992, 1995). We do not pay for superior outcomes in diabetic patient care—we pay for visits, drugs, scans, and procedures.

Appropriateness

For optimal technology use, a thoughtfully engineered healthcare system must ensure that a patient receives no more and no less than the right care; that is, a patient must receive appropriate care. For instance, some estimate that 30 to 40 percent of imaging procedures in the United States are unnecessary (Thrall, 2004; Tosczak, 2004). General Electric has calculated that poor quality costs that company $127 million per year, $60 million of which is attributed to radiology overuse (de Brantes, 2003).

Technology must also be managed after acquisition. Here is an important role for a common outpatient/inpatient EHR (and the instant peer review and communication it affords), standard order sets, decision support, and clinical prediction rules. These resources can address the issues of misuse and underuse of technology. Overuse, in part, results from a systems issue due to financial conflict of interest (i.e., nonsalaried physicians working in a production model). The lack of integrated practice models also has led many technology-intensive areas to be viewed as service areas (e.g., labs, radiology, gastroenterology). When the primary or specialty physician orders a test, it is nearly always completed, regardless of whether it is necessary and whether it is even the appropriate test given the patient's condition. Through greater communication and integration, these support areas can consult with and educate the ordering physicians on the most appropriate tests or modalities.

Appropriate use of technology can be driven by standard evidence-based work manifested by best-practice order sets and decision support. A logical place to start is where we have the most solid evidence supporting optimal care. One example is clinical prediction rules. Using the Canadian computed tomography (CT) head rule, neurosurgical intervention is still optimized with a sensitivity of 100 percent, yet CT imaging for minor head trauma is reduced by more than a third (Smits et al., 2005). High-value technology management requires methodically identifying the right patient and selectively rendering the right care.

The current public environment reinforced by third-party payment for health care has led to high patient expectations regarding the use of technology, in particular imaging and pharmaceuticals. More is typically seen as better. The constant barrage of pharmaceutical and imaging advertisements on television and in print leads patients to pressure physicians toward increased use of higher-cost—although not necessarily more effective—diagnostics and treatment. The ramifications may be manifest in the variability in the cost of care during the last 2 years of life, which varies by a factor of more than 2 from one region of the country to another (Wennberg et al., 2007a, 2007b).

Reliability

Rational incentives from a healthcare system that rewards appropriate use are necessary, but insufficient. If there is no market force that rewards reliability in the context of appropriate use, we will fall short of optimal technology management and high reliability. If an operation is appropriate but injures the patient, we fall short. If magnetic resonance imaging of the spine was appropriate but misinterpreted, we fall short.

Technology management involves managing technology in terms of not only volume, but also reliability (e.g., accuracy, safety). The median accuracy for mammography interpretation in the United States is 66 percent. To increase the median accuracy by 5 points to 71 percent, the bottom 30 percent of radiologists—approximately 6,000 in number—would need to be excluded from practice or improve their performance (Beam et al., 2003). The system today rewards only volume. The practitioner with a 90 percent accuracy rate is paid the same as one with a 40 percent accuracy rate.

If healthcare providers, including residents and fellows, are placed in environments where we know their rate of medical errors will increase, we are falling short of optimal technology management. If we fail to train providers to work in teams where we know their reliability and safety will be enhanced, we are falling short of optimal technology management. Forty percent of residents report making serious medical errors (Mizrahi, 1984). A healthcare provider who has been up for 24 hours is as impaired as someone with a blood alcohol content of 0.08 percent, legally drunk in many states (Dawson and Reid, 1997). We have designed many of our systems for suboptimal technology use.

Simulation is a discipline that has been applied by other industries, including commercial aviation, for a long time. It is now being embraced by medicine. At our institution, we have a simulation center in which we have more than 5,000 learner experiences each year. We expect all medical students to have simulation center competency before their internship year. Before residents and fellows start their jobs at the Mayo Clinic, they must demonstrate competency in an online safety module. Before a central line is placed by any resident or fellow, he or she must first demonstrate competency in a simulated environment with a cross-functional team. Optimal management of technology must include attention not just to its appropriateness, but also to the reliability of its use.

Diffusion

Effective and efficient technology management to support high-reliability patient care requires a nimble and effective diffusion of best practices as well as safety nets, both within an organization and nationwide. Unfortunately, to this point diffusion of best practices for technology use has proved slow and inconsistent (Ting et al., 2008; Wennberg et al., 2007a, 2007b).

Social engineering is an important dimension of high reliability and is requisite for optimal technology management. For an organization to know what its people know, there must be fluid communication and diffusion of best practices and lessons from adverse events, and safety nets must be put in place to prevent harm to patients from technology in the inevitably imperfect hands of even the most competent, conscientious healthcare providers. Many institutions aspire to become learning organizations. Our design employs 100-day enterprise teams in which colleagues work collaboratively across the 5 states of our organization. A chief event officer has responsibility for actively diffusing the lessons from significant adverse events involving harm and for ensuring that each of our 22 hospitals has a safety net in place that takes into account the lessons and systems of the other 21 hospitals. Our social engineering includes face-to-face meetings, committees, and the expectation that colleagues at each site will collaborate and incorporate best practices into their own organization (Leach and Philibert, 2006).

An important catalyst for diffusion is transparency. Our efforts at transparency include an enterprise-quality dashboard that displays outcomes, safety, and service using common definitions and processes (Swensen and Cortese, 2008).

Technology itself can play an important role in technology management. IT may serve important roles in optimizing the appropriate use of technology. It may be designed to fill expected knowledge gaps at the point of care. One example is push technology for providers who "don't know what they don't know," with concise recommended care and expert contact information. We have developed an enterprise learning system that, for selected conditions, can help close the knowledge gap. For instance, a patient with an electrocardiogram indicating long-QT syndrome may receive a variety of treatments based on the particular practitioner and that practitioner's knowledge gap. Today, whenever long-QT syndrome is identified on an outpatient electrocardiogram, a semiurgent notification is sent to the point of care with a link to our enterprise learning system, where instructions for the appropriate care, including antibiotic risks, are delivered with a closed-loop feedback auditable system.

There are also situations in which practitioners know that they lack expertise in treating a condition. In such cases, instead of push technology, practitioners can be directed to a central knowledge repository to learn how best to treat that condition. Today, a knowledge repository could be a textbook, a phone call to a colleague, or the Internet browser for an online search. We are developing a technology called Ask Mayo Expert that makes available the agreed-upon standard best practice, salient risks, and references, along with frequently asked questions and appropriate medical specialty contact information. This is a step toward the most appropriate and reliable use of technology, as well as toward high-reliability patient care.

IT will become an even more important tool as its use expands in health care. It will allow for better analysis of practice patterns and improved research on the most effective approaches, and it will ultimately serve as a critical mechanism for effectively implementing the best practices among the front-line staff caring for patients.

Social Capital

Key to a comprehensive technology management strategy and integral to high-reliability patient care is a conscious investment in social capital (i.e., the active connections among colleagues caring for patients). Social capital investments move an organization from a collection of individuals toward an agile, coherent collective mind.

Optimal organizational learning requires fluent communication of three types: (1) intrateam, (2) interteam and intrasite, and (3) interteam and intersite. The networks must be purposely engineered and nurtured; they must engage research, administrative, and education colleagues. Several aspects of social engineering are worthy of exploration: transparency, teamwork training, horizontal infrastructure, and cross-functional, team-based simulation training. A fundamental tactic in this cultural transformation is the training of health care's youngest learners, medical and nursing students and residents, *together* on cross-functional teams.

An integrated medical practice with organized care coordination is an ecosystem well suited to learning. An integrated practice offers a community in which the interests of medical staff, medical school, and hospital leadership are not competing but aligned. It is a structure in which inpatient–outpatient care is seen as a continuum. The hospital is viewed not as a centerpiece, but often as the safety net for insufficient chronic and preventive outpatient care.

Technology management should be approached in a manner that leverages and creates social capital. Decisions should be made with an organizational perspective by cross-functional, physician-led teams. Allocations should be evidence driven, peer reviewed, and based on merit from the patients' perspective. Individual departments should be advocates and technology experts, not decision makers (because in most organizations the different departments have a financial conflict of interest).

Conclusion

To achieve the goals of technology management and highly reliable patient care, the healthcare industry must foster systems change that leads to continuous learning. Whether the opportunity is a pharmaceutical device or a service, five perspectives need to be addressed to ensure the best outcome:

1. *Policy*—Pay for value, not volume.
2. *Appropriateness*—There are three opportunities for improvement: over-, under-, and mis-utilization.
3. *Reliability*—Appropriate matching of patient needs with technology is futile if there is an inaccurate diagnosis or a complication.
4. *Diffusion*—The disciplined spread of best practices must be actively managed.
5. *Social capital*—Active interpersonal connections facilitate best use of technology across an organization and the industry.

A LEARNING SYSTEM FOR IMPLEMENTATION OF ELECTRONIC HEALTH RECORDS

David C. Classen, M.D., M.S., Jane B. Metzger, and Emily Welebob, R.N., M.S., Computer Sciences Corporation, University of Utah School of Medicine

Over the past decade, many hospitals and ambulatory care sites have implemented EHR systems to improve the quality and safety of patient care. Yet recent studies reveal that, despite considerable investment in these systems, many organizations have thus far made only limited use of their most powerful capabilities to improve the quality and safety of care (Crosson et al., 2007; Nebeker et al., 2005; Simon et al., 2007; Walsh et al., 2008). This paper reviews current approaches to evaluating the contributions of EHR systems to improving clinical performance and describes a new simulation tool that is designed to help organizations evaluate the effectiveness of currently implemented EHR capabilities in meeting quality and safety goals. The problem of the underuse of EHR capabilities exists in all types of care settings, and the simulation tool can assist in several of these settings. However, this discussion is focused in particular on the hospital environment, where the simulation tool is first being applied. The paper also describes how hospitals have applied the knowledge gained from use of this simulation tool.

The EHR for the hospital is a set of interrelated clinical applications. The process of implementing the EHR involves adding new IT support in increments over many years in a series of projects. One promise of EHR systems is that they can improve the safety of medication use in the hospital, both at the point at which medications are ordered and when they are administered. The unsafe use of medications is not the only safety problem in the healthcare system, but it is certainly one of the most significant contributors to *preventable* adverse events. Hence much research on causes, consequences, and ways to avoid incidents of unsafe care has been focused in this area (Bates et al., 1995, 1998; Classen et al., 1991, 1992a, 1992b, 1997; Evans et al., 1994; Leape et al., 1995).

Achieving a reliably safer way to manage medications in the hospital is a major challenge that involves policies, processes, procedures, IT, and a transformational level of change in all of these areas. Furthermore, the changes must be made in concert. Engineers tend to think in terms of process, and this is one way to approach the issue of medication management. From a process perspective, medication management is multidisciplinary and highly complex. Interestingly enough, in most hospitals medication management is carried out largely with manual processes once the medications leave the pharmacy. Even if the process of providing medications goes well, every step of the manual processes must include redundancies (e.g., verification of medication order transcription each shift, double sign-off and signatures on intravenous pump settings and high-risk medications) and must be monitored prospectively because there are so many opportunities for things to go wrong. Attempts to improve medication management must be undertaken with great care and attention to the many process details to avoid inadvertently introducing new opportunities for errors (Ash et al., 2004).

Many studies have shown that the use of medications in the hospital is very risky for patients (Adams et al., 2008; Bates et al., 1995; Kaushal et al., 2001). Efforts to improve the safety of the medication process should initially be focused on the errors that harm patients rather than on those that do not, even though the latter are far more numerous. When medication-related adverse events are subjected to root-cause analysis, nearly 60 percent are found to originate during the prescribing and transcription steps (Leape et al., 1995).

This finding explains the priority placed on computerized physician order entry (CPOE), which can provide a significant additional safety net during physician ordering and eliminate the need for transcription. CPOE software comes with a set of decision support tools that each hospital can use (Metzger and Turisco, 2001). However, doing so involves instituting new accountabilities and processes for using these tools, and the extent of use of CPOE software varies considerably among hospitals. Hence studies of the impacts of CPOE on patient safety also show variable and often disappointing results (Bates, 1998; Classen et al., 1997; Han et al., 2005; Kilbridge et al., 2001; Koppel et al., 2005).

One study of a CPOE system at Brigham and Women's Hospital in Boston showed a significant decrease in medication errors but a significantly smaller decrease in actual harm to patients (Bates, 1998). A study at another hospital found a much larger decrease in adverse drug events with CPOE (Evans et al., 1998). A study in a pediatric hospital showed that the introduction of CPOE had reduced nonintercepted, serious medication errors by 7 percent, but there was no change in the rate of injuries that resulted from errors. As these studies show, having CPOE in place and operational does not improve safety uniformly, nor does it ensure that the potential contributions to medication safety are being well leveraged.

Given the drive for improvements in medication safety, the limited number of ways to evaluate this aspect of CPOE and other modules of the inpatient EHR, as shown in Table 5-1, is somewhat surprising. One approach that first became available in 2007 is certifying inpatient EHR vendor products on the shelf (Metzger et al., 2007). This approach provides a "seal of approval" showing buyers that the software product incorporates certain essential capabilities, including many related to CDS. Another approach to evaluating these EHR systems occurs in certain pay-for-performance initiatives, which use simple questionnaires to gather information about structural measures—use of IT and certain capabilities—although these initiatives are limited and somewhat embryonic.

Other high-level approaches to evaluating EHR systems are included in the CPOE standards from the National Quality Forum and the Leapfrog Group, which address a limited number of issues related to how the systems are used. The Leapfrog Group's standard requires physicians and other licensed prescribers to enter more than 75 percent of medication orders electronically, and it also requires that CDS be capable of intercepting at least 50 percent of common, avoidable adverse drug events (Kilbridge et al., 2006b). Until very recently, hospitals self-certified the status of CPOE use as part of the Leapfrog annual survey (Metzger et al., 2008).

Only two of the available evaluation methods can provide hospitals with feedback concerning how well CPOE capabilities are being used to improve medication safety. System use monitoring, although essential for managing CDS, provides insight only into the CDS tools in use, not into gaps in the coverage of common, preventable medication adverse events. Furthermore, the necessary reports are not easily obtained from all of the CPOE products in the marketplace. Because of time and cost, evaluation studies are infrequent and, even in hospitals with a research capacity, focus on limited areas of impact. Evaluation studies also often take years to complete. The simulation tool developed in support of the Leapfrog CPOE standard fills this void.

The Leapfrog CPOE standard has always required proof of the ability of the implemented CPOE to intercept at least 50 percent of the common,

TABLE 5-1 Available Methods for Evaluating the Performance of Computerized Provider Order Entry

Certification of inpatient computerized provider order entry (CPOE) and clinical decision support as part of certification of the inpatient electronic health record (EHR)	Commission for Certification of Health Information Technology	Information for purchasers concerning necessary capabilities in off-the-shelf products
Leapfrog Standards, National Quality Forum (NQF) Safe Practices	The Leapfrog Group, NQF	Voluntary self-certification of adoption of CPOE, including clinical decision support
Structural measures in pay-for-performance programs	Various payer-sponsored programs	Voluntary self-certification of use of EHRs (sometimes including specific features)
System use monitoring	EHR-provided reports	Provides information about use of order sets and instances of, and responses to, clinical decision support
Evaluation study	Research study exploring hypotheses about potential impacts of CPOE and other applications that build the inpatient EHR	Documents the type and extent of change in hypothesized change areas
Measurement of performance	Process and outcomes measures concerning inpatient care	Provides evidence of the combined effects of improvements in clinical practice and processes, including use of information technology when applicable

preventable medication errors that harm patients (The Leapfrog Group, 2008). The simulation tool that makes this possible has been in development since 2001 and recently became available as part of the Leapfrog survey process (Kilbridge et al., 2001, 2006a, 2006b; Metzger et al., 2008). The objective in developing this tool was to provide a credible, remote CPOE evaluation methodology for hospitals to use to assess and self-report the status of CDS tool use. The resulting evaluation tool provides overall scoring for incorporation into the Leapfrog survey results, as well as a status report back to the hospital (Metzger et al., 2008). (Another version of the tool supporting a similar assessment of implemented ambulatory EHRs will be made available at a future date.)

The evaluation simulates physician order writing in CPOE, using test patients and a set of test orders. It is a Web-based application, and hospital teams obtain instructions and report results through the Web, as described in Table 5-2. The test addresses ten categories of problem medication orders identified in numerous research studies as the frequent causes of medication-related adverse events and unnecessary costs (duplicate laboratory testing), as shown in Table 5-3. The evaluation also considers nuisance alerting, which is a major barrier to physician adoption. During development, reliability testing, and piloting, the assessment tool has been exercised in approximately 20 hospitals. The experience of two case studies is described in Boxes 5-1 and 5-2.

Thus far, the team has learned four major lessons while developing and testing the CPOE evaluation tool:

1. Although not all vendor tools are created equal, the use of medication-related decision support depends more on the effort applied to using the tools than on the specific vendor solution. Some hospitals overcome limitations of the CDS toolset with local software customizations.
2. CDS toolsets in CPOE products now in the marketplace do not address the full range of types of problem medication orders that can lead to patient harm, and many hospitals do not implement the full set of available tools because of usability or manageability issues.
3. The CDS toolset in CPOE has been applied most aggressively in those hospitals with an advanced, enterprise-wide approach to standards for clinical process and practice, including leadership and significant participation by physicians. In this setting, CDS is directly linked to ongoing quality improvement.
4. Smaller hospitals that are part of health systems typically benefit from all of the resources and expertise applied to medication safety and CPOE implementation at the health system level and are generally ahead of their peer institutions that undertake these projects on their own.

In every hospital where the evaluation tool has been employed during its long development process, the physician CPOE leaders and other team members have gained knowledge about gaps in CDS coverage of important order categories in addition to confirming what some already knew about CDS usage. The increased insight now available to other hospitals through use of the CPOE simulation tool promises to spur significant progress on the long journey that remains until the full potential of CPOE is realized to help prevent medication-related adverse drug events.

TABLE 5-2 Leapfrog Computerized Provider Order Entry Evaluation Tool Procedure

Steps in the Evaluation Procedure	Activities
Register for the computerized provider order entry (CPOE) evaluation	• Obtain the password used to participate in the Leapfrog survey • Sign on to the Web application • Enter hospital information • Sign up for adult or pediatric evaluation • Assemble teams for patient set-up and order entry • Ensure that the test system mirrors the production system, or make plans to use the production system
Download test patient information (e.g., age, weight, allergies, lab values)	• When ready to begin set-up for the sample test or full evaluation, sign on to the Web application • Print the list of test patients • Set up test patients • Ensure that patients are "active" (may require nursing unit and bed before orders can be written and signed)
Download test orders	• When ready to begin the sample test or full evaluation, sign on to the Web application • Print test orders, instructions, and answer sheets • Ensure that the physician performing the evaluation has system authorizations required for order entry in CPOE (may be a test user)

BREAKOUT SESSION:
CAPTURING MORE VALUE IN HEALTH CARE

During a breakout session, participants broke into small groups to discuss how to capture more value in health care. They were asked to discuss three issues: (1) how much more value (health returned for dollars invested) could be obtained through the application of systems engineering principles in health care, (2) which one area had the potential for the greatest value to be returned from applying these principles, and (3) which actions could do the most to facilitate the needed changes. The main points of their discussions were reported back to the entire group.

In response to the question of how much value could be obtained from

TABLE 5-2 Continued

Steps in the Evaluation Procedure	Activities
Enter orders into the CPOE application	• Enter test orders for specified test patients • Sign every test order (or pair of orders) • Record the system responses on the answer sheet • Discontinue each test order (or pair of orders)
Enter and submit results	• Sign on to the Web application • Submit information from the answer sheet as instructed
Scoring	• Use automatic scoring of success in providing decision support to avert common, harmful medication errors for each order category and the evaluation overall
Reporting	• Print or view the feedback report immediately available (scores for each order category) • Aggregate the score available for posting along with hospital survey results

SOURCE: Reprinted with permission from Patient Safety & Quality Healthcare. Metzger et al., 2008.

the application of systems engineering principles in health care, respondents began by pointing out that the definition of value was problematic. They discussed the fact that value is hard to measure because it is composed of different components that are measured in different ways, including safety, quality and cost. Some groups concluded that value can be construed as a measure with many definitions, and the particular definition used will depend on the stakeholder's point of view. One group identified the problem of not having a common definition of value among stakeholders as one of the barriers to a patient-centered healthcare system and pointed to the need to align the value space as an interesting point for potential follow-up and additional research. The work of the Commonwealth Commission on High

TABLE 5-3 Medication Order Categories in the Leapfrog Computerized Provider Order Entry Evaluation

Order Category	Description	Examples
Therapeutic duplication	Medication with therapeutic overlap with another new or active order; may be same drug, within drug class, or involve components of combination products	Codeine and Tylenol #3
Single and cumulative dose limits	Medication with a specified dose that exceeds recommended dose ranges or that will result in a cumulative dose that exceeds recommended ranges	Ten-fold excess dose of Methotrexate
Allergies and cross-allergies	Medication for which patient allergy has been documented or allergy to other drug in same category has been documented	Penicillin prescribed for patient with documented penicillin allergy
Contraindicated route of administration	Order specifying a route of administration (e.g., oral, intramuscular, intravenous) not appropriate for the identified medication	Tylenol to be administered intravenously
Drug–drug and drug–food interactions	Medication that results in a known, dangerous interaction when administered in combination with a different medication in a new or existing order for the patient or results in an interaction in combination with a food or food group	Digoxin and quinidine

TABLE 5-3 Continued

Order Category	Description	Examples
Contraindication/dose limits based on patient diagnosis	Medication either contraindicated based on patient diagnosis or diagnosis affects appropriate dosing	Nonspecific beta blocker in patient with asthma
Contraindication dose limits based on patient age and weight	Medication either contraindicated for this patient based on age and weight or for which age and weight must be considered in appropriate dosing	Adult dose of antibiotic in a newborn
Contraindication/dose limits based on laboratory studies	Medication either contraindicated for this patient based on laboratory studies or for which relevant laboratory results must be considered in appropriate dosing	Normal adult dose regimen of renally eliminated medication in patient with elevated creatinine
Contraindication/dose limits based on radiology studies	Medication contraindicated for this patient based on interaction with contrast medium in recent or ordered radiology study	Medication prescribed known to interact with iodine to be used as contrast medium in ordered head computed tomography exam
Corollary	Intervention that requires an associated or secondary order to meet the standard of care	Prompt to order drug levels when ordering aminoglycoside
Cost of care	Test that duplicates a service within a time frame in which there are typically minimal benefits from repeating the test	Repeat test for digoxin level within 2 hours

SOURCE: Reprinted with permission from Patient Safety & Quality Healthcare. Metzger et. al., 2008.

BOX 5-1
Use of Simulation Tool to Evaluate
Computerized Physician Order Entry:
Case Study 1

The Setting
- Academic medical center
- Commercially available computerized provider order entry (CPOE) in use for many years

Lessons Learned
- Verified poor results in some areas: drug–lab, drug–disease, dose limits
- Surprising results in drug–drug and drug–allergy interaction checking
- Pointed out new areas to pursue: wrong route, corollary orders, duplicate test

Actions Taken
- Initiated pharmacy review of preconfigured allergy and drug–drug alerts
- Planned to reduce redundant drug–drug alerting by building from the ground up
- Reviewed important food allergies and how to handle
- Began pharmacy/physician review of circumstances in which corollary orders are important
- Began work with third-party drug knowledge vendor on content needed for dosing-related messages
- Plan to incorporate new functions into next big rebuild of CPOE

Performance Healthcare Systems[3] was cited as an important reference in defining of policy areas that could affect significant cost savings in the system as a way of approaching increased value. Other groups took a pragmatic approach to the question of how much more value could be obtained and based their estimation on the figures presented during the workshop, which had suggested the existence of up to 50 percent waste in the current system. Based on this, they concluded that it was reasonable to assume that a doubling of value was attainable through the application of systems engineering principles. They went on to identify some of the key changes that would be needed to bring about this increased value. These included a realignment of payment incentives away from volume of services, the institution of a comprehensive EHR and health IT system for greater efficiency and as a

---

[3] For more information, see http://www.commonwealthfund.org/Content/Program-Areas/Commission-on-a-High-Performance-Health-System.aspx.

BOX 5-2
Use of Simulation Tool to Evaluate
Computerized Physician Order Entry:
Case Study 2

The Setting
- A 750-bed academic medical center where computerized provider order entry (CPOE) is in use house-wide
- Very proud of work and accomplishments in safety and quality

Lessons Learned
- Only order category covered was drug–allergy checking
- Some categories (patient-specific dose checking based on renal status, weight) being done in pharmacy application, but not delivered to physicians

Actions Taken
- Evaluated order categories in simulation tool against local experience (pharmacist interventions) to assign priorities for advancing clinical decision support (CDS) in CPOE
- Launched aggressive effort to advance CDS

source of data for continuous learning and improvement, and, finally, better systems integration.

Breakout groups were also asked to identify the area in which the greatest value could be returned. Participants pointed to several areas within the healthcare system that were discussed during the workshop and also to some themes that appeared in several presentations. The major area identified was the use of health IT systems in the form of EHRs and a coordinated system for the transfer of knowledge and communication of best practices, as well as a resource for research and improvement. Participants pointed to these information systems as potential conduits for better systemic coordination and informed decision making as a way to increase value.

The area of health provider education was also cited as one that could yield increased value. Participants pointed to the various workshop presentations that touched on the need for change in the culture of the healthcare system and suggested that modifying the way that caregivers are trained would be one way to initiate these changes. They identified several potential modifications to training, including greater interdisciplinary exposure and more emphasis on the team-based nature of modern health care.

Increasing the use of a collaborative approach among caregivers and between disciplines was identified as another area that should be targeted for increasing value. Increasing efficiency and efficacy through better integration of systems was also discussed, along with the adoption of practices that translate to use and evaluation as a part of execution.

Groups further identified the area of payment as one with great potential to extract increased value. They suggested that incentives be realigned in order to promote best practices instead of favoring greater volume, which the current fee-for-service compensation system rewards.

In response to the question of what actions could do the most to facilitate the changes needed to capture more value in health care, participants returned to some of the areas and themes mentioned previously and described strategies that could be taken to carry out these actions. Participants noted that the particular approach to reform is itself an important consideration. They suggested that reform start with easy, manageable issues and then progress to broader, more difficult reforms. This two-tiered approach would allow for a demonstration of the potential for improvement within the system, and it would give those orchestrating the reform the opportunity to get greater buy-in from stakeholders. One group described the necessity to be prepared to undergo constant evolution and to not have a predetermined end state.

Several groups mentioned the need to encourage a more collaborative approach to the care process and to involve multidisciplinary groups. Participants mentioned the need to overcome barriers created by the current culture in order to allow for more integrated care; reforming the models of education for healthcare providers would be one way to approach this problem. The need for greater collaboration between process engineers and medical professionals was also mentioned as an area for action in achieving higher value from health care. Groups discussed what steps might be taken to encourage greater interdisciplinary research, including changing the way engineers and health professionals are educated and developing funding mechanisms. Specific suggestions included the creation of a master's of engineering in engineering and healthcare systems and the establishment of combined interdisciplinary institutes for research and practice.

Changes in the availability, implementation, and application of EHRs and health IT were discussed as ways to better communicate best practices, to allow for better analysis of process and outcomes data that could be fed back and used to improve the system, and to create better continuity of care. One group described the health IT system as the glue that ties everything together and makes it act like a system. In order to achieve connectedness, however, interfaces between technology and users need to be redesigned to allow for ease of use and seamless integration into the care process. Steps in creating a successful health IT system will include using simulation to validate the systems before implementation and inculcating the expectation that systems will improve with use and learning over time.

Use of data from health IT systems to model and optimize care processes would be a natural application of systems engineering to health care. One of the groups discussed the value of examining existing processes to get a better understanding of what needs to be done, what may be done better, and what may not need to be done at all and then using this evaluation as a basis to reengineer systems.

Several groups shared ideas for specific projects or approaches that could take the field further down the path to greater value. Exploiting the EHR system as a resource for research through data mining was one suggestion. Another was to combine healthcare economics models with process engineering models in order to get a better grasp on measuring value and outlining strategies for further action. One group recommended subjecting healthcare processes in which engineering is particularly experienced, such as resource allocation and queuing prioritization, to more rigorous study through the lens of operations research. Additionally, there was widespread support for an effort to clarify nomenclature between the two fields in order to simplify future collaboration. Development of best practices that incorporate systems engineering principles was discussed, as well as the creation of a web portal for the dissemination of these best practices; this portal could be supervised by a joint IOM/National Academy of Engineering committee or subcontracted to a university. Participants suggested that the financial engineering community should be engaged to design more effective incentives for wellness was suggested. Finally, several groups reiterated the need to better define value in the context of a learning healthcare system and from the perspective of all of the stakeholders involved. This would allow the creation of processes that measure value and make it possible to include value in decision-making processes.

REFERENCES

Adams, M., D. Bates, and G. Coffman. 2008. *Saving lives, saving money. The imperative for computerized physician order entry in Massachusetts hospitals.* Cambridge: Massachusetts Technology Collaborative and New England Healthcare Institute.

AMIA (American Medical Informatics Association). 2006. *A roadmap for national action on clinical decisions support.* https://www.amia.org/files/cdsroadmap.pdf (accessed January 28, 2010).

Ash, J. S., P. N. Gorman, V. Seshadri, and W. R. Hersh. 2004. Computerized physician order entry in U.S. Hospitals: Results of a 2002 survey. *Journal of the American Medical Informatics Association* 11(2):95–99.

Bates, D. W. 1998. Drugs and adverse drug reactions: How worried should we be? *Journal of the American Medical Association* 279(15):1216–1217.

Bates, D. W., D. J. Cullen, N. Laird, L. A. Petersen, S. D. Small, D. Servi, G. Laffel, B. J. Sweitzer, B. F. Shea, R. Hallisey, M. V. V. R. Nemeskal, P. Hojnowski-Diaz, R. Stephen Petrycki, M. Cotugno, H. Patterson, B. F. Shea, M. Hickey, S. Kleefield, J. Cooper, D. J. Cullen, E. Kinneally, R. Nemeskal, B. J. Sweitzer, S. D. Small, H. J. Demonaco, M. D. Clapp, R. Hallisey, T. Gallivan, J. Ives, K. Porter, B. T. Thompson, G. Laffel, J. R. Hackman, and A. Edmondson. 1995. Incidence of adverse drug events and potential adverse drug events. Implications for prevention. ADE Prevention Study Group. *Journal of the American Medical Association* 274(1):29–34.

Bates, D. W., L. L. Leape, D. J. Cullen, N. Laird, L. A. Petersen, J. M. Teich, E. Burdick, M. Hickey, S. Kleefield, B. Shea, M. Vander Vliet, and D. L. Seger. 1998. Effect of computer-ized physician order entry and a team intervention on prevention of serious medication errors. *Journal of the American Medical Association* 280(15):1311–1316.

Beam, C. A., E. F. Conant, E. A. Sickles, and S. P. Weinstein. 2003. Evaluation of proscrip-tive health care policy implementation in screening mammography. *Radiology* 229(2): 534–540.

CBO (Congressional Budget Office). 2008. *Technological change and the growth of health care spending (Pub. No. 2764)*. Washington, DC: CBO.

Classen, D. C., J. P. Burke, S. L. Pestotnik, R. S. Evans, and L. E. Stevens. 1991. Surveillance for quality assessment: IV. Surveillance using a hospital information system. *Infection Control and Hospital Epidemiology* 12(4):239–244.

Classen, D. C., R. S. Evans, S. L. Pestotnik, S. D. Horn, R. L. Menlove, and J. P. Burke. 1992a. The timing of prophylactic administration of antibiotics and the risk of surgical-wound infection. *New England Journal of Medicine* 326(5):281–286.

Classen, D. C., S. L. Pestotnik, R. S. Evans, and J. P. Burke. 1992b. Description of a computer-ized adverse drug event monitor using a hospital information system. *Hospital Pharmacy* 27(9):774, 776-779, 783.

Classen, D. C., S. L. Pestotnik, R. S. Evans, J. F. Lloyd, and J. P. Burke. 1997. Adverse drug events in hospitalized patients. Excess length of stay, extra costs, and attributable mortal-ity. *Journal of the American Medical Association* 277(4):301–306.

Crosson, J. C., P. A. Ohman-Strickland, K. A. Hahn, B. DiCicco-Bloom, E. Shaw, A. J. Orzano, and B. F. Crabtree. 2007. Electronic medical records and diabetes quality of care: Results from a sample of family medicine practices. *Annals of Family Medicine* 5(3):209–215.

Dawson, D., and K. Reid. 1997. Fatigue, alcohol and performance impairment. *Nature* 388(6639):235.

de Brantes, F. 2003. Bridges to excellence: A program to start closing the quality chasm in healthcare. *Journal for Healthcare Quality* 25(2):2, 11.

Evans, R. S., S. L. Pestotnik, D. C. Classen, S. D. Horn, S. B. Bass, and J. P. Burke. 1994. Preventing adverse drug events in hospitalized patients. *Annals of Pharmacotherapy* 28(4):523–527.

Evans, R. S., S. L. Pestotnik, D. C. Classen, T. P. Clemmer, L. K. Weaver, J. F. Orme, Jr., J. F. Lloyd, and J. P. Burke. 1998. A computer-assisted management program for antibiotics and other antiinfective agents. *New England Journal of Medicine* 338(4):232–238.

Han, Y. Y., J. A. Carcillo, S. T. Venkataraman, R. S. Clark, R. S. Watson, T. C. Nguyen, H. Bayir, and R. A. Orr. 2005. Unexpected increased mortality after implementation of a commer-cially sold computerized physician order entry system. *Pediatrics* 116(6):1506–1512.

Hillman, B. J., C. A. Joseph, M. R. Mabry, J. H. Sunshine, S. D. Kennedy, and M. Noether. 1990. Frequency and costs of diagnostic imaging in office practice—a comparison of self-referring and radiologist-referring physicians. *New England Journal of Medicine* 323(23):1604–1608.

Hillman, B. J., G. T. Olson, P. E. Griffith, J. H. Sunshine, C. A. Joseph, S. D. Kennedy, W. R. Nelson, and L. B. Bernhardt. 1992. Physicians' utilization and charges for outpatient diagnostic imaging in a medicare population. *Journal of the American Medical Association* 268(15):2050–2054.

Hillman, B. J., G. T. Olson, R. W. Colbert, and L. B. Bernhardt. 1995. Responses to a payment policy denying professional charges for diagnostic imaging by nonradiologist physicians. *Journal of the American Medical Association* 274(11):885–887.

IOM (Institute of Medicine) 1997. *Computer-based patient record: An essential technology for health care* (revised edition). 1997. Washington, DC: National Academy Press.

_____. 2001. *Crossing the quality chasm: A new health systems for the 21st century.* Washington, DC: National Academy Press.

_____. 2003. *Health professions education: A bridge to quality.* Washington, DC: The National Academies Press.

_____. 2007. *The learning healthcare system: Workshop summary.* Washington, DC: The National Academies Press

Kaushal, R., D. W. Bates, C. Landrigan, K. J. McKenna, M. D. Clapp, F. Federico, and D. A. Goldmann. 2001. Medication errors and adverse drug events in pediatric inpatients. *Journal of the American Medical Association* 285(16):2114–2120.

Kilbridge, P., D. C. Classen, and E. Welebob. 2001. *Overview of the Leapfrog Group test standard for computerized physician order entry.* Report by first consulting group to the Leapfrog Group. http://www.leapfroggroup.org/media/file/Leapfrog-CPOE_Evaluation2.pdf (accessed June 21, 2010).

Kilbridge, P. M., D. C. Classen, D. W. Bates, and C. R. Denham. 2006a. The national quality forum safe practice standard for computerized physician order entry: Updating a critical patient safety practice. *Journal of Patient Safety* 2:183–188.

Kilbridge, P. M., E. M. Welebob, and D. C. Classen. 2006b. Development of the leapfrog methodology for evaluating hospital implemented inpatient computerized physician order entry systems. *Quality and Safety in Health Care* 15(2):81–84.

Koppel, R., J. P. Metlay, A. Cohen, B. Abaluck, A. R. Localio, S. E. Kimmel, and B. L. Strom. 2005. Role of computerized physician order entry systems in facilitating medication errors. *Journal of the American Medical Association* 293(10):1197–1203.

Leach, D. C., and I. Philibert. 2006. High-quality learning for high-quality health care: Getting it right. *Journal of the American Medical Association* 296(9):1132–1134.

Leape, L. L., D. W. Bates, D. J. Cullen, J. Cooper, H. J. Demonaco, T. Gallivan, R. Hallisey, J. Ives, N. Laird, G. Laffel, R. Nemeskal, L. A. Petersen, K. Porter, D. Servi, B. F. Shea, S. D. Small, B. J. Sweitzer, B. T. Thompson, M. Vander Vliet, ADE Prevention Study Group, D. Bates, P. Hojnowski-Diaz, S. Petrycki, M. Cotugno, H. Patterson, M. Hickey, S. Kleefield, E. Kinneally, M. D. Clapp, J. R. Hackman, and A. Edmondson. 1995. Systems analysis of adverse drug events. ADE Prevention Study Group. *Journal of the American Medical Association* 274(1):35–43.

The Leapfrog Group. 2008. *Factsheet: Computer physician order entry.* http://www.leapfroggroup.org/media/file/FactSheet_CPOE.pdf (accessed June 21, 2010).

Masys, D. 2007. *AMIA informatics 2007 year in review.* http://dbmichair.mc.vanderbilt.edu/amia2007/ (accessed January 28, 2010).

Metzger, J., and F. Turisco. 2001. *Computerized physician order entry: A look at the vendor marketplace and getting started.* The Leapfrog Group. http://www.informatics-review.com/thoughts/cpoe-leap.html (accessed June 21, 2010).

Metzger, J., E. Welebob, M. Del Beccaro, and C. Spurr. 2007. Taking the measure of inpatient EHRs. Hospitals inch closer to certified products. *Journal of the American Health Information Management Association* 78(6):24–30; quiz, 33–24.

Metzger, J. B., E. Welebob, F. Turisco, and D. C. Classen. 2008. The Leapfrog Group's CPOE standard and evaluation tool. *Patient Safety & Quality Healthcare* 5(4):22–25. www. psqh.com/julaug08/cpoe.html (accessed January 27, 2009).

Mizrahi, T. 1984. Managing medical mistakes: Ideology, insularity and accountability among internists-in-training. *Social Science & Medicine* 19(2):135–146.

Nebeker, J. R., J. M. Hoffman, C. R. Weir, C. L. Bennett, and J. F. Hurdle. 2005. High rates of adverse drug events in a highly computerized hospital. *Archives of Internal Medicine* 165(10):1111–1116.

Simon, S. R., R. Kaushal, P. D. Cleary, C. A. Jenter, L. A. Volk, E. J. Orav, E. Burdick, E. G. Poon, and D. W. Bates. 2007. Physicians and electronic health records: A statewide survey. *Archives of Internal Medicine* 167(5):507–512.

Smits, M., D. W. Dippel, G. G. de Haan, H. M. Dekker, P. E. Vos, D. R. Kool, P. J. Nederkoorn, P. A. Hofman, A. Twijnstra, H. L. Tanghe, and M. G. Hunink. 2005. External validation of the Canadian CT head rule and the New Orleans criteria for CT scanning in patients with minor head injury. *Journal of the American Medical Association* 294(12):1519–1525.

Swensen, S. J., and D. A. Cortese. 2008. Transparency and the "end result idea." *Chest* 133(1):233–235.

Thrall, J. H. 2004. The emerging role of pay-for-performance contracting for health care services. *Radiology* 233(3):637–640.

Ting, H. H., H. M. Krumholz, E. H. Bradley, D. C. Cone, J. P. Curtis, B. J. Drew, J. M. Field, W. J. French, W. B. Gibler, D. C. Goff, A. K. Jacobs, B. K. Nallamothu, R. E. O'Connor, and J. D. Schuur. 2008. Implementation and integration of prehospital ECGs into systems of care for acute coronary syndrome: A scientific statement from the American Heart Association Interdisciplinary Council on Quality of Care and Outcomes Research, Emergency Cardiovascular Care Committee, Council on Cardiovascular Nursing, and Council on Clinical Cardiology. *Circulation* 118(10):1066–1079.

Tosczak, M. 2004. UnitedHealth trying to limit imaging use. *The Business Journal* December 24. http://triad.bizjournals.com/triad/stories/2004/12/27/story2.html (accessed May 31, 2010).

Walsh, K. E., C. P. Landrigan, W. G. Adams, R. J. Vinci, J. B. Chessare, M. R. Cooper, P. M. Hebert, E. G. Schainker, T. J. McLaughlin, and H. Bauchner. 2008. Effect of computer order entry on prevention of serious medication errors in hospitalized children. *Pediatrics* 121(3):e421–e427.

Wennberg, J. E., E. S. Fisher, J. S. Skinner, and K. K. Bronner. 2007a. Extending the P4P agenda, part 2: How Medicare can reduce waste and improve the care of the chronically ill. *Health Affairs (Millwood)* 26(6):1575–1585.

Wennberg, J. E., A. M. O'Connor, E. D. Collins, and J. N. Weinstein. 2007b. Extending the P4P agenda, part 1: How Medicare can improve patient decision making and reduce unnecessary care. *Health Affairs (Millwood)* 26(6):1564–1574.

6

Next Steps:
Aligning Policies with
Leadership Opportunities

INTRODUCTION

Appropriate to the title of the workshop, Engineering a Learning Healthcare System: A Look at the Future, the final session was devoted to exploring critical policy areas that must be engaged in order to advance engineering approaches to transformational changes in health care, including those that might trigger "disruptive innovations." Five panelists provided context and policy recommendations, drawing from widely varying experiences in academic medical centers, community hospitals, integrated care delivery organizations, ambulatory clinics, and skilled nursing facilities: Paul F. Conlon, senior vice president for Clinical Quality and Patient Safety at Trinity Health; Denis A. Cortese, president and chief executive officer of the Mayo Clinic; Mary Jane Koren, assistant vice president of The Commonwealth Fund; Louise L. Liang, senior vice president of quality and clinical systems support for Kaiser Foundation Health Plan and Kaiser Foundation Hospitals; and Douglas W. Lowery-North, vice chair of clinical operations at Emory Healthcare Department of Emergency Medicine.

Each panelist offered brief reflections on his or her vision for changes in practice, policy, and culture. Recurring themes included the need for delivery of best practices, both clinical and administrative; process standardization and improvement at care interfaces; and leveraging human capital.

PROCESS STANDARDIZATION AND IMPROVEMENT

Interfaces

A key element of the panel's discussion was the notion of interfaces between engineers and providers, and among multiple processes. Cortese discussed the importance of medical school admissions selection criteria to ensure that medical education and training include fundamental engineering concepts. He provided the Mayo medical school as an example of a medical school where the size will not increase until the training program adds incrementally to historical practices. American health care is not lacking for resources, Conlon said. Those resources are probably abundant, but they suffer from poor distribution and use. He spoke of the importance of the intersection of engineering with health care in helping to build an understanding of the systems we use for creating the product that at this point is so rife with inefficiency and waste.

Lowery-North also highlighted the gap in uptake of healthcare engineers. He attributed it to language differences between medicine and health care. Fortifying the interface between health care and engineering will provide additional perspectives on the opportunities in health care for accelerated improvement. Cortese said that healthcare educators need to ensure there is a basic understanding of systems engineering in their programs and that their students, the future healthcare practitioners, need to understand how to handle data, turn it into information, and turn that information into knowledge, as well as effective communication tools. Cortese also indicated that engineering schools can play an important role in integrating health information training into engineering curriculums and master's and postgraduate programs through relationships developed with academic medical centers. The Regenstrief Institute at Purdue has one such program; other examples can be found at Georgia Tech, the University of Wisconsin, and North Carolina State.

Systems Improvement

The roles of the federal government and the private sector could be to create multidisciplinary centers to address issues of quality, value, and waste. Such centers could link the work of researchers, practitioners, educators, and engineers, and could include both basic and applied research, according to Cortese. The centers could demonstrate and disseminate tools, technologies, and knowledge, and they could perhaps identify a federal agency to take a lead role. Perhaps the government and private sources could ensure stable and adequate funding. Such an approach could help overcome barriers to the application of systems engineering, information technologies (ITs), and communication technologies, and it could play an important role in educating students. Public education would also have a role. If health care is to be improved through engineering, the government has to work to improve public education.

Reflecting on the intersection of engineering and healthcare delivery and on the kind of policies needed to help increase value, Conlon proposed using technology to hardwire some best clinical practices. For example, if a patient anywhere in a system is identified as being at risk for ulcers or falling, the act of entering that information in the electronic health record (EHR) could trigger a set of evidence-based nursing orders designed to mitigate against those risks. Individual nurses would have the opportunity to modify those orders as appropriate. Using technology to facilitate co-ordination of care is vitally important, yet Conlon expressed concern over the debate with IT vendors about whether they are implementing the right information in the right systems for the changes needed.

Liang addressed the measurements, measuring systems, and metrics used by large health plans and purchasers to identify process measures, all of them driven by claims data. Such data are available, Liang noted, but the measures only feed current activities instead of encouraging better outcomes or processes. Data collection is time intensive, Liang noted, and she urged an examination of the benefits provided vs. the burden created in achieving those benefits. Cortese added another layer by challenging the Joint Commission to completely change the way it does business and instead become a conduit for sharing information—a reporting center that could encourage the learning process throughout health care.

Another basic challenge to system improvement is the adoption of health IT. For example, nursing homes have not been at the technological forefront in terms of IT, Koren said. Although the homes are starting to use IT, it is a disruptive innovation, and too many of them see it as something that you buy, you plug in, and then you teach somebody to press the button. Few vendors engage the possibilities of IT as a change management tool. Therefore, Koren said, we need to think about teaching nursing homes how to do things like process mapping and workflow design and to use those tools to optimal advantage. And because doctors often do not like to go to nursing homes, more effective ways are needed to use telehealth and telemonitoring tools to ensure that patients get the best medical care even at those times when a physician is not present.

Delivery of Value

Koren also highlighted some opportunities for skilled nursing care facilities to increase the value derived from services. She urged the audience to consider the best ways to design facilities, employing engineering systems insights that support caring for a frail, usually older population. Cortese followed up on this line of thinking by advocating that the federal government simply pay for value, a policy proposal that has gained significant traction as offering an alternative to reimbursement. Liang discussed the idea of generating value through the creation and use of medical knowledge, and she noted the significant workshop conversation about the barrier of financial incentives. Right now the healthcare system pays for activity and, as expected, activity is the result. However, value, quality, service, and better outcomes should be the focus of reimbursement.

For full attainment of the value potential, Liang said that better use of informatics is needed, and this means that the federal government needs to do more to address in a straightforward fashion the privacy concerns of institutions and patients that arise from the use of information for clinical knowledge generation. In light of the recent challenges experienced by other institutions, she said, legitimate privacy concerns need to be clarified in order to allow and support full leverage of the significant information becoming available to the healthcare community.

LEVERAGING PEOPLE FOR HEALTHCARE IMPROVEMENT

Culture and the Learning Process

Culture is generally the most important barrier to change, Cortese observed, and this is especially true with health care. Lowery-North cautioned against losing the component of human systems engineering when evaluating engineering approaches to culture change. Organizational composition, diffusion of innovation, and change management strategies are areas in which health care continues to lag behind other sectors, Lowery-North said, and this is probably why it has been so difficult to effect change. The pharmaceutical sales industry can offer insight into how to change physician behavior, panelists said. Examining the experiences of that group of people may offer some lessons about how to change the behaviors of physicians, who in practice may have little, if any, incentive to change. Cortese noted that one facet of necessary cultural change is found in the current emphasis on research and even teaching over patient care. In academic centers, most often the motivator is research; many academic medical centers exist because of research. If someone has full funding, they get a tenured position; if they lose funding, they are often required to dedicate more time to teaching. In the face of such concerns, it is unfortunately the case that medical care is totally secondary. Rather than separate the two, Cortese said, what is important is to draw research and patient care closer together so that every patient experience becomes a learning opportunity.

Conlon identified the omnipresent measurement culture, monitoring the effectiveness of the healthcare system and identifying opportunities for improvement, as a barrier to change, explaining that the growing burden of data capture is potentially beginning to exceed the value of information. That is a problem because nurses and physicians spend too much time marking off checklists in order to be able to prove, for example, that ACE inhibitors or beta-blockers were used properly. This is a great opportunity to automate that data capture—and correspondingly shift the culture—so that practitioners can devote more of their time directly to patient care.

Conlon noted that EHR implementation is about more than simply documenting health information in EHRs; it can serve as a catalyst to really transform how we deliver care. The records provide the opportunity to actually look at processes of care and to redesign them. Liang also offered a word of caution by citing the work of Ronald Heifetz, who wrote *Leadership Without Easy Answers*: "One of the most common leadership mistakes is expecting technical solution to solve adaptive problems" (Heifetz, 1994).

Liang also argued that cultural challenges are a major issue everywhere, even in the Kaiser Permanente system in which physicians and nurses are more aligned than perhaps anywhere else. The fact remains that the fundamental guild or craftsman culture of healthcare professionals is still a significant problem, Liang said. For Kaiser, the biggest factor enabling that culture change has been the availability of transparent, specific data that are comparable across the organization and which allow different locations of care to see what is possible in other parts of the organization and what is possible in terms of national benchmarking—as well as where their individual performances stand. That information needs to be made available, but it also needs to be combined with good evidence about the right pathway and with contextual knowledge about how the clinic next door does so much better. Such context is not necessarily found in the data; the data say where to go look, where to have the conversations about exactly what someone is doing that could offer lessons to others.

Occasionally it takes people time to accept the data. There are times when some physicians and departments have to go through a dialogue of "The data [are] wrong, my patients are sicker, you just don't understand," but eventually they come to accept the system. Kaiser has seen a huge decrease in its variation and a large improvement overall, Liang said, based fundamentally on the availability of the data to identify issues and help people grapple with the fact that, at the moment, everything is not possible.

Communicating With and Engaging Patients

Communication was a central point of discussion in the final session of the workshop. Three primary communication themes arose: (1) interoperability of systems in order to facilitate communication, (2) communication between care team members, and (3) enlisting the patient in support of knowledge development.

Noting the lack of portability of patient records among care settings, patients, and providers, Conlon discussed the predominance of incompatible software that effectively precludes information sharing. There is a great policy opportunity for consistency in the interoperability of these systems and in the exchange of the information associated with them. Conlon also urged the adoption of policies that enable information to follow patients and to exist in a form that can be easily shared and transferred, regardless of location. Liang added that the federal government should set interoperability standards, particularly in areas that hold outstanding promise, such as home monitoring and other similar medical devices, as well as standards that will help give all patients the right to take their medical records with them. Right now these records can be provided in print, on a compact disc, or on a memory stick, but that is still a far cry from what it should be. Lowery-North emphasized that developing interoperability standards will be critical. A favorable factor is that physician practitioners are gradually migrating to larger group settings, which are more likely to adopt information systems that have interoperability standards because they are more likely to have been created with a systems engineering approach in mind.

Another area with policy implications is the team nature of health care; however, we are not teaching people to work in teams, according to Koren. Educational policy is needed to make sure that we have people who are skilled and working in an interdisciplinary or multidisciplinary manner. Moving doctors into such teams is an innate problem because, for example, doctors typically don't like to go to nursing homes. These teams are largely led by nurses, with paraprofessionals working at the bottom. An issue, therefore, is how we can integrate those paraprofessionals into that team. We need engineering to help us think about how to bring workers into that team and effectively listen to the knowledge being generated at the front lines of care. How do we best use that knowledge to make the system better and more responsive to what people want?

Finally, it was noted that if patients are to become more engaged in the research process, several rules will have to change. Privacy remains a barrier to knowledge generation from patient data, yet the concerns are largely perceptual in nature. Research is an opportunity to shift the culture in health care through getting people to understand that research in the name of patient care improvement is legitimate, publishable, hypothesis-testing research.

RECURRING THEMES FOR ROUNDTABLE ATTENTION

The presentations and discussions within the workshop zeroed in on a number of specific ideas and themes concerning the best ways to use engineering to improve healthcare delivery. In addition, they provided a variety of insights into engineering approaches to dealing with systems complexity and identified critical areas needing attention in health care. The recurring themes of discussion throughout the 2 days of the workshop are summarized below. While perhaps intuitively obvious—hence the reason for their recurrence—they were nonetheless noted as worthy of attention and engagement by the Roundtable members.

- *The system's processes must be centered on the right target—the patient.* Patient-centered care was defined in the 2001 Institute of Medicine (IOM) report *Crossing the Quality Chasm* as providing care that is respectful of and responsive to individual patient preferences, needs, and values and ensuring that patient values guide all clinical decisions (IOM, 2001). However, health care is by nature highly complex, involving multiple participants and parallel activities that sometimes take on a character of their own, independent of patient needs or desires. Throughout several sessions, workshop participants emphasized the need to ensure that processes support patients—and that patients are not forced into processes. Patient needs and perspectives must be at the center of all process design, technology application, and clinician engagement.
- *System excellence is created by the reliable delivery of established best practice.* Identifying and embedding practices that work best, and developing the system processes to ensure their delivery every time, help to define excellence in system performance and to focus the system on delivering the best possible care for patients. In health care, establishing practices from the best available evidence and building them as routines into practice patterns, as well as developing systems to document results and update best practices as the evidence evolves, will integrate some of the best elements from the engineering disciplines into healthcare issues. Participants often cited the need for better integration of the development and communication of best practices in healthcare systems, as well as the need for process systems to track care details and outcomes, with feedback for practice refinement and better patient outcomes.
- *Complexity compels reasoned allowance for tailored adjustments.* Established routines may need circumstance-specific adjustments related to differences in the appropriateness of established health-

care regimens for various individuals, variations in caregiver skill, the evolving nature of the science base—or all three. Mass customization and other engineering practices can help assure a consistency that can accelerate the recognition of the need for tailoring and delivering the most appropriate care—with the best prospects for improved outcomes—for the patient. Participants pointed to the need for the development of a system of care flexible enough to incorporate these considerations and to leverage the lessons learned from their employment in a process of continuous learning.

- *Learning is a non-linear process.* The focus on an established hierarchy of scientific evidence as a basis for evaluation and decision making cannot fully accommodate the fact that much of the sound learning in complex systems occurs in local and individual settings. Participants cited the need to bridge the gap between dependence on formal trials, such as randomized controlled trials, and the experience of local improvement in order to speed learning and avoid impractical costs.

- *Emphasize interdependence and tend to the process interfaces.* A system is most vulnerable at links between critical processes. In health care, attention to the nature of relationships and hand-offs between elements of the patient care and administrative processes is therefore vital and a crucial component of focusing the process on the patient experience and improving outcomes.

- *Teamwork and cross-checks trump command and control.* Especially in systems designed to guarantee safety, system performance that is effective and efficient requires careful coordination and teamwork as well as a culture that encourages parity among all those with established responsibilities. During the workshop, several examples were cited of other industries that have used systems design and social engineering to better integrate and strengthen their systems processes with great improvements in efficiency and safety.

- *Performance, transparency, and feedback serve as the engine for improvement.* Continuous learning and improvement in patient care requires transparency in processes and outcomes as well as the ability to capture feedback and make adjustments.

- *Expect errors in the performance of individuals, perfection in the performance of systems.* Human error is inevitable in any system, and should be assumed. On the other hand, safeguards and designed redundancies can deliver perfection in system performance. Mapping processes, embedding prompts, cross-checks, and information loops can assure best outcomes and allow human capacity to focus on what can not be programmed—compassion and individual patient needs. Several workshop presentations shared success stories and lessons learned from other industries, such as the automotive and airline industries, that have effectively incorporated this strategy.

- *Align rewards on the key elements of continuous improvement.* Incentives, standards, and measurement requirements can serve as powerful change agents. Therefore, it is vital that they be carefully considered and directed to the targets most important to improving the patient and provider experiences. Participants noted that it is vital that incentives be carefully considered and directed to the targets most important to improving the efficiency, effectiveness, and safety of the system—and ultimately patient outcomes—as well as taking into consideration the patient and provider experiences.
- *Education and research can facilitate understanding and partnerships between engineering and the health professions.* The relevance of systems engineering principles to health care and the impressive transformation brought to other industries, speaks to the merits of developing common vocabularies, concepts, and ongoing joint education and research activities that help generate stronger questions and solutions. Workshop participants pointed to the dearth of training opportunities bridging these two professions and spoke of the need to encourage greater collaborative work between them.
- *Foster a leadership culture, language, and style that reinforce teamwork and results.* Positive leadership cultures foster and celebrate consensus goals, teamwork, multidisciplinary efforts, transparency, and continuous monitoring and improvement. In citing examples of successful learning systems, participants highlighted the need for a supportive and integrated leadership.

AREAS FOR INNOVATION AND COLLABORATIVE ACTION

Presentations and discussions during the workshop offered insight into the opportunities for Roundtable members to consider possible follow-up actions for ongoing multi-stakeholder involvement to advance the integration of engineering sciences into healthcare systems improvement.

Discussions during the breakout sessions provided the opportunity for workshop attendees, in both the health and engineering fields, to engage with each other and identify novel opportunities for innovative work that might yield breakthroughs that capture more value in health care. Participants felt that the opportunities were great for various engineering approaches to streamline processes and improve efficiency, but they struggled with the ambiguity of the definition of value in health care. The result was that they largely referred back to themes covered in the workshop presentations and summarized elsewhere in this summary. This suggests that there is still much work to do in laying a foundation at the intersection of engineering and health care if drilling down with greater specificity is to add substantially to value.

That said, workshop participants identified several areas for collaborative work that merit follow-up. With particular emphasis on the need for ongoing means of communication and collaboration that will bring better perspective and nurtured understanding from the two fields, areas mentioned for possible Roundtable follow-up include the following:

1. *Clarify terms:* The ability of healthcare professionals to draw upon relevant and helpful engineering principles for system improvement could be facilitated by a better mutual understanding of the terminology. A collaborative effort by the IOM and the National Academy of Engineering could create a targeted glossary and develop potentially bridging terminology for use as appropriate.

2. *Identify best practices:* Three areas of systems orientation are particularly important to improving the efficiency and effectiveness of health care: (1) focusing the system elements more directly on the key outcome—the patient experience, (2) ensuring transparency in the performance of the system and its players and components, and (3) establishing a culture that emphasizes teamwork, consistency, and excellence. Progress could be accelerated by identifying and disseminating examples of best practices from health care and from engineering on each of these dimensions.

3. *Explore health professions education change:* In the face of a rapidly changing environment in health care—expanding diagnostic and treatment options, much greater knowledge available, movement beyond the point at which any one individual can personally hold all the information necessary, and IT that opens new capabilities—changes to the education of health professionals can advance caregiver skills in knowledge navigation, teamwork, patient–provider partnership, and process awareness.

4. *Advance the science of payment for value:* With cost increases in health care consistently outstripping gains in performance by most measures, progress toward counteracting this trend could be achieved with a stronger focus on ways to enhance both health and economic returns from healthcare investments. This could include work in the areas of understanding, measuring, and providing incentives for value in health care.

5. *Explore fostering the development of a science of waste assessment and engagement:* Similarly, and directly related, an exploration of the elements of inefficiency in health care, how to define and mea-

sure waste, and how to mobilize responses to eliminating waste could contribute to increasing value within healthcare systems.

6. *Support the development of a robust health IT system:* The development of a health IT system, designed with systems-related continuous improvement principles in mind, must lie at the core of an efficient, effective learning system. Beginning with challenges to EHR adoption, much work remains in order to achieve such a system that allows for continuous learning; permits data sharing, including the construction of databases; employs consistent standards; and addresses privacy and security concerns. Health IT is a natural place for collaborative work between engineers and caregivers, beginning with better resolution of barriers to the achievement of such a system through the employment of both expert lenses.

As healthcare and engineering professionals consider these areas for collaboration and innovation, it is important to emphasize that the focus of all the engineering applications to health care discussed in the workshop was, ultimately, improving patient outcomes. The reforms that were discussed are all focused on to bringing the right care to the right person at the right time at the right price. The essential questions are straightforward: Can it work? Will it work—for *this* patient, in *this* setting? Do the benefits outweigh any harms? Do the benefits justify the costs? Do the reforms offer important advantages over existing alternatives?

If full advantage is to be taken of this potential, much work remains to bridge the gaps between the professions of health care and engineering. As the problems within healthcare systems become increasingly better defined, the opportunity increases for true collaborative approaches that go beyond joint acknowledgment and parallel approaches. This workshop, while limited by the chosen areas of emphasis and the specific backgrounds of the participants, identified a number of important prospects for advancing the discussion and sharing of ideas as a more frequent and routine activity.

Better coordination, collaboration, public–private partnerships, and priority setting are central challenges for the U.S. healthcare system. The discussions summarized in this report highlight engineering's potential contribution to progress toward the Roundtable membership's concept of a learning health system with a stated goal: that by the year 2020, 90 percent of clinical decisions will be supported by accurate, timely, and up-to-date clinical information and will reflect the best available evidence.

REFERENCE

Heifetz, R. A. 1994. *Leadership without easy answers*. Cambridge, MA: Belknap Press of Harvard University Press.

IOM (Institute of Medicine). 2001. *Crossing the quality chasm: A new health systems for the 21st century*. Washington, DC: National Academy Press.

Appendixes

Appendix A

Workshop Agenda

Engineering a Learning Healthcare System:
A Look at the Future

A Learning Healthcare System Workshop
Roundtable on Evidence-Based Medicine
The Institute of Medicine (IOM)
… *in cooperation with* …
the National Academy of Engineering (NAE)

April 29–30, 2008
The Keck Center of The National Academies
Washington, DC 20001

Issues Motivating the Discussion

1. Health care is substantially underperforming on most dimensions: effectiveness, appropriateness, safety, cost, efficiency, and value.
2. Increasing complexity in health care is likely to accentuate current problems unless reform efforts go beyond financing to foster significant changes in the culture, practice, and delivery of health care.
3. Extensive administrative and clinical data collected in healthcare settings are largely unused for new insights on the effectiveness of healthcare interventions and systems of care.
4. If the effectiveness of health care is to keep pace with the opportunity of diagnostic and treatment innovation, system design and information technology must be structured to ensure application of the best evidence, continuous learning, and research insights generated as a natural by-product of the care process.
5. Engineering principles are at the core of a learning healthcare system—one structured to keep the patient constantly in focus, while continuously improving quality, safety, knowledge, and value in health care.

6. Impressive transformations have occurred through systems and process engineering in service and manufacturing sectors—e.g., banking, airline safety, automobile manufacturing.
7. Despite the obvious differences that exist in the dynamics of mechanical vs. biological and social systems, the current challenges in health care necessitate an entirely fresh view of the organization, structure, and function of the delivery and monitoring processes in health care.
8. Taking on the challenges in health care offers the engineering sciences an opportunity to test, learn, and refine approaches to understanding and improving innovation in complex adaptive systems.

DAY ONE

8:30　WELCOME AND INTRODUCTIONS
*Denis A. Cortese, Mayo Clinic and Roundtable on
Evidence-Based Medicine (IOM)
William B. Rouse, Georgia Institute of Technology and Planning
Committee Chair (NAE)*

8:45　KEYNOTES: 1. LEARNING OPPORTUNITIES FOR HEALTH CARE
　　　　　　　　2. TEACHING OPPORTUNITIES FROM ENGINEERING
Opening keynote speakers will address some of the key systemic shortfalls and challenges in health care today, reflecting on the changes needed and how systems engineering might help foster a healthcare system that delivers the care we know works and that learns from the care delivered.
*Brent C. James, Intermountain Healthcare (IOM)
W. Dale Compton, Purdue University (NAE)*

9:45　SESSION 1: ENGAGING COMPLEX SYSTEMS THROUGH ENGINEERING CONCEPTS
How do the various engineering disciplines (e.g., systems engineering, industrial engineering, operations research, human factors engineering, financial engineering, risk analysis) engage system complexity, and how might this perspective inform and improve health care? What can we learn from the contrasts?
Chair: Paul H. O'Neill, Value Capture, LLC
➤ *Systems engineering perspectives*
  William B. Rouse, Georgia Institute of Technology (NAE)
➤ *Engineering systems analysis tools*
  Richard C. Larson, Massachusetts Institute of Technology (NAE)

[10:35–10:55 Break]

> *Engineering systems design tools*
  James M. Tien, University of Miami (NAE)
> *Engineering systems control tools*
  Harold W. Sorenson, University of California, San Diego

Panel discussion to follow

12:00   Lunch

1:00   Session 2: Healthcare System Complexities, Impediments, and
        Failures
        What are the multiple healthcare system components and
        processes that affect the generation and application of evidence,
        and which inefficiencies, impediments, structural barriers, and
        failures are most acutely in need of attention and correction?
        How might systems engineering address these issues?
        *Chair and Introduction: Cato T. Laurencin, University of
        Virginia Health Systems (IOM)*
        > *Healthcare culture*
          William W. Stead, Vanderbilt University Medical Center
(IOM)
        > *Diagnostic and treatment technologies*
          Rita F. Redberg, University of California, San Francisco
        > *Clinical data systems and clinical decision support*
          Michael D. Chase, Kaiser Permanente Colorado
        > *Care coordination and linkage*
          Amy L. Deutschendorf, Johns Hopkins Hospital and Health
          System
        > *Administrative and business systems*
          Ralph W. Muller, University of Pennsylvania Health System
        > *Information and knowledge development*
          Eugene C. Nelson, Dartmouth–Hitchcock Medical Center

Panel discussion to follow

[3:15–3:30 Break]

3:30   Session 3: Case Studies in Transformation Through Systems
        Engineering
        How has systems engineering been successfully used in certain
        industries and sectors? Which key lessons best apply in the

transformation of a sociologically and technologically complex healthcare arena? Are there examples of successful applications to health care? What are some key lessons from other sectors and service industries in managing complexity?

    Chair: Carmen Hooker Odom, Milbank Memorial Fund

> *Airline safety*
> *John J. Nance, formerly of National Patient Safety Foundation*
> *Alcoa reorientation*
> *Earnest J. Edwards, formerly of Alcoa*
> *Veterans Health Affairs*
> *Kenneth W. Kizer, Medsphere Systems Corporation (IOM)*
> *Ascension Health*
> *David B. Pryor, Ascension Health*

Panel discussion to follow

5:15   DAY'S SUMMARY AND FRAMEWORK DISCUSSION
What framework might illustrate ways in which lessons from engineering could map onto healthcare systems?
    Paul H. O'Neill, Value Capture, LLC, and
    William B. Rouse, Georgia Institute of Technology (NAE)

5:30   RECEPTION

DAY TWO

8:00   WELCOME AND RECAP OF THE FIRST DAY
William B. Rouse, Georgia Institute of Technology and Planning Committee Chair (NAE)

8:15   SESSION 4: FOSTERING SYSTEMS CHANGE TO DRIVE CONTINUOUS LEARNING IN HEALTH CARE
The IOM *Learning Healthcare System* workshop publication identified several common characteristics of a learning healthcare organization, including culture that emphasizes transparency and learning through continuous feedback loops, care as a seamless team process, best practices that are embedded in system design, information systems that reliably deliver evidence and capture results, and results that are bundled to improve the level of practice and the state of the science. What do feedback and

performance improvement look like for each topic below, and how can impediments be turned into enablers?
Chair: Richard C. Larson, Massachusetts Institute of Technology (NAE)

> *Learning-, team-, and patient-oriented culture*
  Steven J. Spear, Massachusetts Institute of Technology
> *Knowledge development, access, and use*
  Donald E. Detmer, American Medical Informatics Association (IOM)
> *Technologies management*
  Stephen J. Swensen, Mayo Clinic
> *Information systems organization and management*
  David C. Classen, Computer Sciences Corporation

Panel discussion to follow

[10:00–10:30 BREAK]

10:30   BREAKOUT SESSION: CAPTURING MORE VALUE IN HEALTH CARE
         Five groups to meet and discuss three questions:
         > At a macro level, what's your best guess on *how much more value* (health returned for money invested) could be obtained through application of systems engineering principles in health care?
         > If you had to identify *one area in which the greatest value* could be returned, what would that be?
         > What are the *actions*, taken by whom, that could do the most to facilitate the needed changes?
         Breakout Chairs
         > Kenneth Boff, Room 205
         > Richard C. Larson, Room 206
         > William B. Rouse, Room 204
         > Harold W. Sorenson, Room 208
         > James M. Tien, Room 213

11:45   LUNCH AVAILABLE (OUTSIDE ROOM 100)

1:00   BREAKOUT SESSION REPORTS

1:45   SESSION 5: OBSERVATIONS ON INITIATING SYSTEMS CHANGE IN HEALTH CARE
         Donald M. Berwick, Institute for Healthcare Improvement (IOM)

2:15   SESSION 6: NEXT STEPS: ALIGNING POLICIES WITH LEADERSHIP
         OPPORTUNITIES
         What are the key policy priorities if the best and most applicable
         lessons from the engineering sciences are to be applied in
         bringing about the necessary transformational changes? A panel
         of leaders from key settings will offer brief (5-minute) reflections
         on the policy and related culture changes necessary, followed by
         an interactive discussion.
         *Chair: Donald M. Berwick, Institute for Healthcare Improvement
         (IOM)*
         ➤ *Academic medical centers*
         Denis A. Cortese, Mayo Clinic (IOM)
         ➤ *Community hospital settings*
         Paul F. Conlon, Trinity Health
         ➤ *Integrated healthcare delivery organizations*
         Louise L. Liang, Kaiser Permanente
         ➤ *Small ambulatory care settings*
         Douglas W. Lowery-North, Emory University
         ➤ *Skilled nursing facilities*
         Mary Jane Koren, The Commonwealth Fund

Panel discussion to follow

4:30   CONCLUDING SUMMARY REMARKS AND ADJOURNMENT
         *Denis A. Cortese, Mayo Clinic and Roundtable on
         Evidence-Based Medicine (IOM)*
         J. Michael McGinnis, IOM

Planning Committee:
William B. Rouse. Ph.D., M.S. *(Chair),* Georgia Institute of Technology
Jerome H. Grossman, M.D., Harvard University
Brent C. James, M.D., M.Stat., Intermountain Healthcare, Inc.
Helen S. Kim, M.B.A., Gordon and Betty Moore Foundation
Cato T. Laurencin, M.D., Ph.D., University of Virginia
The Honorable Paul H. O'Neill, Value Capture, LLC

Appendix B

Biographical Sketches of
Workshop Participants

Donald M. Berwick, M.D., M.P.P., is president and chief executive officer (CEO) of the Institute for Healthcare Improvement. Dr. Berwick is clinical professor of pediatrics and health care policy at the Harvard Medical School and professor of health policy and management at the Harvard School of Public Health. He is also a pediatrician, an associate in pediatrics at Boston's Children's Hospital, and a consultant in pediatrics at Massachusetts General Hospital. Dr. Berwick has published more than 130 scientific articles in numerous professional journals on subjects relating to healthcare policy, decision analysis, technology assessment, and healthcare quality management. Books he has coauthored include *Curing Health Care; New Rules: Regulation, Markets and the Quality of American Health Care; and Cholesterol, Children, and Heart Disease: An Analysis of Alternatives.* From 1987 through 1991 Dr. Berwick was cofounder and coprincipal investigator for the National Demonstration Project on Quality Improvement in Health Care. He is a past president of the International Society for Medical Decision Making. He is an elected member of the Institute of Medicine (IOM), and since 2002 has served on the IOM's Governing Council and as the liaison to the IOM's Global Health Board. Dr. Berwick was appointed by President Clinton to serve on the Advisory Commission on Consumer Protection and Quality in the Healthcare Industry in 1997 and 1998. In 2005, in recognition of his exemplary work for the National Health Service in the United Kingdom, he was appointed honorary Knight Commander of the Most Excellent Order of the British Empire—the highest award given to non-British citizens. A summa cum laude graduate of Harvard College, Dr.

Berwick holds a Master's in Public Policy from the John F. Kennedy School of Government and an M.D. cum laude from Harvard Medical School.

Michael D. Chase, M.D., is the associate medical director of quality for Kaiser Permanente of Colorado. In this role, he oversees programs in quality, prevention, chronic care, patient safety, risk management, and research. In addition, Dr. Chase is the executive medical group sponsor of HealthConnect, the Kaiser Permanente electronic medical record, which was implemented in fall 2004. Dr. Chase has been with the Permanente Medical group since 1986 and continues to be a practicing internist. His past areas of interest and experience have included guideline development, pharmacy issues, leading clinical medical education for staff, teaching of medical students and residents, and development and use of clinical registries. He is a past department chief of internal medicine. In 1998 he was instrumental in the implementation of the first electronic medical record at Kaiser Permanente Colorado in 1998, for which he won the Nicholas E. Davies Award.

David C. Classen, M.D., M.S., is the chief medical officer at First Consulting Group and leads First Consulting's safety and quality of healthcare initiatives and consulting practice in this area. Dr. Classen is also an associate professor of medicine at the University of Utah and a consultant in infectious diseases at the University of Utah School of Medicine in Salt Lake City. He was the chair of Intermountain Healthcare's Clinical Quality Committee for Drug Use and Evaluation and was the initial developer of patient safety research and patient safety programs at Intermountain Healthcare. In addition, he developed, implemented, and evaluated a computerized physician order entry program at the Latter-Day Saints Hospital that significantly improved the safety of medication use. He was a member of the IOM committee that created *National Healthcare Quality*. He also chaired the Federal Safety Taskforce: Quality Interagency Coordination Taskforce/ Institute for Healthcare Improvement (IHI) Collaborative on Improving Safety in High Hazard Areas. He was co-chair of the IHI's Collaborative on Perioperative Safety. Dr. Classen currently chairs the Surgical Safety Collaborative at the IHI and is also a faculty member of the IHI/National Health Foundation Safer Patients Initiative in the United Kingdom. Dr. Classen is a developer of the "trigger tool methodology" at the IHI for the improved detection of adverse events. It is being used by more than 150 healthcare organizations throughout the United States and Europe. He received his M.D. from the University of Virginia School of Medicine and a M.Sc. in medical informatics from the University of Utah School of Medicine. He served as chief medical resident at the University of Connecticut. He is board certified in internal medicine and infectious diseases.

W. Dale Compton, Ph.D., is the Lillian M. Gilbreth Distinguished Professor (Emeritus) of Industrial Engineering at Purdue University. His early research was in physics, focusing on condensed matter, and was carried out first at the U.S. Naval Research Laboratory and later, for 9 years, at the University of Illinois, where he was a faculty member. The final 5 years at Illinois were spent as a professor of physics and director of the Coordinated Science Laboratory—an interdisciplinary engineering research laboratory. Upon moving to the Ford Motor Company Research Laboratories in 1970, his activities changed from doing research to managing research and development, and his last 13 years were spent as vice president of research. The research laboratories were involved in nearly all aspects of the technology that goes into the development and manufacture of a car or truck. After 2 years as the first Senior Fellow of the National Academy of Engineering (NAE), Dr. Compton joined the School of Industrial Engineering at Purdue. His current research deals with the creation and use of metals and alloys having a nanocrystalline microstructure. He is a member of St. Vincent Hospital (Indianapolis) Quality Committee of the Board of Directors and a past member of the IHI National Advisory Committee on Pursuing Perfection. Since 2000 he has served as home secretary for the NAE.

Paul F. Conlon, Pharm.D., J.D., is currently senior vice president for clinical quality and patient safety at Trinity Health and a member of the Trinity Health Senior Leadership Council. Dr. Conlon is also a clinical assistant professor of pharmacy at the University of Michigan. He is responsible for improving, measuring, monitoring, and reporting on clinical quality and patient safety for Trinity Health. He interacts with many parties interested in clinical quality, including employer groups, providers, trade associations, and insurers. Prior to joining the corporate office, he held a variety of positions within Mercy Health Services, which merged with the Holy Cross Health Care System in 2000 to become Trinity Health. He has been a clinical pharmacist in critical care and infectious disease, led an inpatient pharmacy department, has been the director of pharmacy for a large health maintenance organization (HMO), and was the director for clinical quality support for a large teaching hospital. He also has been a clinical pharmacist for the University of Michigan renal transplant team and continues as a College of Pharmacy faculty member. He serves on numerous community, state, and national clinical quality improvement groups and has been a healthcare consultant to the General Motors Corporation. Dr. Conlon has authored articles on a wide range of topics, from clinical pharmacokinetics to healthcare administration. He received his Pharm.D. from the University of Michigan and his J.D. from the University of Detroit. Dr. Conlon also completed a residency in hospital pharmacy at the University of Michigan.

He is licensed to practice pharmacy in Massachusetts and Michigan and to practice law in Michigan.

Denis A. Cortese, M.D., is president and CEO of the Mayo Clinic and chair of its executive committee. He has been a member of the board of trustees since 1997, and he previously served on that board from 1990 to 1993. Following service in the U.S. Naval Corps, he joined the staff of Mayo Clinic in Rochester, Minnesota, in 1976 as a specialist in pulmonary medicine. He was a member of the board of governors in Rochester before moving to Mayo Clinic in Jacksonville, Florida, in 1993. From 1999 to 2002 he served as chair of the board of governors at Mayo Clinic and chair of the board of directors at St. Luke's Hospital in Jacksonville, FL. He is a director and former president of the International Photodynamic Association and has been involved in the bronchoscopic detection, localization, and treatment of early-stage lung cancer. He is a member of the Healthcare Leadership Council and the Harvard/Kennedy School Healthcare Policy Group, and is a former member of the Center for Corporate Innovation. He served on the steering committee for the RAND Ix Project, "Using Information Technology to Create a New Future in Healthcare," and the Principals Committee of the National Innovation Initiative. He also is a charter member of the Advisory Board of World Community Grid and a founding member of the American Medical Group Association Chairs/Presidents/CEOs Council. Dr. Cortese is a graduate of Temple Medical School, completed his residency at the Mayo Graduate School of Medicine, and is a professor of medicine in the Mayo Clinic College of Medicine. Dr. Cortese is a member of the IOM, a Fellow of the Royal College of Physicians in England, and an honorary member of the Academia Nacional de Mexicana (Mexico).

Donald E. Detmer, M.D., M.A., is president and CEO of the American Medical Informatics Association. He is also a professor of medical education in the Department of Public Health Sciences at the University of Virginia and visiting professor at the College of Healthcare Information Management Executives, University College of London. Dr. Detmer is a member of the IOM as well as a lifetime associate of the National Academies, a fellow of the American Association for the Advancement of Science (AAAS) as well as the American Colleges of Medical Informatics, Sports Medicine, and Surgeons. In addition to co-chairing the Blue Ridge Academic Health Group, he chairs the Board of MedBiquitous. He is treasurer of the Council of Medical Specialty Societies. Dr. Detmer is past chair of the Board on Health Care Services of the IOM, the National Committee on Vital and Health Statistics, and the Board of Regents of the National Library of Medicine. He was a commissioner on the President's recent Commission on Systemic Interoperability. He chaired the 1991 IOM study, *The*

Computer-Based Patient Record, and coedited the 1997 version of the same report. He was a member of the committee that developed the IOM reports *To Err Is Human* and *Crossing the Quality Chasm*. From 1999 to 2003 he was the Dennis Gillings Professor of Health Management at Cambridge University and is a lifetime member of Clare Hall College, Cambridge. His education includes an M.D. from the University of Kansas, with subsequent training at the National Institutes of Health (NIH), the Johns Hopkins Hospital, Duke University Medical Center, the IOM, and Harvard Business School. His M.A. is from the University of Cambridge.

Amy L. Deutschendorf, M.S., R.N., A.P.R.N., is the senior director for clinical resource management at Johns Hopkins Hospital and Health System; the principal of Clinical Resource Consultants, LLC; and a faculty associate of John Hopkins University School of Nursing. Ms. Deutschendorf has more than 30 years of management, staff education and development, and consulting experience, including advanced nursing practice, administration, clinical care delivery design, nurse leadership development, and corporate regulatory compliance. She began her career as a clinical nurse specialist in medicine and oncology and has been the senior director for nursing practice, education, and research and care management at Johns Hopkins Bayview Medical Center. She has provided clinical, management and strategic consultation services nationally to academic medical institutions and has developed and implemented innovative strategies for patient care models to improve patient satisfaction, quality, and safety. She has published and presented nationally on a variety of topics affecting patient outcomes, including risk reduction strategies, professional nursing advancement, patient care delivery, and current healthcare trends. She holds an M.S. in nursing from the University of Maryland and a B.S. in nursing from Case Western Reserve University.

Earnest J. Edwards, M.B.A., is a retired senior vice president and controller of Alcoa, Inc. During his 34-year Alcoa career, he held a number of finance and accounting positions and served as general manager of Alcoa's information technology function before becoming controller. With Alcoa's reorganization and reorientation through quantum change in the early 1990s, he successfully led the finance organization through a major restructuring of the controllership and financial management functions to become more efficient, effective, and value adding. He is currently active in several community and educational organizations. He is vice chair of the board and chair of the finance committee of Martha Jefferson Health Service, Charlottesville, VA; vice rector of the board of visitors and chairman of the finance committee at Virginia State University, Petersburg, VA; director of the Pittsburgh Theological Seminary Board, and director emeritus of LaRoche College Board, Pittsburgh, PA. He received his B.S. in Accounting from Virginia State University and his M.B.A. from Duquesne University. He has been an active member of the Financial Executive International organization and chaired its Technical Committee on Corporate Reporting, which is an active participant in the Accounting Standards Setting and Reporting Process of the Financial Accounting Standards Board and Securities and Exchange Commission. He was named one of America's 10 most influential corporate figures in the accounting field by *Accounting Today* magazine in 1990. Prior to Alcoa, he was a commissioned officer in the Air Force.

Brent C. James, M.D., M.Stat., is executive director of the Institute for Health Care Delivery Research and vice president of medical research and continuing medical education at Intermountain Healthcare, Inc. Based in Salt Lake City, Utah, Intermountain Healthcare is an integrated system of 23 hospitals, almost 100 clinics, more than 450 physicians, and an HMO/PPO insurance plan jointly responsible for more than 450,000 covered lives. Dr. James is known internationally for his work in clinical quality improvement, patient safety, and the infrastructure that underlies successful improvement efforts, such as culture change, data systems, payment methods, and management roles. Before coming to Intermountain, he was an assistant professor in the Department of Biostatistics at the Harvard School of Public Health, providing statistical support for the Eastern Cooperative Oncology Group, and staffed the American College of Surgeons' Commission on Cancer. He holds faculty appointments at the University of Utah School of Medicine, Harvard School of Public Health, Tulane University School of Public Health and Tropical Medicine, and the University of Sydney, Australia, School of Public Health. He is also a member of the National Academy of Sciences/IOM. Dr. James holds B.S. degrees in computer science (electrical engineering) and medical biology, an M.D. (completed residency training in general surgery and oncology), and an M.Stat. degree from the University of Utah.

Kenneth W. Kizer, M.D., M.P.H., is chairman of Medsphere Systems Corporation, Inc., the leading provider of U.S. open-source healthcare information technology. Among other positions, he previously served as president and CEO of Medsphere; founding president and CEO of the National Quality Forum, a Washington, DC-based private, nonprofit healthcare quality improvement and consensus standards-setting organization; under secretary for health in the U.S. Department of Veterans Affairs and CEO of the Veterans Healthcare System, for which he is widely credited with being the chief architect and engineer of the radical transformation undertaken in the latter 1990s; director of the California Department of Health Services; and director of the California Emergency Medical Services Authority. Board certified in six medical specialties and subspecialties, Dr. Kizer practiced emergency medicine and medical toxicology in both academic and private practice settings. He graduated with honors from Stanford University and the University of California, Los Angeles (UCLA), holds two honorary doctorates, and is the recipient of numerous honors and awards, including the Earnest A. Codman Award from the Joint Commission on the Accreditation of Healthcare Organizations, the Gustav O. Leinhard Award from the IOM, the Justin Ford Kimball Innovator Award from the American Hospital Association, the Nathan Davis Award for Executive Excellence from the American Medical Association, and the Jean Spencer Felton Award for Excellence in Scientific Writing. Dr. Kizer is a member of Alpha Omega Alpha National Honor Medical Society, Delta Omega National Honorary Public Health Society, and the IOM, and he has been selected as 1 of the 100 Most Powerful People in Health Care by *Modern Healthcare* magazine. He has authored more than 400 publications in the medical and healthcare literature.

Mary Jane Koren, M.D., M.P.H., assistant vice president of The Commonwealth Fund, joined the fund in 2002 and leads the Picker/Commonwealth Program on Quality of Care for Frail Elders. Dr. Koren, an internist and geriatrician, began her academic career at Montefiore Medical Center, Bronx, New York, where she helped establish one of the early geriatric fellowship programs in New York, practiced in both nursing home and homecare settings, and was the associate medical director of the Montefiore Home Health Care Agency. She later joined the faculty of Mount Sinai's Department of Geriatrics and served as associate chief of staff for extended care at the Bronx Veterans Administration Medical Center. Leaving academic practice, she was appointed as director of the New York State Department of Health's Bureau of Long Term Care Services, where she ran the nursing home survey and certification programs, led the state's implementation of the *Omnibus Budget Reconciliation Act of 1987* (the Nursing Home Reform Law), and participated in many of the state's long-term care policy initiatives. Following that, she served as principal clinical coordinator for the New Jersey Peer Review Organization, which directed the Federal Health Care Quality Improvement Program. In 1993 she joined the Fan Fox and Leslie R. Samuels Foundation, first as an advisor and later as vice president of a grantmaking program in the field of health services and aging. Throughout her career she has been active as a health services researcher in the area of long-term care quality.

Richard C. Larson, Ph.D., is founding director of the Center for Engineering System Fundamentals at Massachusetts Institute of Technology (MIT).

He received his Ph.D. from MIT, where he is Mitsui Professor in the Department of Civil and Environmental Engineering and in the Engineering Systems Division. The majority of his career has focused on operations research as applied to services industries. He is the author, coauthor, or editor of six books and the author of numerous scientific articles, primarily in the fields of urban service systems, queuing, logistics, disaster management, disease dynamics, dynamic pricing of critical infrastructures, and workforce planning. From 1993 to 1994 he served as president of the Operations Research Society of America, and in 2005 he served as president of the Institute for Operations Research and the Management Sciences, also known as INFORMS. For more than 15 years Dr. Larson was codirector of the MIT Operations Research Center. He is a member of the NAE and is an INFORMS Founding Fellow. He has been honored with the INFORMS President's Award and the Kimball Medal. In recognition of his research on pandemic influenza and healthcare systems analysis, he has recently been requested to join the IOM Board on Health Sciences Policy. He is founding director of the Learning International Networks Consortium (LINC), an MIT-based international project that has held four international symposia and sponsored a number of initiatives in Africa, China, and the Middle East. On behalf of LINC, his recent foreign trips have been to China, Japan, Senegal, Iran, Indonesia, Algeria, Pakistan, Jordan, Kuwait, and the United Arab Emirates. From 1999 through 2004, Dr. Larson served as founding codirector of the forum "The Internet and the University."

Louise L. Liang, M.D., is senior vice president of quality and clinical systems support at Kaiser Foundation Health Plan and Kaiser Foundation Hospitals, which she joined in 2002. Working with leaders throughout Kaiser Permanente, she oversees the national quality agenda to ensure that members receive excellent care and service. She was responsible for the development and implementation of the organization-wide electronic health record and administrative systems to support the continuity and quality of care as well as efficient business functions. Prior to her role at Kaiser Permanente, Dr. Liang served as the chair on the IHI Board of Directors. From 1997 to 2001, Dr. Liang served as the chief operating officer and medical director of Group Health Cooperative of Puget Sound and as the founding CEO and president of Group Health Permanente, its affiliated medical group. Previously she held various leadership positions in hospital, health plan, and public policy settings. Dr. Liang served on the Malcolm Baldrige National Quality Award Panel of Judges during 1998 and 1999, on the Leadership Council of the American Association of Health Plans during 2000 and 2001, and on various other boards and committees.

Douglas W. Lowery-North, M.D., joined Emory University's faculty in 1995 and worked as the medical director of the new Emory University Hospital Emergency Department. Dr. Lowery-North is currently vice chair of clinical operations/Emory Healthcare in Emory's Department of Emergency Medicine. He is responsible for the strategic management of emergency care provided at the Emory University Hospital Emergency Department (ED) (annual census 28,000), Emory Crawford Long Hospital ED (annual census 55,000), and Emory Johns Creek Hospital ED (opened in February 2007). Clinically, his interests include cardiovascular and transplant-related emergencies, point-of-care ED ultrasound and echocardiography (he is rarely seen in the ED without his ultrasound machine in tow), quality management and performance improvement in the ED, and informatics and knowledge management in the healthcare setting. He is also a student at the Emory Rollins School of Public Health, where he is completing his M.S. in public health informatics. He loves teaching and has received several prestigious teaching awards, including the American College of Emergency Physicians (ACEP) National Teaching Award as well as the Dean's Teaching Award at Emory University and the Emory Emergency Medicine Residency Teacher of the Year Award. He teaches regularly at the ACEP Teaching Fellowship. He graduated from Vanderbilt Medical School in 1987 and was awarded the Dean's Award for Excellence in Medical Education. He completed his residency training in emergency medicine at UCLA Medical Center and the Robert Geffen School of Medicine at UCLA.

J. Michael McGinnis, M.D., M.P.P., is a long-time contributor to national and international health policy leadership. Dr. McGinnis is now a senior scholar at the IOM and executive director of the IOM Roundtable on Value & Science-Driven Health Care. He is also an elected member of the IOM. He previously was senior vice president at the Robert Wood Johnson Foundation (RWJF) and, unusual for political appointees, held continuous appointment through the Carter, Reagan, Bush, and Clinton administrations, with responsibility for coordinating activities and policies in disease prevention and health promotion. Programs and policies created and launched at his initiative include the Healthy People process-setting national health objectives, the U.S. Preventive Services Task Force, *Dietary Guidelines for Americans* (with the U.S. Department of Agriculture), *Ten Essential Services of Public Health*, the RWJF Health and Society Scholars Program, the RWJF Young Epidemiology Scholars Program, and the RWJF Active Living family of programs. Internationally, he chaired the World Bank/European Commission Task Force on postwar reconstruction of the health sector in Bosnia, and worked both as field epidemiologist and state coordinator for the World Health Organization's successful smallpox eradication program in India.

Ralph W. Muller, M.A., is chief executive officer of the University of Pennsylvania Health System (UPHS), a $2.7 billion enterprise that includes three fully owned and two joint venture hospitals, a faculty practice plan, a primary-care provider network, multispecialty satellite facilities, home care, hospice care, and long-term care. Prior to joining UPHS, he was the president and CEO of the University of Chicago Hospitals and Health System. From 2001 to 2002, he was a visiting fellow at the Kings Fund in London. From 1985 to 1986 Mr. Muller served as deputy dean of the Division of the Biological Sciences at the Pritzker School of Medicine at the University of Chicago. Before joining the university, Mr. Muller held senior positions with the Commonwealth of Massachusetts, including service as deputy commissioner of the Massachusetts Department of Public Welfare, where he was responsible for the state's major welfare programs, including Medicaid. He is a director of the National Committee for Quality Assurance and a commissioner of the Joint Commission. He has served as commissioner on the Medicare Payment Advisory Commission, chair of the Association of American Medical Colleges, chair of the Council of Teaching Hospitals and Health Systems, and vice chair of the University Healthsystems Consortium. He is a Fellow of the AAAS. He received his bachelor's degree in economics from Syracuse University and his master's degree in government from Harvard University.

John J. Nance, J.D., is a founding member of the National Patient Safety Foundation at the American Medical Association. He is also a decorated Air Force officer and pilot and is one of the pioneers of the safety revolution in professional communication, teamwork, and leadership known in aviation as crew resource management. Mr. Nance's current work focuses on improving health care from patient safety to practice satisfaction with hospitals and clinics nationwide. He focuses on leadership and the human propensity for mistakes, even among the most tenured professionals. Mr. Nance is also an author and a broadcast analyst on medical and patient safety and aviation safety with ABC World News and Good Morning America.

Eugene C. Nelson, D.Sc., M.P.H., is professor of community and family medicine at Dartmouth Medical School and director of quality administration for the Dartmouth–Hitchcock Medical Center. He is a senior scientist at the Dartmouth Institute for Health Policy and Clinical Practice. Dr. Nelson is a national leader in healthcare improvement and the development and application of measures of system performance, health outcomes, and patient and customer perceptions. In the early 1990s Dr. Nelson and his colleagues at Dartmouth began developing clinical microsystem thinking. His work to develop the "clinical value compass" and "whole system measures" to assess healthcare system performance have made him a well-recognized quality and value measurement expert. He is the recipient of the Joint Commission's Ernest A. Codman Award for his work on outcomes measurement in health care. Dr. Nelson has been a pioneer in bringing modern quality improvement thinking into the mainstream of health care. He helped launch the IHI and served as a founding board member. He has authored more than 100 articles and monographs and is the first author of 2 recent books, *Quality by Design: A Clinical Microsystems Approach* and *Practice-Based Learning and Improvement: A Clinical Improvement Action Guide: Second Edition.* He received an M.P.H. from Yale University and a D.Sc. from Harvard University.

Paul H. O'Neill, M.P.A., was the 72nd Secretary of the U.S. Department of the Treasury, serving from 2001 to 2002. Mr. O'Neill was chair and CEO of Alcoa from 1987 to 1999, and he retired as chair at the end of 2000. Prior to joining Alcoa, he was president of International Paper Company from 1985 to 1987 and had previously served as vice president from 1977 to 1985. He worked as a computer systems analyst with the U.S. Veterans Administration from 1961 to 1966 and served on the staff of the U.S. Office of Management and Budget (OMB) from 1967 to 1977, with the last 3 years as OMB's deputy director. He received a bachelor's degree in economics from Fresno State College in California and a master's degree in public administration from Indiana University.

David B. Pryor, M.D., is the chief medical officer of Ascension Health, the largest not-for-profit healthcare delivery system in the United States. Prior to joining Ascension Health, Dr. Pryor was senior vice president and chief information officer for Allina Health System in Minneapolis. Earlier, Dr. Pryor was president of the New England Medical Center Hospitals in Boston. He spent the first 15 years of his career at Duke University Medical Center, where he served as director of the cardiology consultation service, the section on clinical epidemiology and biostatistics, the Duke Database for Cardiovascular Disease, and clinical program development. Dr. Pryor has participated on numerous national and international committees. He has also served as an advisor to a number of developing companies. In addition to his position at Ascension Health, Dr. Pryor's academic appointments include consulting associate professor of medicine at Duke University Medical Center and adjunct professor at Saint Louis University School of Public Health.

Rita F. Redberg, M.D., M.Sc., is a cardiologist specializing in outcomes research and heart disease in women. Dr. Redberg has written, edited, and contributed to many books, including *You Can Be a Woman Cardiologist,*

Heart Healthy: The Step-by-Step Guide to Preventing and Healing Heart Disease, and *Coronary Disease in Women: Evidence-Based Diagnosis and Treatment,* and she has written more than 100 peer-reviewed journal articles. She serves on numerous technology assessment forums, such as the Center for Medical Technology Policy, California Technology Assessment Forum, and the Institute for Clinical and Economic Research Board, and she was a member of the Medicare Coverage Advisory committee. She earned her M.D. from the University of Pennsylvania School of Medicine. She completed her residency in Internal Medicine at Columbia–Presbyterian Medical Center in New York, where she went on to complete a fellowship in cardiology. Then she completed a fellowship in noninvasive cardiology at Mount Sinai Medical Center, also in New York. In addition, Dr. Redberg has an M.Sc. in health policy and administration from the London School of Economics. She recently completed an RWJF Health Policy Fellowship.

William B. Rouse, Ph.D., M.S., is the executive director of the Tennenbaum Institute at the Georgia Institute of Technology. He is also a professor in the College of Computing and School of Industrial and Systems Engineering. Dr. Rouse has written hundreds of articles and book chapters, and has authored many books, including, most recently, *People and Organizations: Explorations of Human-Centered Design, Essential Challenges of Strategic Management,* and the award-winning *Don't Jump to Solutions.* He is editor of *Enterprise Transformation: Understanding and Enabling Fundamental Change,* coeditor of *Organizational Simulation: From Modeling & Simulation to Games & Entertainment,* coeditor of the best-selling *Handbook of Systems Engineering and Management,* and editor of the eight-volume series *Human/Technology Interaction in Complex Systems.* Among many advisory roles, he has served as chair of the Committee on Human Factors of the National Research Council, as a member of the U.S. Air Force Scientific Advisory Board, and as a member of the Department of Defense Senior Advisory Group on Modeling and Simulation. Dr. Rouse is a member of the NAE as well as a fellow of four professional societies: the Institute of Electrical and Electronics Engineers, the International Council on Systems Engineering, the Institute for Operations Research and Management Science, and the Human Factors and Ergonomics Society.

Harold W. Sorenson, Ph.D., is a founding faculty member of the University of California, San Diego (UCSD) and is currently a professor of mechanical and aerospace engineering at the Jacobs School of Engineering. From 1989 to 2001 Dr. Sorenson served as senior vice president and general manager for the MITRE Corporation, a nonprofit organization that applies systems engineering and advanced technologies to address challenges in system development and enterprise modernization for the defense and intelligence communities as well as for the Federal Aviation Administration and the Internal Revenue Service. He returned to the UCSD campus in 2003 as faculty director of the graduate program in architecture-based enterprise systems engineering being developed by the Jacobs School of Engineering and the Rady School of Management. A long-time scientific and technology advisor to the U.S. defense and intelligence communities, he chaired the Air Force Scientific Advisory Board from 1990 to 1993 and was the chief scientist of the U.S. Air Force from 1985 to 1988. Dr. Sorenson is a fellow of the Institute of Electrical and Electronics Engineers (IEEE) and of the AAAS. He is a recipient of the IEEE Centennial Medal, two Exceptional Civilian Service awards and a Meritorious Civilian Award from the Air Force, the Director's Award from the Defense Intelligence Agency, the Benjamin H. Gold Medal for Engineering from the Armed Forces Communications and Electronics Association, and the Air Force Association's Doolittle Award.

Steven J. Spear, D.B.A., M.S., M.S., is a researcher, writer, public speaker, educator, and consultant who works with organizations to create competitive advantage through the strength of their internal operations, managing complex design, production, and administrative processes for exceptional performance. The primary theme is strongly coupling doing work with learning how to do that work ever better, thereby achieving unmatchable combinations of quality, safety, responsiveness, efficiency, and flexibility. His articles about Toyota have been award winners and best sellers; those about healthcare quality and medical education have appeared in *Annals of Internal Medicine*, *Academic Medicine*, and other medical journals, and he is the author of many case studies. A book based on his research, *The High-Velocity Edge*, was published by McGraw Hill in 2010. At MIT Spear teaches an introduction to lean manufacturing and six sigma for students in the Leaders for Manufacturing and Systems Design and Management programs. At the IHI, he has been involved in a number of projects to raise the quality of care by introducing systems management principles from non-healthcare exemplars. He also teaches at Harvard Medical School and School of Public Health programs. Previously, he was an assistant professor at Harvard Business School for 6 years. Dr. Spear played an integral role in developing the Alcoa business system and the Perfecting Patient Care program of the Pittsburgh Regional Healthcare Initiative. Alcoa's annual reports detailed hundreds of millions of dollars in savings and other gains, and Pittsburgh hospitals have generated reductions of 50 to 90 percent in afflictions such as hospital-acquired infections, along with other gains in quality of care and quality of work. He also worked for the investment bank Prudential-Bache, the U.S. Congress Office of Technology Assessment, and the University of Tokyo. Spear's doctorate is from Harvard Business School and his two master's degrees—in management and mechanical engineering—are from MIT.

William W. Stead, M.D., is associate vice chancellor for strategy/transformation and director of the Informatics Center at Vanderbilt University Medical Center. He serves as chief information officer of the medical center and chief information architect for the university. His interest in computer-based patient records and systems to support practice dates to 1968. At Vanderbilt his team has translated biomedical informatics research into novel approaches to information infrastructure to reduce implementation costs and barriers to adoption. The resulting enterprise-wide electronic patient chart and communication/decision support tools strengthen his current focus on system-supported, evidence-based practice and research leading toward personalized medicine. Dr. Stead is McKesson Foundation Professor of Biomedical Informatics and professor of medicine. He is a founding fellow of both the American College of Medical Informatics and the American Institute for Engineering in Biology and Medicine and an elected member of both the IOM and the American Clinical and Climatological Association. He was the first recipient of the Lindberg Award for Innovation in Informatics and is the 2007 recipient of the Collen Award for Excellence in Medical Informatics. He was the founding editor-in-chief of the *Journal of the American Medical Informatics Association*, served as chair of the Board of Regents of the National Library of Medicine and as a Presidential appointee to the Commission on Systemic Interoperability, and serves on the Computer Science and Telecommunication Board of the National Research Council and is chair of its Committee on Engaging the Computer Science Research Community in Health Care Informatics. He is a member of the Tennessee eHealth Advisory Council. Dr. Stead received his B.A. and M.D. from Duke University, where he also completed training in internal medicine and nephrology.

Stephen J. Swensen, M.D., M.M.M., the Mayo Clinic director for quality. He is professor of radiology in the Mayo Clinic College of Medicine. He served as chair of the Department of Radiology from 1998 to 2006 and was education program director in the preceding 5 years. He is a member of the Mayo Clinic Management Oversight Group and Clinical Practice Committee. He is past president of the Society of Thoracic Radiology and the Fleischner Society. He has chaired the American College of Radiology's Quality Metrics Committee and the Radiological Society of North America's Continuous Quality Improvement Initiative. Dr. Swensen has been principal investigator on three NIH grants. He has authored 2 books and more than 100 peer-reviewed articles. Dr. Swensen received his M.D. from the University of Wisconsin. His residency training was at the Mayo Clinic and his Thoracic Radiology Fellowship was at Harvard Medical School, Brigham and Women's Hospital. In 2004 he received a master's of medical management degree from Carnegie Mellon University's Heinz School of Public Policy and Management.

James M. Tien, Ph.D., is a distinguished professor and the dean of the College of Engineering at the University of Miami, Coral Gables, Florida. He has held leadership positions at Bell Telephone Laboratories, at the RAND Corporation, and at Structured Decisions Corporation (which he cofounded in 1974). He joined the Department of Electrical, Computer and Systems Engineering at Rensselaer in 1977, became acting chair of the department, joined a unique interdisciplinary Department of Decision Sciences and Engineering Systems as its founding chair, and twice served as the acting dean of engineering. Dr. Tien's areas of research interest include the development and application of computer and systems analysis techniques to information and decision systems. He has published extensively, been invited to present many plenary lectures, and been honored with both teaching and research awards, including being elected a fellow of the IEEE, the Institute for Operations Research and the Management Sciences, and the AAAS and being a recipient of the IEEE Joseph G. Wohl Outstanding Career Award, the IEEE Major Educational Innovation Award, the IEEE Norbert Wiener Award, and the IBM Faculty Award. Dr. Tien is also an elected member of the NAE. He received a BEE from Rensselaer Polytechnic Institute and a S.M. and Ph.D. in electrical engineering from MIT.

Appendix C

Workshop Attendee List

Pat Adams
National Pharmaceutical Council

Mahdu Agarwal
Department of Veterans Affairs

John Agos
sanofi-aventis

Brian Arndt
University of Wisconsin

Neeraj Arora
National Cancer Institute (NIH)

Judith Bader
National Cancer Institute (NIH)

Rachel Behrman
Food and Drug Administration

Rami Ben-Joseph
sanofi-aventis

Stefano Bertuzzi
National Institutes of Health

Donald M. Berwick
Institute for Healthcare
    Improvement

Doug Bodner
Georgia Institute of Technology

Douglas Boenning
U.S. Department of Health and
    Human Services

Kenneth Boff
Georgia Institute of Technology

Marilyn Sue Bogner
Institute for the Study of Human
    Error, LLC

Rosemary Botchway
Primary Care Coalition of
    Montgomery County

Lynda Bryant-Comstock
GlaxoSmithKline

Randy Burkholder
PhRMA

Betsy Carrier
National Association of Public
    Hospitals

Linda Carter
Johnson & Johnson

Michael D. Chase
Kaiser Permanente Colorado

Xuanhong Cheng
Lehigh University

David C. Classen
Computer Sciences Corporation

Emily Clements
Pfizer, Inc.

Andrew Cohen
AGC & Associates

Perry Cohen
Parkinson Pipeline Project

Zohara Cohen
National Institute of Biomedical
    Imaging and BioEngineering
    (NIH)

W. Dale Compton
Purdue University

Paul F. Conlon
Trinity Health

Denis A. Cortese
Mayo Clinic

David Cowan
Georgia Institute of Technology

Tapas Das
University of South Florida

Dave Davis
Association of American Medical
    Colleges

Donald E. Detmer
American Medical Informatics
    Association

Amy L. Deutschendorf
Johns Hopkins Hospital and
    Health System

Deirdre DeVine
Evidence-Based Practice Systems

Louis Diamond
Thomson Healthcare

Molla Donaldson
MSD Healthcare

Denise Dougherty
Agency for Healthcare Research
    and Quality

Andrea Douglas
PhRMA

Reena Duseja
University of Pennsylvania

Ria Eapen
National Consumers League

Earnest J. Edwards
Alcoa, Inc.

Noel Eldridge
Department of Veterans Affairs

Maggie Elestwani
Memorial Hermann–Texas Medical
    Center

Henry Ernstthal
Ernstthal & Associates

Lynn Etheredge
George Washington University

Craig Feied
Microsoft

Karen Feinstein
Pittsburgh Regional Health
    Initiative

Rosemarie Filart
National Center for Research
    Resources (NIH)

David Fornet
Memorial Hermann–Texas Medical
    Center

Kathleen Frisbee
Department of Veterans Affairs

Jean Paul Gagnon
sanofi-aventis

William Galey
Howard Hughes Medical Institute

Rajesh Ganesan
George Mason University

Barry Gershon
Wyeth Pharmaceuticals

Michael Gillam
Microsoft

Mark Gorman
National Coalition for Cancer
    Survivorship

Tina Grande
Healthcare Leadership Council

Barbara Greenan
American College of Cardiology

Robert Greenes
Arizona State University

Atul Grover
Association of American Medical
    Colleges

Kiran Gupta
Harvard Medical School

Jan Heinrich
Health Policy R&D

Alejandra Herr
Avalere Health, LLC

Michael Hewitt
Memorial Hermann–Texas Medical
    Center

Barbara Hirsch
Nurse Attorney

Carmen Hooker Odom
Milbank Memorial Fund

Han-Yao Huang
Merck, Inc.

Belinda Ireland
BJC HealthCare

Brent C. James
Intermountain Healthcare, Inc.

Robert Kambic
Centers for Medicare & Medicaid
    Services

Elisabeth Kato
Hayes, Inc.

John J. Kelly
Abington Memorial Hospital

Bette Keltner
Georgetown University

Kenneth W. Kizer
Medsphere Systems Corporation,
    Inc.

Ronald Klar
Health Services Analysis, Inc.

Kathleen Klink
Office of Senator Hillary Clinton

Diane Kollar
Georgia Institute of Technology

Mary Jane Koren
The Commonwealth Fund

Hanns Kuttner
University of Michigan

Arnold Kuzmack
Food and Drug Administration

Mollie Lane
Senate Finance Committee

William Lang
American Association of Colleges
    of Pharmacy

Richard C. Larson
Massachusetts Institute of
    Technology

Cato T. Laurencin
University of Virginia Health
    System

Eva Lee
Georgia Institute of Technology

Jason Lee
New England Healthcare Institute

Michelle Leff
National Institute on Drug Abuse
    (NIH)

Anna Legreid Dopp
Office of Senator Joe Lieberman

Dan Leonard
National Pharmaceutical Council

Odette Levesque
Department of Veterans Affairs

Louise L. Liang
Kaiser Permanente

Keith Lind
AARP

John Linehan
Northwestern University

Douglas W. Lowery-North
Emory University

James Luo
National Institute of Biomedical
Imaging and BioEngineering
(NIH)

Brian Maloney
AstraZeneca Pharmaceuticals

Norman Marks
Food and Drug Administration

Karen Matsuoka
U.S. House of Representatives,
Ways and Means Committee

Michael Mayo-Smith
Department of Veterans Affairs

Audrey McDowell
U.S. Department of Health and
Human Services

Linda McKibben
The McKibben Group, LLC

Kathryn McLaughlin
America's Health Insurance Plans

Robert Mechanic
Brandeis University

Nancy Miller
National Institutes of Health

Kunal Mitra
American Medical Association

Ralph W. Muller
University of Pennsylvania Health
System

Ken Musselman
Regenstrief Center for Healthcare
Engineering

John J. Nance
National Patient Safety Foundation

Eugene C. Nelson
Dartmouth–Hitchcock Medical
Center

John O'Donnell
AstraZeneca Pharmaceuticals

Paul H. O'Neill
Value Capture, LLC

Eduardo Ortiz
National Heart Lung and Blood
Institute (NIH)

Steve Pelletier
Pelletier Editorial

Eleanor M. Perfetto
Pfizer, Inc.

Susan Pingleton
Association of American Medical
Colleges

David B. Pryor
Ascension Health

Barbra Rabson
Massachusetts Health Quality
Partners

John Rayburn
Healthcare Leadership Council

Rita F. Redberg
University of California, San
  Francisco

Nancy Ridenour
U.S. House of Representatives

Proctor Reid
National Academy of Engineering

John Ring
American Heart Association

Nuala Ronan
Databean, LLC

Shaina Rood
Avalere Health, LLC

William B. Rouse
Tennenbaum Institute

Patricia Rowell
Department of Veterans Affairs

Francois Sainfort
University of Minnesota

Karen Sanders
American Psychiatric Association

Adam L. Scheffler
Freelance

Karen Sepucha
Massachusetts General Hospital

Nicoleta Serban
Georgia Institute of Technology

Brenda Sheingold
George Mason University

Sharon Siler
Avalere Health, LLC

Rebecca Singer Cohen
United Biosource Corporation

Jamie Skipper
U.S. House of Representatives

Ken Skodacek
Medical Device Consultant

Harold W. Sorenson
University of California, San Diego

Steven J. Spear
Massachusetts Institute of
  Technology

William W. Stead
Vanderbilt University Medical
  Center

Melissa Stegun
George Washington University

Elise Stein
U.S. Senate Committee on Finance

Lisa Summers
National Partnership for Women
  and Families

Nancy Sung
Burroughs Wellcome Fund

Jeff Swarz
National Cancer Institute

Stephen J. Swensen
Mayo Clinic

James M. Tien
University of Miami

Deborah Trautman
Office of Speaker Nancy Pelosi

Sylvia Trujillo
American Medical Association

William Turner
Office of Senator Barack Obama

Craig Umscheid
University of Pennsylvania Health
System

Shaokui Wei
Food and Drug Administration

Kimberly Westrich
National Pharmaceutical Council

Kendal Williams
University of Pennsylvania Health
System

Reginald Williams
Avalere Health, LLC

Steve Witz
Regenstrief Center for Healthcare
Engineering

Hui-Hsing Wong
U.S. Department of Health and
Human Services

Janet Wright
American College of Cardiology

Jonelle Wright
University of Miami Miller School
of Medicine

John Yeh
The National Academies/USAID/
U.S. State Department

Teresa Zayas-Caban
Agency for Healthcare Research
and Quality

Jose Zayas-Castro
University of South Florida

Judith Zboyovski
Veterans Health Administration

Laura Zick
Eli Lilly and Company

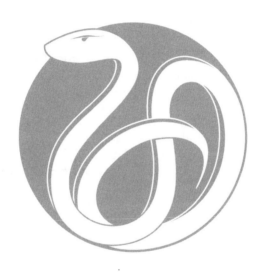